Biomechanical Analysis in Physical Activity and Sports

Biomechanical Analysis in Physical Activity and Sports

Guest Editor
Pedro Miguel Forte

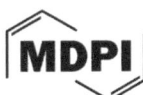

Basel • Beijing • Wuhan • Barcelona • Belgrade • Novi Sad • Cluj • Manchester

Guest Editor
Pedro Miguel Forte
Sports
Higher Institute of Educational Sciences of the Douro
Penafiel
Portugal

Editorial Office
MDPI AG
Grosspeteranlage 5
4052 Basel, Switzerland

This is a reprint of the Special Issue, published open access by the journal *Journal of Functional Morphology and Kinesiology* (ISSN 2411-5142), freely accessible at: www.mdpi.com/journal/jfmk/special_issues/0YVTYI86LU.

For citation purposes, cite each article independently as indicated on the article page online and as indicated below:

Lastname, A.A.; Lastname, B.B. Article Title. *Journal Name* **Year**, *Volume Number*, Page Range.

ISBN 978-3-7258-3908-7 (Hbk)
ISBN 978-3-7258-3907-0 (PDF)
https://doi.org/10.3390/books978-3-7258-3907-0

© 2025 by the authors. Articles in this book are Open Access and distributed under the Creative Commons Attribution (CC BY) license. The book as a whole is distributed by MDPI under the terms and conditions of the Creative Commons Attribution-NonCommercial-NoDerivs (CC BY-NC-ND) license (https://creativecommons.org/licenses/by-nc-nd/4.0/).

Contents

About the Editor vii

Pedro Forte
Special Issue "Biomechanical Analysis in Physical Activity and Sports"
Reprinted from: *J. Funct. Morphol. Kinesiol.* **2025**, *10*, 116, https://doi.org/10.3390/jfmk10020116   1

Marie Adelaide Nicolas-Peyrot, Yves Lescure, Eleonore Perrin, Magdalena Martinez-Rico, Corentin Travouillon, Gabriel Gijon-Nogueron and Eva Lopezosa-Reca
Optimizing Running Mechanics, Effects of Cadence, Footwear, and Orthoses on Force Distribution: A Quasi-Experimental Study
Reprinted from: *J. Funct. Morphol. Kinesiol.* **2025**, *10*, 89, https://doi.org/10.3390/jfmk10010089 .   4

Cristiana Mercê, Keith Davids, Rita Cordovil, David Catela and Marco Branco
Learning to Cycle: Why Is the Balance Bike More Efficient than the Bicycle with Training Wheels? The Lyapunov's Answer
Reprinted from: *J. Funct. Morphol. Kinesiol.* **2024**, *9*, 266, https://doi.org/10.3390/jfmk9040266 .   17

Julio Martín-Ruiz, Ignacio Tamarit-Grancha, Carlos Cordente-Martínez, Raúl Santamaría-Fernández, Concepción Ros Ros and Laura Ruiz-Sanchis
Design of a Freely Accessible Web Application (Instrument for the Measurement of Balance in Primary Education, IMEP) for the Assessment of Static and Dynamic Balance in Children Aged 6–9 Years Based on Force Platforms
Reprinted from: *J. Funct. Morphol. Kinesiol.* **2024**, *9*, 281, https://doi.org/10.3390/jfmk9040281 .   35

Mafalda P. Pinto, Daniel A. Marinho, Henrique P. Neiva, Tiago M. Barbosa and Jorge E. Morais
Insights on the Selection of the Coefficient of Variation to Assess Speed Fluctuation in Swimming
Reprinted from: *J. Funct. Morphol. Kinesiol.* **2024**, *9*, 129, https://doi.org/10.3390/jfmk9030129 .   50

Luka Pezelj, Boris Milavić and Mirjana Milić
Anthropometric and Somatotype Profile of Elite Finn Class Sailors
Reprinted from: *J. Funct. Morphol. Kinesiol.* **2024**, *9*, 121, https://doi.org/10.3390/jfmk9030121 .   59

Esteban Aedo-Muñoz, Jorge Pérez-Contreras, Alejandro Bustamante-Garrido, David Arriagada-Tarifeño, Jorge Cancino-Jiménez, Manuel Retamal-Espinoza, et al.
Is Countermovement Jump an Indirect Marker of Neuromuscular Mechanism? Relationship with Isometric Knee Extension Test
Reprinted from: *J. Funct. Morphol. Kinesiol.* **2024**, *9*, 242, https://doi.org/10.3390/jfmk9040242 .   70

André B. Peres, Tiago A. F. Almeida, Danilo A. Massini, Anderson G. Macedo, Mário C. Espada, Ricardo A. M. Robalo, et al.
Similarity Index Values in Fuzzy Logic and the Support Vector Machine Method Applied to the Identification of Changes in Movement Patterns During Biceps-Curl Weight-Lifting Exercise
Reprinted from: *J. Funct. Morphol. Kinesiol.* **2025**, *10*, 84, https://doi.org/10.3390/jfmk10010084 .   80

James M. Wakeling, Stanislava Smiešková, Matej Vajda and Jan Busta
A Comparison of Paddle Forces between Whitewater and Flatwater Training in C1 Canoe Slalom
Reprinted from: *J. Funct. Morphol. Kinesiol.* **2024**, *9*, 167, https://doi.org/10.3390/jfmk9030167 .   98

Gennaro Boccia, Paolo Riccardo Brustio, Luca Beratto, Ilaria Peluso, Roberto Ferrara, Diego Munzi, et al.
Upper-Limb Muscle Fatigability in Para-Athletes Quantified as the Rate of Force Development in Rapid Contractions of Submaximal Amplitude
Reprinted from: *J. Funct. Morphol. Kinesiol.* **2024**, *9*, 108, https://doi.org/10.3390/jfmk9020108 . **106**

María Alejandra Camacho-Villa, Jhon Hurtado-Alcoser, Andrés Santiago Jerez, Juan Carlos Saavedra, Erika Tatiana Paredes Prada, Jeimy Andrea Merchán, et al.
Handgrip Strength and Upper Limb Anthropometric Characteristics among Latin American Female Volleyball Players
Reprinted from: *J. Funct. Morphol. Kinesiol.* **2024**, *9*, 168, https://doi.org/10.3390/jfmk9030168 . **120**

Sophia Stasi, Georgios Papagiannis, Athanasios Triantafyllou, Panayiotis Papagelopoulos and Panagiotis Koulouvaris
Post-Arthroplasty Spatiotemporal Gait Parameters in Patients with Hip Osteoarthritis or Developmental Dysplasia of the Hip: An Observational Study
Reprinted from: *J. Funct. Morphol. Kinesiol.* **2024**, *9*, 110, https://doi.org/10.3390/jfmk9030110 . **131**

Krystof Volesky, Jan Novak, Michael Janek, Jakub Katolicky, James J. Tufano, Michal Steffl, et al.
Assessing the Test-Retest Reliability of MyotonPRO for Measuring Achilles Tendon Stiffness
Reprinted from: *J. Funct. Morphol. Kinesiol.* **2025**, *10*, 83, https://doi.org/10.3390/jfmk10010083 . **143**

Drew Commandeur, Marc Klimstra, Ryan Brodie and Sandra Hundza
A Comparison of Bioelectric and Biomechanical EMG Normalization Techniques in Healthy Older and Young Adults during Walking Gait
Reprinted from: *J. Funct. Morphol. Kinesiol.* **2024**, *9*, 90, https://doi.org/10.3390/jfmk9020090 . . **157**

Filipa Cardoso, Ricardo Cardoso, Pedro Fonseca, Manoel Rios, João Paulo Vilas-Boas, João C. Pinho, et al.
Changing the Mandibular Position in Rowing: A Brief Report of a World-Class Rower
Reprinted from: *J. Funct. Morphol. Kinesiol.* **2024**, *9*, 153, https://doi.org/10.3390/jfmk9030153 . **168**

About the Editor

Pedro Miguel Forte

Pedro Miguel Gomes Forte completed his Ph.D. in Sports Sciences in 2018 at the University of Beira Interior, Master's degree in Exercise and Health in 2014 at the Polytechnic Institute of Bragança, and Bachelor's degree in Sports in 2012 at the Polytechnic Institute of Bragança. He is currently attending a Ph.D. program in Biomechanics and Bioengineering Applied to Health at the University of Alcalá. He works as Associate Professor at the Higher Institute of Educational Sciences of Douro, Invited Adjunct Teacher at the Polytechnic Institute of Bragança School of Education, and Coordinating Researcher at CI-ISCE. He is also a member of the Research Center for Active Living and Wellbeing (LiveWell). He has published more than 200 works. Throughout his career, he has collaborated with more than 350 co-authors on scientific papers.

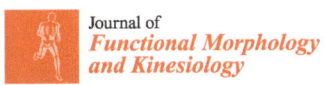

Editorial

Special Issue "Biomechanical Analysis in Physical Activity and Sports"

Pedro Forte [1,2,3]

1. Department of Sports, Higher Institute of Educational Sciences of the Douro, 4560-708 Penafiel, Portugal; pedromiguel.forte@gmail.com or pedromiguel.forte@iscedouro.pt
2. Department of Sports Sciences, Instituto Politécnico de Bragança, 5300-253 Bragança, Portugal
3. Research Center for Active Living and Wellbeing, Instituto Politécnico de Bragança, 5300-253 Bragança, Portugal

Citation: Forte, P. Special Issue "Biomechanical Analysis in Physical Activity and Sports". *J. Funct. Morphol. Kinesiol.* 2025, 10, 116. https://doi.org/10.3390/jfmk10020116

Received: 26 March 2025
Accepted: 28 March 2025
Published: 30 March 2025

Citation: Forte, P. Special Issue "Biomechanical Analysis in Physical Activity and Sports". *J. Funct. Morphol. Kinesiol.* 2025, 10, 116. https://doi.org/10.3390/jfmk10020116

Copyright: © 2025 by the author. Licensee MDPI, Basel, Switzerland. This article is an open access article distributed under the terms and conditions of the Creative Commons Attribution (CC BY) license (https://creativecommons.org/licenses/by/4.0/).

1. Introduction

Biomechanics plays a vital role in helping us understand how the human body moves, especially in the context of sports and physical activity. By applying principles from physics and engineering, biomechanical analysis allows us to study the forces acting on the body. This is incredibly valuable not only for enhancing athletic performance but also for health and physical activity-related analysis. Recent technological advances, including motion capture systems, force plates, electromyography (EMG), and computational fluid dynamics, have provided us with powerful tools for measuring and modeling movement with unparalleled precision [1–3]. These technologies have been adopted across various sports, including running, cycling, and swimming, helping athletes and coaches in enhancing their performance techniques [2,3]. In addition, the emergence of wearable technology and artificial intelligence (AI) has further advanced real-time analysis capabilities. Today, athletes can receive immediate feedback through sensors embedded in their gear, allowing them to adjust their technique on the spot, which also plays a big part in preventing injuries [1].

Despite significant advances in sports biomechanics, several key gaps remain to be addressed. One of the major challenges is translating findings from controlled laboratory environments into real-world sports settings. While many studies have contributed to our understanding, they do not always reflect the complex, dynamic conditions of actual performance [4,5]. To overcome these challenges, there is a need for more field-based research that integrates biomechanical assessments into both training and competitive environments [5]. Another limitation is the narrow focus on elite athletes. Research often overlooks recreational athletes, children, older adults, and individuals with disabilities [6]. It is essential to expand our studies to include these groups to develop more inclusive and broadly applicable training programs [7]. Furthermore, while many biomechanical interventions show immediate benefits, there is a need for long-term studies that evaluate how these changes influence injury risk and athletic development over time [1,4].

In practical terms, the applications of biomechanics are vast. By examining joint angles, muscle activation, and force distribution, biomechanists and healthcare professionals can identify inefficiencies in movement and develop personalized training plans [8]. For instance, runners can benefit from gait retraining programs that not only improve efficiency but also help prevent common overuse injuries. Furthermore, insights from biomechanics inform rehabilitation processes, ensuring that injured athletes return to sport safely and effectively [4]. Additionally, this area plays a crucial role in improving sports equipment design. Whether it is running shoes or adaptive equipment for athletes with disabilities, biomechanics ensures that these tools are optimized for comfort and performance [2]. Finally, coaches are increasingly leveraging biomechanical data to personalize exercises and improve techniques, addressing each athlete's specific strengths and areas for improvement [9].

Looking ahead, the future of biomechanics lies at the intersection of technology and interdisciplinary collaboration. AI-powered models are set to enhance how we analyze human movement, facilitating the delivery of personalized training and immediate feedback [2]. We also anticipate the emergence of more portable and user-friendly wearable sensors, enabling high-quality biomechanical assessments in real-world settings and enhancing the applicability of research findings to actual conditions [10].

In addition, exploring how the nervous system interacts with biomechanics may result in more effective rehabilitation strategies, especially for athletes recovering from neurological injuries [11]. This approach will help ensure biomechanics contributes to a more inclusive and forward-thinking sporting environment [12].

The recently published Special Issue, "*Biomechanical Analysis in Physical Activity and Sports*", brings attention to the exciting ways biomechanics shapes the future of sports and exercise. As new technologies facilitate the study of bodily movements, there is an increasing need to connect research with real-world applications in sports, fitness, or athletics. This Special Issue allows researchers, coaches, and sports professionals to share novel insights, practical solutions, and creative collaborations that enhance athlete performance, safety, and training effectiveness. It presents a valuable chance to explore the impact of biomechanics on movement and competitive performance.

2. Biomechanical Analysis in Physical Activity and Sports

This Special Issue on Biomechanical Analysis in Physical Activity and Sports presents a comprehensive collection of studies that collectively contribute to a more applied understanding of human movement in sports performance and clinical contexts. The research published here spans several key thematic areas, including neuromuscular function, gait analysis, anthropometry, sport-specific techniques, motor learning, and methodological innovation, each offering relevant contributions to the scientific community and practitioners working in the field.

Biomechanical Analysis in Physical Activity and Sports provides valuable insights into age-related changes in neuromuscular control and gait patterns to rehabilitation practices, helping to refine strategies for patients recovering from surgery and anatomic pathologies, improving their mobility and quality of life [13]. Finally, it offers a novel approach to assessing speed fluctuation in swimming, which is integral for performance optimization in aquatic sports, providing athletes and coaches with valuable insights into pacing strategies [14].

The contributions to this Special Issue reflect the multidimensional nature of biomechanical analysis in sport and physical activity. The integration of new technologies, interdisciplinary methods, and population-specific considerations showcases the maturity and continued evolution of the field. These papers deepen the scientific understanding of movement and offer practical applications for coaches, clinicians, and practitioners seeking to enhance performance and wellbeing across diverse populations.

Conflicts of Interest: The author declares no conflicts of interest.

References

1. Alzahrani, A.; Ullah, A. Advanced Biomechanical Analytics: Wearable Technologies for Precision Health Monitoring in Sports Performance. *Digit. Health* **2024**, *10*, 20552076241256745. [CrossRef]

2. Wang, Y.; Shan, G.; Li, H.; Wang, L. A Wearable-Sensor System with AI Technology for Real-Time Biomechanical Feedback Training in Hammer Throw. *Sensors* **2023**, *23*, 425. [CrossRef]
3. Wang, X.; Liu, R.; Zhang, T.; Shan, G. The Proper Motor Control Model Revealed by Wheelchair Curling Quantification of Elite Athletes. *Biology* **2022**, *11*, 176. [CrossRef]
4. Erdmann, W.; Aschenbrenner, P.; Kowalczyk, R.; Urbański, R. University Laboratory of Biomechanics and Sport Analytics and Engineering in Gdansk as an Important Science Institution. *MOJ Appl. Bionics Biomech.* **2020**, *4*, 8–13. [CrossRef]
5. Hara, Y.; Silva, A.; Sá, K.; Carpes, F.; Rossato, M. Sport Biomechanics before and after the Rio 2016 Paralympic Games. *Rev. Bras. Med. Esporte* **2024**, *30*, e2022_0001. [CrossRef]
6. Lopes, J.; Guimarães, K.; Lopes, S.; Pérego, S.; Andrade, C. Analysis of Biomechanics in Athletes with Disabilities: A Systematic and Narrative Review. *Fisioter. Mov.* **2023**, *36*, e36201. [CrossRef]
7. Li, L.; Ren, F.; Baker, J. The Biomechanics of Shoulder Movement with Implications for Shoulder Injury in Table Tennis: A Mini-Review. *Appl. Bionics Biomech.* **2021**, *2021*, 9988857. [CrossRef]
8. Wan, B.; Gao, Y.; Wang, Y.; Zhang, X.; Li, H.; Shan, G. Hammer Throw: A Pilot Study for a Novel Digital-Route for Diagnosing and Improving Its Throw Quality. *Appl. Sci.* **2020**, *10*, 1922. [CrossRef]
9. Yao, J.; Guo, N.; Xiao, Y.; Li, Z.; Li, Y.; Pu, F.; Fan, Y. Lower Limb Joint Motion and Muscle Force in Treadmill and Over-Ground Exercise. *Biomed. Eng. Online* **2019**, *18*, 89. [CrossRef]
10. Knudson, D. Association of ResearchGate Research Influence Score with Other Metrics of Top Cited Sports Biomechanics Scholars. *Biomed. Hum. Kinet.* **2023**, *15*, 57–62. [CrossRef]
11. Manolachi, V.; Potop, V.; Chernozub, A.; Khudyi, O.; Delipovici, I.; Eshtayev, S.; Mihailescu, L. Theoretical and Applied Perspectives of the Kinesiology Discipline in the Field of Physical Education and Sports Science. *Phys. Educ. Stud.* **2022**, *26*, 316–324. [CrossRef]
12. Chen, C. Biomechanical Process of Skeletal Muscle under Training Condition Based on 3D Visualization Technology. *J. Healthc. Eng.* **2022**, *2022*, 2656405. [CrossRef] [PubMed]
13. Stasi, S.; Papagiannis, G.; Triantafyllou, A.; Papagelopoulos, P.; Koulouvaris, P. Post-Arthroplasty Spatiotemporal Gait Parameters in Patients with Hip Osteoarthritis or Developmental Dysplasia of the Hip: An Observational Study. *J. Funct. Morphol. Kinesiol.* **2024**, *9*, 110. [CrossRef] [PubMed]
14. Pinto, M.P.; Marinho, D.A.; Neiva, H.P.; Barbosa, T.M.; Morais, J.E. Insights on the Selection of the Coefficient of Variation to Assess Speed Fluctuation in Swimming. *J. Funct. Morphol. Kinesiol.* **2024**, *9*, 129. [CrossRef] [PubMed]

Disclaimer/Publisher's Note: The statements, opinions and data contained in all publications are solely those of the individual author(s) and contributor(s) and not of MDPI and/or the editor(s). MDPI and/or the editor(s) disclaim responsibility for any injury to people or property resulting from any ideas, methods, instructions or products referred to in the content.

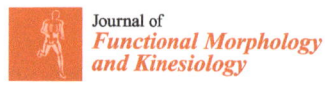

Article

Optimizing Running Mechanics, Effects of Cadence, Footwear, and Orthoses on Force Distribution: A Quasi-Experimental Study

Marie Adelaide Nicolas-Peyrot [1,2], Yves Lescure [1,2], Eleonore Perrin [2], Magdalena Martinez-Rico [3], Corentin Travouillon [4], Gabriel Gijon-Nogueron [5,*] and Eva Lopezosa-Reca [5]

[1] Facultad Ciencias de la Salud, Universidad de Malaga, 29017 Malaga, Spain; ma-nicolaspeyrot@ecole-rockefeller.com (M.A.N.-P.); yves-lescure@ecole-rockefeller.com (Y.L.)
[2] Department of Podologie, Ecole Rockefeller, 69008 Lyon, France; eleonore-perrin@ecole-rockefeller.com
[3] Department of Health Sciences, Faculty of Nursing and Podiatry, Industrial Campus of Ferrol, Universidad de da Coruña, 15001 Ferrol, Spain; magdalenamr96@gmail.com
[4] TRINOMA Co., 48800 Villefort, France; corentin.travouillon@gmail.com
[5] Department Nursing and Podiatry, Universidad de Malaga, 29017 Malaga, Spain; evalopezosa@uma.es
* Correspondence: gagijon@uma.es

Citation: Nicolas-Peyrot, M.A.; Lescure, Y.; Perrin, E.; Martinez-Rico, M.; Travouillon, C.; Gijon-Nogueron, G.; Lopezosa-Reca, E. Optimizing Running Mechanics, Effects of Cadence, Footwear, and Orthoses on Force Distribution: A Quasi-Experimental Study. *J. Funct. Morphol. Kinesiol.* **2025**, *10*, 89. https://doi.org/10.3390/jfmk10010089

Academic Editor: Pedro Miguel Forte

Received: 30 December 2024
Revised: 5 March 2025
Accepted: 7 March 2025
Published: 10 March 2025

Citation: Nicolas-Peyrot, M.A.; Lescure, Y.; Perrin, E.; Martinez-Rico, M.; Travouillon, C.; Gijon-Nogueron, G.; Lopezosa-Reca, E. Optimizing Running Mechanics, Effects of Cadence, Footwear, and Orthoses on Force Distribution: A Quasi-Experimental Study. *J. Funct. Morphol. Kinesiol.* **2025**, *10*, 89. https://doi.org/10.3390/jfmk10010089

Copyright: © 2025 by the authors. Licensee MDPI, Basel, Switzerland. This article is an open access article distributed under the terms and conditions of the Creative Commons Attribution (CC BY) license (https://creativecommons.org/licenses/by/4.0/).

Abstract: Background: Running is a popular physical activity known for its health benefits but also for a high incidence of lower-limb injuries. This study examined the effects of three biomechanical interventions—cadence adjustments, footwear modifications, and foot orthoses—on plantar pressure distribution and spatiotemporal running parameters. **Methods**: A quasi-experimental, repeated-measures design was conducted with 23 healthy recreational runners (mean age 25, mean BMI 22.5) who ran at least twice per week. Five conditions were tested: baseline (C0), increased cadence (C1), orthoses (C2), low-drop footwear (C3), and a combination of these (C4). Data were collected on a Zebris treadmill, focusing on rearfoot contact time, peak forces, and stride length. **Results**: Increasing cadence (C1) reduced rearfoot impact forces (−81.36 N) and led to a shorter stride (−17 cm). Low-drop footwear (C3) decreased rearfoot contact time (−1.89 ms) and peak force (−72.13 N), while shifting pressure toward the midfoot. Orthoses (C2) effectively redistributed plantar pressures reducing rearfoot peak force (−41.31 N) without changing stride length. The combined intervention (C4) yielded the most pronounced reductions in peak forces across the rearfoot (−183.18 N) and forefoot (−139.09 N) and increased midfoot contact time (+5.07 ms). **Conclusions**: Increasing cadence and low-drop footwear significantly reduced impact forces, improving running efficiency. Orthoses effectively redistributed plantar pressures, supporting individualized injury prevention strategies. These findings suggest that combining cadence adjustments, footwear modifications, and orthoses could enhance injury prevention and running efficiency for recreational runners.

Keywords: running; biomechanics; cadence; foot orthoses; plantar pressure

1. Introduction

Running holds an essential place in the sporting landscape and continues to attract an increasing number of participants worldwide, with more than 600 million people engaging in this activity. In recent years, its popularity has surged, particularly due to its accessibility and widely recognized health benefits. A 2022 report by World Athletics highlighted a 30% increase in running participation over the past decade, driven by urban running events and the rise of fitness culture [1,2]. In France alone, 25% of the population (12.4 million people) participate in running, underscoring its widespread appeal [3].

Beyond its popularity, running is associated with both physical and mental health benefits, including improved cardiovascular health, weight management, and stress reduction [4]. However, it also presents a notable risk of musculoskeletal injuries, with an annual incidence ranging from 19.4% to 79.3% among runners [5]. The most common injuries affect the lower limbs [6,7], particularly the knee, leg, and foot, resulting from multifactorial causes, including training errors, biomechanical characteristics, and environmental factors.

The most prevalent injuries include patellofemoral pain syndrome (PFPS), iliotibial band syndrome (ITBS), Achilles tendinopathy, and stress fractures. These injuries not only hinder performance but may also lead to long-term health consequences. Studies indicate that up to 50% of runners experience recurrent injuries within a year of returning to activity [8]. For instance, PFPS is often linked to patellar misalignment and muscle imbalances [9,10], ITBS is associated with excessive friction between the iliotibial band and femur [11,12], Achilles tendinopathy results from repetitive strain, and stress fractures are common in runners who dramatically increase their training volume [13,14].

These injury risks highlight the need for targeted biomechanical interventions that address improper force distribution and suboptimal spatiotemporal parameters during running [15,16]. Risk factors such as inappropriate training loads and biomechanical abnormalities (e.g., overpronation, excessive hip adduction) have been implicated, though their direct relationship with injuries remains debated [17–20].

Recent research emphasizes the role of running technique, particularly cadence and foot strike patterns, in modulating injury risk. A low cadence or pronounced rearfoot strike has been associated with increased knee and hip loading, contributing to PFPS and ITBS [21,22]. Consequently, running retraining has emerged as a promising strategy for reducing injury risk by optimizing biomechanical parameters and redistributing forces away from vulnerable structures [23,24].

While previous studies have examined cadence modification, footwear adjustments, and orthoses separately, little is known about their combined effects on running mechanics. Understanding these interactions could improve injury prevention and rehabilitation strategies. While studies have examined their separate effects, limited evidence exists on their synergistic impact [25,26].

This study aims to assess both the individual and combined effects of these interventions on key biomechanical parameters, such as cadence, stride length, and force distribution. By addressing this gap in the literature, this research seeks to provide evidence-based recommendations for optimizing running mechanics, reducing injury risk, and enhancing performance.

Biomechanical running analysis, including detailed stride assessment and correction of abnormalities, has shown promise in injury prevention. Advanced tools, such as the Zebris instrumented treadmill, allow for real-time plantar pressure analysis, identifying spatiotemporal gait parameters and force distribution patterns. These include cadence, stride length, rearfoot–midfoot–forefoot contact time, and peak force distribution, essential for designing targeted interventions to correct biomechanical inefficiencies [27].

Several biomechanical interventions have been proposed to mitigate injury risk, including cadence modifications, footwear adjustments, and foot orthoses [28,29]. Increasing cadence (typically by 5–10%) has been shown to reduce stride length, vertical oscillations, and braking forces during ground contact [30,31]. Similarly, low-drop footwear promotes midfoot or forefoot strikes, shifting mechanical loads away from the knee [32,33]. Foot orthoses modify plantar pressure distribution and foot structure deformation, but their precise effects remain uncertain—especially when combined with other interventions [34,35].

This study seeks to provide a comprehensive understanding of these biomechanical interventions and their potential for reducing injury risk and enhancing running performance. The findings will offer valuable insights for clinicians and sports scientists in optimizing running mechanics and promoting long-term athlete health.

2. Methods

2.1. Protocol and Registration

This study complied with all STROBE guidelines [29]. This study was conducted in accordance with the Declaration of Helsinki on Ethical Principles for Medical Research Involving Human Subjects and was approved by the Ethics Committee of the University of Malaga (CEUMA 206-2023-H) in Spain [30]. Data confidentiality was also ensured. Data collection and storage adhered to strict confidentiality protocols. To ensure data confidentiality, all personal identifiers were removed or anonymized. Participant data were securely stored in an encrypted database, accessible only to the research team. No data will be publicly shared but may be made available upon reasonable request, in compliance with legal and ethical regulations.

2.2. Design

A quasi-experimental design with repeated measures was chosen for this study. This approach allowed for the evaluation of multiple interventions within the same group of participants, thereby reducing inter-individual variability and increasing statistical power. While randomized controlled trials (RCTs) are often considered the gold standard for reducing bias, a quasi-experimental design was deemed more practical due to logistical constraints, such as the difficulty of recruiting a large number of participants for multiple randomized groups.

Additionally, this design enabled the assessment of combined interventions (e.g., cadence adjustment, footwear modification, and orthotics), which would be challenging to implement in a traditional RCT framework. To address potential sources of bias, strict control over experimental conditions was maintained, including standardized warm-up protocols, rest periods, and environmental factors.

Each participant was randomly assessed under the following five conditions (Table 1):

- C0 (Reference Condition): Rearfoot-to-toe drop of 10 mm, no cadence adjustment, no orthotics.
- C1 (Cadence only): 10 mm rearfoot-to-toe drop, 10% increase in cadence, no orthotics.
- C2 (Plantar orthoses): 10 mm rearfoot-to-toe drop and Alain Lavigne Inversion Foot Orthoses (ALIFOrthoses) [31].
- C3 (Asics Noosa shoe): 5 mm rearfoot-to-toe drop, no orthotics. The low drop favors a plantar attack on the forefoot or midfoot, which can modify the forces exerted on the rearfoot compared to high-drop shoes [32].
- C4 (Cross-interventions): 10% increase in cadence, ALIFOrthoses, 5-mm rearfoot-to-toe drop.

Table 1. Each condition's key features.

Condition	Footwear	Drop	Cadence	Orthoses
C0 (Reference)	Control shoes	10 mm	No adjustment (0%)	None
C1 (Cadence only)	Control shoes	10 mm	+10%	None
C2 (Plantar orthoses)	Control shoes	10 mm	No adjustment (0%)	ALIFOrthoses
C3 (Asics Noosa)	Asics NOOSA	5 mm	No adjustment (0%)	None
C4 (Cross-interventions)	Asics NOOSA	5 mm	+10%	ALIFOrthoses

2.3. Participants

A total of 23 healthy recreational runners (mean age: 25 ± 4.5 years, BMI: 22.5 ± 1.34) were recruited. Participants were required to run at least twice weekly and have no history of lower-limb injuries in the past six months. All participants were at least 18 years old and could follow the study instructions.

Inclusion criteria:

- Age ≥ 18 years.
- Recreational running activity of at least 2 sessions per week (running 5 km in under 25 min).
- Habitual use of running shoes with a 10 mm drop.
- Willingness and ability to adhere to the study protocol.

Exclusion criteria:

- Degenerative diseases of the bones and joints (diagnosed based on medical history).
- Surgery of the lower limbs.
- Recent knee or ankle injuries or serious foot injuries that may have left morphological changes.
- Painful skin conditions (e.g., calluses, plantar warts).
- Lower-limb injuries in the past 6 months (verified by self-report).

These criteria ensured the selection of a homogeneous population, minimizing potential biases linked to biomechanical disorders or adaptations.

After receiving detailed information about the study aims and procedures, each participant signed an informed consent form.

The experimental measurements were carried out at the R&D laboratory of the Rockefeller School in Lyon (8th arrondissement) between February and November 2024. The laboratory was equipped to maintain controlled environmental conditions, optimizing data reliability.

2.4. Procedure

The running shoes used in the study were ASICS NOOSA, featuring a 5 mm rearfoot-to-toe drop and a weight of 255 g (men's size 9). They incorporated FlyteFoam® (Onitsuka Co., Ltd., Kobe, Japan) midsole technology for lightweight cushioning with organic fibers to enhance durability. The outsole was made of wet grip rubber and was designed to provide excellent traction on wet surfaces, while the upper part comprised a no-sew, breathable mesh for superior comfort (Figure 1).

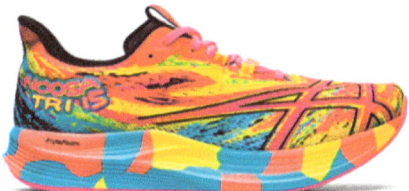

Figure 1. Profile view of the Noosa model from Asics.

The foot orthoses were thermoformed "Alain Lavigne Inversion Foot Orthoses" (ALI-FOrthoses) [31], designed with a full-length medial wedge and a Shore A hardness of 35. The orthoses included a supinating rearfoot wedge, medial arch support, supinated forefoot wedge, and a lateral stabilizing wedge for enhanced support and alignment (Figure 2).

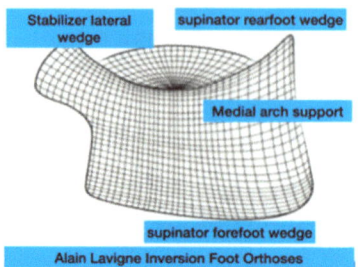

Figure 2. Front view of Alain Lavigne Inversion Foot Orthoses design.

2.5. Experimental Conditions

The Zebris treadmill was selected for its unique ability to measure plantar pressure distribution and spatiotemporal parameters in real time. The key features include a matrix of capacitive pressure sensors under the tread, which provides high-resolution data on force distribution and gait dynamics. This system allows precise speed adjustments (0.2–24 km/h in 0.1 km/h increments) and real-time data visualization, making it ideal for analyzing running mechanics under controlled conditions.

Before starting the experimental conditions, the participants completed a 5 min warm-up period on the Zebris treadmill at a self-selected speed while wearing their own shoes. This was performed to ensure participant comfort and achieve a stable running state, thereby reducing potential variability during the trials, in line with the recommendations of similar studies.

To minimize fatigue as a confounding factor, rest periods of five minutes were implemented between conditions. During this time, participants remained seated, hydrated, and refrained from physical activity.

Each participant ran at a fixed speed of 12 km/h on a Zebris treadmill, which was selected for its high-resolution plantar pressure measurement and spatiotemporal parameter analysis.

Each participant performed test runs under the five distinct experimental conditions described above, each performed at a constant speed of 12 km/h. This speed was chosen based on its relevance to recreational runners because it represents a moderate pace that is achievable for most participants while allowing for detailed biomechanical analysis. However, this fixed speed may limit the external validity of the findings for runners who typically train at significantly faster or slower paces.

Biomechanical data from the Zebris treadmill is collected using a matrix of capacitive pressure sensors integrated under the tread. These sensors continuously measure the pressure exerted by the feet on the tread surface. They are individually calibrated to ensure high accuracy [33,34]. Data were acquired via sensors that recorded the variations in pressure as the subject ran on the treadmill. The data include information on the distribution of plantar pressure, phases of contact (rearfoot, midfoot, and toes), and zones of maximum pressure [34].

The measurements were transmitted in real time to a computer to ensure synchronization with the software. This dedicated software interprets and displays data in real time in the form of color-coded plantar pressure maps and spatiotemporal parameters, such as cadence, step length, contact time, etc., to analyze balance and stability [35].

The data are then recorded for in-depth analysis. The software generates graphs, tables, and detailed reports. The results are stored and can be compared across multiple trials or subjects to assess progress or detect asymmetries [33].

Each condition consisted of two minutes of running: the first minute was for familiarization and the second minute for data collection.

2.6. Sample Size

The required sample size was calculated using a 95% confidence level and 80% power based on the effect size derived from preliminary data. The study concluded that 24 participants per group were required to achieve the study objectives. However, due to recruitment challenges, the final sample size was limited to 23 participants. This discrepancy may slightly reduce the statistical power of the study, potentially increasing the risk of Type II errors (false negatives). Nevertheless, the repeated-measures design mitigates this limitation by increasing the sensitivity to detect within-subject differences.

2.7. Statistical Analysis

A repeated-measures ANOVA was chosen because each participant underwent all five conditions, allowing us to account for within-subject variability and enhance statistical power by using each individual as their own control. Before analysis, we checked normality to verify the normality of data distribution ($p > 0.01$). In cases where normality assumptions were violated, non-parametric tests (e.g., Wilcoxon signed-rank test) were applied to assess the effects across conditions while controlling for inter-individual variability. The Kolmogorov–Smirnov test was conducted to verify the normality of data distribution ($p > 0.01$). In cases where normality assumptions were violated, non-parametric tests (e.g., Wilcoxon signed-rank test) were applied.

Descriptive statistics were expressed as means and standard deviations, with 95% confidence intervals. Statistical significance was set at $p < 0.05$, and all analyses were performed using MATLAB (R2021a, 8.3.0.532, The MathWorks Inc., Natick, MA, USA), which was chosen for its robust handling of complex biomechanical data and capability to run post hoc comparisons with appropriate corrections for multiple testing.

3. Results

The study included 23 recreational runners with an average age of 25 years (SD = 4.5) and a BMI of 22.5 (SD = 1.34). Participants ran at least twice per week and had no history of lower-limb surgery or injuries in the past six months. To facilitate results interpretation, key findings are summarized before each table.

3.1. Overview of Key Findings

- Cadence adjustment (C1) and the combined intervention (C4) showed the most pronounced reductions in rearfoot peak force, while footwear changes primarily influenced midfoot contact time.
- The combined intervention (C4) produced the largest reduction in rearfoot impact (-139.09 N, $p < 0.001$), suggesting it may be the most effective strategy for minimizing joint stress in runners.
- Footwear modification (C3) led to an increase in midfoot contact time (+1.98 ms), while orthoses (C2) redistributed plantar pressure with a moderate effect on rearfoot force.
- Stride length and step length were significantly reduced under conditions C1 and C4, suggesting a more compact and controlled gait pattern.

3.2. Spatiotemporal and Force Distribution Comparisons

A detailed comparison of spatiotemporal parameters and force distribution across conditions is presented in Table 2.

Table 2. Comparison of spatiotemporal parameters and force distribution across different running conditions.

Parameter	C0 (Mean ± SD)	C1 (Mean ± SD)	C2 (Mean ± SD)	C3 (Mean ± SD)	C4 (Mean ± SD)	Δ (vs. C0)	p-Value	Effect Size (Cohen's d)
Rearfoot contact time (ms)	42.22 ± 3.45	42.00 ± 5.34	41.00 ± 4.23	44.11 ± 2.87	41.83 ± 3.76	−1.22 (C2), +1.89 (C3)	<0.001 *	0.45 (C2), 0.61 (C3)
Midfoot contact time (ms)	51.45 ± 2.3	53.28 ± 2.67	53.27 ± 4.22	53.43 ± 3.29	56.52 ± 3.98	+1.83 (C1), +5.07 (C4)	<0.001 *	0.48 (C1), 0.89 (C4)
Forefoot contact time (ms)	79.4 ± 4.32	80.45 ± 3.4	80.09 ± 2.39	78.5 ± 4.2	79.02 ± 3.1	+1.01 (C1), −0.94 (C3)	<0.001 *	0.35 (C1), 0.38 (C3)
Rearfoot peak force (N)	461.08 ± 76.5	379.72 ± 67.8	419.77 ± 38.8	388.95 ± 54.4	321.99 ± 59.2	−81.36 (C1), −139.09 (C4)	<0.001 *	0.55 (C1), 1.02 (C4)
Forefoot peak force (N)	1041.7 ± 86.4	973.65 ± 79.2	1024.48 ± 89.3	976.63 ± 92.2	858.54 ± 85.2	−68.07 (C1), −183.18 (C4)	<0.001 *	0.47 (C1), 1.21 (C4)
Stride length (cm)	240.17 ± 48.2	223.17 ± 37.3	240.12 ± 52.2	237.69 ± 39.1	223.57 ± 42.9	−17.00 (C1), −16.60 (C4)	<0.001 *	0.56 (C1), 0.54 (C4)
Step length (cm)	119.75 ± 16.3	111.41 ± 21.7	119.99 ± 18.4	118.50 ± 19.3	111.67 ± 23.9	−8.34 (C1), −8.08 (C4)	<0.001 *	0.52 (C1), 0.50 (C4)

* Significant; ms milliseconds; cm centimeter; N newton; SD Standard deviation.

3.3. Key Observations

Regarding rearfoot contact time, condition C2 reduced it by 1.22 ms (Cohen's d = 0.45, $p < 0.001$), indicating a moderate effect. In contrast, condition C3 increased rearfoot contact time by 1.89 ms (Cohen's d = 0.61, $p < 0.001$), reflecting a more noticeable change. With respect to the midfoot contact time, C4 had the most substantial impact, increasing this phase by 5.07 ms (Cohen's d = 0.89, $p < 0.001$), suggesting a strong effect.

In terms of peak rearfoot force, all conditions led to a significant reduction, with C4 producing the most pronounced decrease (−139.09 N, Cohen's d = 1.02, $p < 0.001$). Similarly, for peak forefoot force, C4 showed the greatest reduction (−183.18 N, Cohen's d = 1.21, $p < 0.001$), indicating a substantial effect. Finally, regarding stride and step length, both C1 and C4 significantly reduced stride length by −17 cm and −16.6 cm, respectively (Cohen's d = 0.56 and 0.54, $p < 0.05$), suggesting an adaptation toward a more compact running pattern (Figure 3).

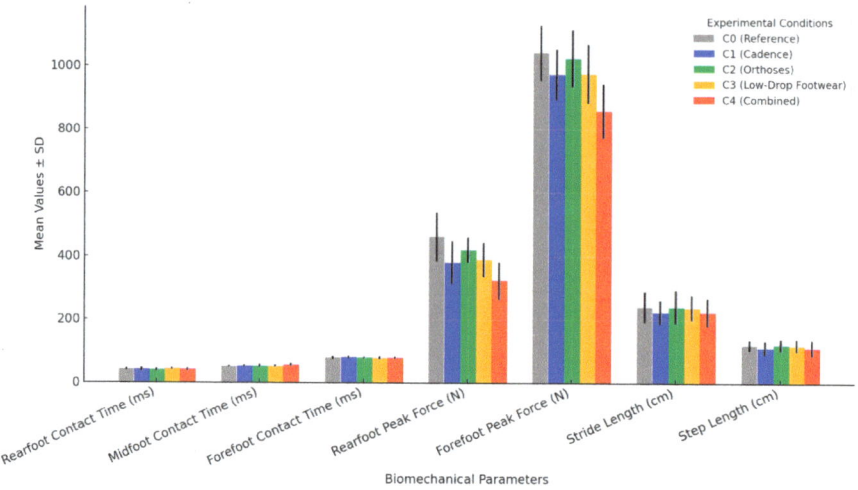

Figure 3. Distribution of biomechanical parameters across different running conditions.

4. Discussion

The aim of our study was to assess the individual and combined effects of different interventions on key spatiotemporal parameters of strength and force distribution. Our findings contribute to the growing body of literature on running biomechanics and provide practical insights for optimizing running mechanics to reduce injury risk and enhance performance.

Regarding the drop of the shoes, these parameters, in the scientific literature, are influenced by the various experimental conditions. A shoe with a 10 mm drop (C0) favors a rearfoot attack, increasing rearfoot contact time and peak rearfoot force. However, the impact on stride and step length may vary between individuals [36]. Our results align with previous studies, which demonstrated that a higher rearfoot-to-toe drop promotes a rearfoot strike pattern, increasing loading on the knee and hip joints [25,37].

A 10% increase in cadence (C1) generally reduces ground contact time, decreases peak force, and can slightly shorten stride length, improving efficiency and reducing the risk of injury [24]. Increasing cadence by 5–10% significantly reduces impact forces and loading rates, particularly at the knee joint [38].

Inversion foot orthoses (C2) alter the distribution of plantar pressures, influencing peak forces and contact times in different areas of the foot, with varying effects depending on the correction made [39]. Orthotics play a key role in redistributing plantar loads and reducing stress on specific structures, such as the medial tibia and Achilles tendon [40].

The use of shoes with a drop reduced to 5 mm (C3) encourages a midfoot or forefoot attack, reducing rearfoot contact time and peak rearfoot force, while possibly increasing forefoot contact time [36]. Minimalist shoes with low rearfoot-to-toe drops promote a forefoot strike pattern, reducing impact forces at the rearfoot but increasing loading on the forefoot [41]. Finally, a combination of several of these conditions (C4) with a +10% cadence, inversion soles, and shoes with a 5 mm drop can encourage a midfoot attack, reduce ground impact, and optimize force distribution, positively influencing stride and step length [36,39]. A multifactorial approach is essential to address the complex biomechanical demands of running, supporting the need for integrated interventions [42].

This study demonstrates that increasing cadence (C1) significantly reduces stride length and step length, decreases peak force in the rearfoot and forefoot, and increases contact time in the midfoot and forefoot. These findings align with research indicating that increased cadence reduces impact forces and stride length, enhancing running economy and reducing injury risk [43]. Our findings have significant implications for clinical and training practices. For example, increasing cadence (C1) could be particularly beneficial for runners with high injury rates, such as those with patellofemoral pain syndrome (PFPS) or iliotibial band syndrome (ITBS), as it reduces knee-joint loading and impact forces [38].

Alain Lavigne Inversion Foot Orthoses (C2) did not significantly affect stride or step length but reduced peak rearfoot force, with no significant forefoot changes, and increased midfoot and forefoot contact time. This suggests that orthotics redistribute plantar loads, primarily affecting the rearfoot without altering stride length [44]. Alain Lavigne Inversion Foot Orthoses (C2) could be particularly useful for runners with excessive pronation or flat feet as they help redistribute plantar pressures and reduce stress on the medial tibia and Achilles tendon.

Using shoes with a reduced drop (5 mm) (C3) led to moderate reductions in stride and step length, decreased rearfoot and forefoot peak forces, increased midfoot contact time, and reduced forefoot contact time. These effects are consistent with studies showing that a lower shoe drop encourages a midfoot strike, altering impact forces and running mechanics [45].

The combination of these interventions (C4) resulted in pronounced reductions in stride and step length, significant decreases in rearfoot and forefoot peak forces, and increased midfoot contact time, with no changes in forefoot contact. This cumulative effect underscores the benefits of integrated approaches, as highlighted in literature advocating for combined strategies to maximize biomechanical benefits [46].

Overall, the findings corroborate prior research showing that biomechanical adjustments, such as increasing cadence and using reduced-drop shoes, enhance running economy and decrease lower-joint impact forces, reducing injury risk [36,43]. Orthotics contribute by redistributing forces without affecting stride length, supporting existing research on their role in managing plantar load distribution [47]. Specific interventions, like cadence increases (C1) and reduced-drop shoes (C3), could be recommended as non-invasive strategies to reduce mechanical stress on lower joints, benefiting individuals with conditions such as plantar fasciitis, medial tibial stress syndrome, or Achilles tendinopathy [10,48]. ALIFOrthoses (C2) may assist in redistributing plantar loads, aiding in rehabilitation after injuries such as stress fractures or foot deformities (for example, flat or hollow foot) [49].

Combining these interventions (C4) could optimize multiple biomechanical parameters in personalized rehabilitation protocols, particularly for complex cases involving multiple injury risk factors or performance limitations. Furthermore, these strategies can be integrated into motor reprogramming programs to teach optimized running techniques, offering proactive solutions for injury prevention and recurrence [50].

This study has several limitations that should be acknowledged. First, the sample size of 23 participants, although sufficient for detecting significant differences, may limit the generalizability of the findings. A larger sample size would enhance the statistical power and allow for subgroup analyses based on factors such as running experience or injury history.

Second, the short duration of the intervention (two minutes per condition) may not fully capture the long-term effects of these biomechanical adjustments. Future studies should consider longer intervention periods to assess the sustainability of these changes.

Third, the controlled laboratory setting, while ideal for standardizing conditions, may limit the ecological validity of the findings. Running on a treadmill differs from outdoor running in terms of surface variability, environmental factors, and psychological responses. Future research should validate these findings in real-world settings using wearable sensors or outdoor running protocols.

This study paves the way for further research into the multifactorial optimization of running biomechanics. Future studies could explore the longitudinal effects of these combined interventions on sports performance and injury prevention. For example, a six-month follow-up study could assess whether the observed biomechanical changes lead to a reduction in injury rates or improvements in running economy.

Additionally, it would be relevant to evaluate these adjustments in specific populations, such as runners with musculoskeletal injuries, by integrating clinical and functional parameters to assess the benefits on performance and overall health. For instance, runners with a history of stress fractures or Achilles tendinopathy could be targeted to evaluate the effectiveness of reduced-drop shoes and orthotics in reducing recurrence rates.

Another promising direction is the integration of wearable technologies, such as onboard sensors or smart insoles, to provide real-time feedback on running mechanics. These devices could be used to validate treadmill findings in outdoor running conditions and to personalize biomechanical adjustments based on individual needs. For example, a runner with excessive pronation could receive real-time feedback on foot strike patterns and pressure distribution, enabling immediate corrections during training sessions.

Our results indicate that cadence adjustments (+10%) and low-drop footwear (5 mm) can significantly reduce rearfoot impact forces, making them practical, non-invasive interventions for injury prevention. Orthotic modifications, while less influential on stride parameters, effectively redistribute plantar pressures, making them useful for runners with existing biomechanical imbalances:

- Cadence adjustment (+10%) may be particularly beneficial for runners at high risk of overuse injuries (e.g., patellofemoral pain syndrome (PFPS) or iliotibial band syndrome (ITBS)), as it helps reduce knee-joint loading [38].
- Inversion foot orthoses (C2) could be useful for runners with excessive pronation or flat feet, as they aid in redistributing plantar pressures and reducing stress on the medial tibia and Achilles tendon.
- Low-drop footwear (C3) may help runners transition to a midfoot strike, potentially benefiting those with high-impact running mechanics but requiring careful adaptation to avoid excessive forefoot loading.
- Combined interventions (C4) could be recommended for runners needing comprehensive biomechanical optimization, particularly in rehabilitation settings or performance training programs.

5. Conclusions

This study shows that modifying cadence (+10%) and wearing reduced-drop footwear (5 mm) significantly influences running mechanics, particularly by reducing impact forces and altering foot contact durations. ALIF Orthoses (C2) had a limited effect on stride length but significantly redistributed plantar loads, suggesting its role in load management rather than stride modification.

The combined intervention (C4) produced the most pronounced cumulative effects, particularly in reducing impact forces and modifying foot contact durations, reinforcing the benefits of a multifactorial approach in optimizing running biomechanics.

Future research should assess the long-term impact of cadence adjustments and footwear modifications on injury rates, particularly in runners with a history of overuse injuries. Additionally, wearable technology could be leveraged to monitor real-time biomechanical adaptations in natural running environments

Combining these interventions (C4) offers a multi-faceted strategy to enhance running efficiency, optimize biomechanics, and reduce injury risk.

This study highlights the potential of combined biomechanical modifications in enhancing running mechanics and reducing injury risks. By integrating cadence, footwear, and orthotic adjustments, runners and clinicians can implement evidence-based strategies for performance optimization and injury prevention.

Author Contributions: Conceptualization, Y.L., M.A.N.-P. and G.G.-N.; methodology, Y.L., E.L.-R. and G.G.-N.; formal analysis, E.P. and M.M.-R.; data curation, Y.L. and M.A.N.-P.; writing—original draft preparation, Y.L. and G.G.-N.; writing—review and editing, M.A.N.-P., Y.L., E.P., M.M.-R., C.T., G.G.-N. and E.L.-R. All authors have read and agreed to the published version of the manuscript.

Funding: This research received no external funding.

Institutional Review Board Statement: The study was conducted in accordance with the Declaration of Helsinki and approved by the Ethics Committee of the University of Malaga (CEUMA 206-2023-H) (27 February 2024) Spain.

Informed Consent Statement: Informed consent was obtained from all subjects involved in the study.

Data Availability Statement: The data are unavailable due to privacy or ethical restrictions; a statement is still required.

Conflicts of Interest: Author Corentin Travouillon was employed by the company TRINOMA. The remaining authors declare no conflicts of interest.

References

1. The State of Trail Running 2022. RunRepeat—Athletic Shoe Reviews. Available online: https://runrepeat.com/the-state-of-trail-running-2022 (accessed on 26 February 2025).
2. Hebdo N°1760-61-62—Pourquoi Court-On? Courrier International. Available online: https://www.courrierinternational.com/magazine/2024/1760-61-62-magazine (accessed on 26 December 2024).
3. Correia, C.K.; Machado, J.M.; Dominski, F.H.; de Castro, M.P.; de Brito Fontana, H.; Ruschel, C. Risk factors for running-related injuries: An umbrella systematic review. *J. Sport Health Sci.* **2024**, *13*, 793–804. [CrossRef] [PubMed]
4. Aicale, R.; Tarantino, D.; Maffulli, N. Overuse injuries in sport: A comprehensive overview. *J. Orthop. Surg. Res.* **2018**, *13*, 309. [CrossRef]
5. Edwards, W.B. Modeling Overuse Injuries in Sport as a Mechanical Fatigue Phenomenon. *Exerc. Sport Sci. Rev.* **2018**, *46*, 224–231. [CrossRef]
6. Taunton, J.E.; Ryan, M.B.; Clement, D.B.; McKenzie, D.C.; Lloyd-Smith, D.R.; Zumbo, B.D. A retrospective case-control analysis of 2002 running injuries. *Br. J. Sports Med.* **2002**, *36*, 95–101. [CrossRef]
7. Nielsen, R.O.; Cederholm, P.; Buist, I.; Sørensen, H.; Lind, M.; Rasmussen, S. Can GPS be used to detect deleterious progression in training volume among runners? *J. Strength Cond. Res.* **2013**, *27*, 1471–1478. [CrossRef]
8. Lopes, A.D.; Hespanhol Júnior, L.C.; Yeung, S.S.; Costa, L.O.P. What are the main running-related musculoskeletal injuries? A Systematic Review. *Sports Med.* **2012**, *42*, 891–905. [CrossRef] [PubMed]
9. Ferber, R.; Hreljac, A.; Kendall, K.D. Suspected Mechanisms in the Cause of Overuse Running Injuries. *Sports Health* **2009**, *1*, 242–246. [CrossRef] [PubMed]
10. Hreljac, A. Impact and overuse injuries in runners. *Med. Sci. Sports Exerc.* **2004**, *36*, 845–849. [CrossRef]
11. Hespanhol Junior, L.C.; Pena Costa, L.O.; Lopes, A.D. Previous injuries and some training characteristics predict running-related injuries in recreational runners: A prospective cohort study. *J. Physiother.* **2013**, *59*, 263–269. [CrossRef]
12. Napier, C.; Willy, R.W. The Prevention and Treatment of Running Injuries: A State of the Art. *Int. J. Sports Phys. Ther.* **2021**, *16*, 968–970. [CrossRef]
13. van der Worp, M.P.; ten Haaf, D.S.M.; van Cingel, R.; de Wijer, A.; Nijhuis-van der Sanden, M.W.G.; Staal, J.B. Injuries in runners; a systematic review on risk factors and sex differences. *PLoS ONE* **2015**, *10*, e0114937. [CrossRef] [PubMed]
14. Chan, Z.Y.; Zhang, J.H.; Au, I.P.; An, W.W.; Shum, G.L.; Ng, G.Y.; Cheung, R.T. Gait Retraining for the Reduction of Injury Occurrence in Novice Distance Runners: 1-Year Follow-up of a Randomized Controlled Trial. *Am. J. Sports Med.* **2018**, *46*, 388–395. [CrossRef]
15. Napier, C.; Cochrane, C.K.; Taunton, J.E.; Hunt, M.A. Gait modifications to change lower extremity gait biomechanics in runners: A systematic review. *Br. J. Sports Med.* **2015**, *49*, 1382–1388. [CrossRef]
16. Bredeweg, S.W.; Zijlstra, S.; Bessem, B.; Buist, I. The effectiveness of a preconditioning programme on preventing running-related injuries in novice runners: A randomised controlled trial. *Br. J. Sports Med.* **2012**, *46*, 865–870. [CrossRef] [PubMed]
17. de Souza Júnior, J.R.; Rabelo, P.H.R.; Lemos, T.V.; Esculier, J.-F.; Barbosa, G.M.P.; Matheus, J.P.C. Effects of two gait retraining programs on pain, function, and lower limb kinematics in runners with patellofemoral pain: A randomized controlled trial. *PLoS ONE* **2024**, *19*, e0295645. [CrossRef] [PubMed]
18. Kernozek, T.W.; Ricard, M.D. Foot placement angle and arch type: Effect on rearfoot motion. *Arch. Phys. Med. Rehabil.* **1990**, *71*, 988–991.
19. Barton, C.J.; Lack, S.; Hemmings, S.; Tufail, S.; Morrissey, D. The 'Best Practice Guide to Conservative Management of Patellofemoral Pain': Incorporating level 1 evidence with expert clinical reasoning. *Br. J. Sports Med.* **2015**, *49*, 923–934. [CrossRef]
20. Anderson, L.M.; Martin, J.F.; Barton, C.J.; Bonanno, D.R. What is the Effect of Changing Running Step Rate on Injury, Performance and Biomechanics? A Systematic Review and Meta-analysis. *Sports Med. Open* **2022**, *8*, 112. [CrossRef]
21. dos Santos, A.F.; Nakagawa, T.H.; Lessi, G.C.; Luz, B.C.; Matsuo, H.T.; Nakashima, G.Y.; Maciel, C.D.; Serrão, F.V. Effects of three gait retraining techniques in runners with patellofemoral pain. *Phys. Ther. Sport* **2019**, *36*, 92–100. [CrossRef]
22. Boldt, A.R.; Willson, J.D.; Barrios, J.A.; Kernozek, T.W. Effects of medially wedged foot orthoses on knee and hip joint running mechanics in females with and without patellofemoral pain syndrome. *J. Appl. Biomech.* **2013**, *29*, 68–77. [CrossRef]
23. Esculier, J.-F.; Bouyer, L.J.; Dubois, B.; Fremont, P.; Moore, L.; McFadyen, B.; Roy, J.-S. Is combining gait retraining or an exercise programme with education better than education alone in treating runners with patellofemoral pain? A randomised clinical trial. *Br. J. Sports Med.* **2018**, *52*, 659–666. [CrossRef] [PubMed]

24. Musgjerd, T.; Anason, J.; Rutherford, D.; Kernozek, T.W. Effect of Increasing Running Cadence on Peak Impact Force in an Outdoor Environment. *Int. J. Sports Phys. Ther.* **2021**, *16*, 1076–1083. [CrossRef] [PubMed]
25. Daoud, A.I.; Geissler, G.J.; Wang, F.; Saretsky, J.; Daoud, Y.A.; Lieberman, D.E. Foot strike and injury rates in endurance runners: A retrospective study. *Med. Sci. Sports Exerc.* **2012**, *44*, 1325–1334. [CrossRef]
26. Bonacci, J.; Vicenzino, B.; Spratford, W.; Collins, P. Take your shoes off to reduce patellofemoral joint stress during running. *Br. J. Sports Med.* **2014**, *48*, 425–428. [CrossRef] [PubMed]
27. Eslami, M.; Begon, M.; Hinse, S.; Sadeghi, H.; Popov, P.; Allard, P. Effect of foot orthoses on magnitude and timing of rearfoot and tibial motions, ground reaction force and knee moment during running. *J. Sci. Med. Sport* **2009**, *12*, 679–684. [CrossRef]
28. Jor, A.; Lau, N.W.; Daryabor, A.; Koh, M.W.; Lam, W.-K.; Hobara, H.; Kobayashi, T. Effects of foot orthoses on running kinetics and kinematics: A systematic review and meta-analysis. *Gait Posture* **2024**, *109*, 240–258. [CrossRef]
29. Cuschieri, S. The STROBE guidelines. *Saudi J. Anaesth.* **2019**, *13*, S31–S34. [CrossRef]
30. WMA—The World Medical Association-WMA Declaration of Helsinki—Ethical Principles for Medical Research Involving Human Participants. Available online: https://www.wma.net/policies-post/wma-declaration-of-helsinki/ (accessed on 26 December 2024).
31. Lavigne, A.; Lescure, Y.; Delacroix, S. La podologie orthopédique avancée. *Rev. Du Podol.* **2017**, *13*, 8–10. [CrossRef]
32. Nigg, B.M.; Wakeling, J.M. Impact forces and muscle tuning: A new paradigm. *Exerc. Sport Sci. Rev.* **2001**, *29*, 37–41. [CrossRef]
33. Guyot, M. Analyse Baropodométrique Embarquée Après un Programme de Rééducation sur Tapis de Marche dans la Maladie de Parkinson. Ph.D. Thesis, Université de Lorraine, Nancy, France, 2020.
34. Bisiaux, M.; Moretto, P.; Lensel, G.; Thévenon, A. Détermination d'un seuil de pression plantaire attendu: Utilisation de l'approche adimensionnelle pour réduire la variabilité des pressions plantaires Determination of an expected plantar pressure threshold: Dimensionless approach use to reduce the variability of the plantar pressures. *Ann. Readapt. Med. Phys.* **2003**, *46*, 539–544. [CrossRef]
35. Gouelle, A. Analyse des appuis plantaires sur tapis de marche: État actuel et perspectives. In Proceedings of the 35ème Journée Montpelliéraine de Podologie, Médecine et Chirurgie du Pied, Montpellier, France, 7 March 2014.
36. Schubert, A.G.; Kempf, J.; Heiderscheit, B.C. Influence of stride frequency and length on running mechanics: A systematic review. *Sports Health* **2014**, *6*, 210–217. [CrossRef] [PubMed]
37. Ogasawara, I.; Shimokochi, Y.; Konda, S.; Mae, T.; Nakata, K. Effect of Rearfoot Strikes on the Hip and Knee Rotational Kinetic Chain During the Early Phase of Cutting in Female Athletes. *Sports Med. Open* **2021**, *7*, 75. [CrossRef] [PubMed]
38. Lenhart, R.L.; Thelen, D.G.; Wille, C.M.; Chumanov, E.S.; Heiderscheit, B.C. Increasing Running Step Rate Reduces Patellofemoral Joint Forces. *Med. Sci. Sports Exerc.* **2014**, *46*, 557–564. [CrossRef]
39. Nakhaee, M.; Mohseni-Bandpei, M.; Mousavi, M.E.; Shakourirad, A.; Safari, R.; Kashani, R.V.; Mimar, R.; Amiri, H.; Nakhaei, M. The effects of a custom foot orthosis on dynamic plantar pressure in patients with chronic plantar fasciitis: A randomized controlled trial. *Prosthet. Orthot. Int.* **2023**, *47*, 241–252. [CrossRef] [PubMed]
40. Farris, D.; Buckeridge, E.; Trewartha, G.; McGuigan, P. The Effects of Orthotic Heel Lifts on Achilles Tendon Force Strain During Running. *Comp. Biochem. Physiol. Part A: Mol. Integr. Physiol.* **2008**, *150*, S82. [CrossRef]
41. Lieberman, D.E.; Venkadesan, M.; Werbel, W.A.; Daoud, A.I.; D'andrea, S.; Davis, I.S.; Mang'eni, R.O.; Pitsiladis, Y. Foot strike patterns and collision forces in habitually barefoot versus shod runners. *Nature* **2010**, *463*, 531–535. [CrossRef]
42. Bachand, R.; Bazett-Jones, D.M.; Esculier, J.-F.; Fox, C.; Norte, G.E.; Garcia, M.C. The Dogma of Running Injuries: Perceptions of Adolescent and Adult Runners. *J. Athl. Train.* **2024**, *59*, 955–961. [CrossRef]
43. Heiderscheit, B.C.; Chumanov, E.S.; Michalski, M.P.; Wille, C.M.; Ryan, M.B. Effects of step rate manipulation on joint mechanics during running. *Med. Sci. Sports Exerc.* **2011**, *43*, 296–302. [CrossRef]
44. Crago, D.; Bishop, C.; Arnold, J.B. The effect of foot orthoses and insoles on running economy and performance in distance runners: A systematic review and meta-analysis. *J. Sports Sci.* **2019**, *37*, 2613–2624. [CrossRef]
45. Warne, J.P.; Gruber, A.H. Transitioning to Minimal Footwear: A Systematic Review of Methods and Future Clinical Recommendations. *Sports Med. Open* **2017**, *3*, 33. [CrossRef]
46. Cheung, R.T.H.; Davis, I.S. Landing pattern modification to improve patellofemoral pain in runners: A case series. *J. Orthop. Sports Phys. Ther.* **2011**, *41*, 914–919. [CrossRef] [PubMed]
47. Bonanno, D.R.; Murley, G.S.; Munteanu, S.E.; Landorf, K.B.; Menz, H.B. Effectiveness of foot orthoses for the prevention of lower limb overuse injuries in naval recruits: A randomised controlled trial. *Br. J. Sports Med.* **2018**, *52*, 298–302. [CrossRef] [PubMed]
48. Willy, R.W.; Davis, I.S. The effect of a hip-strengthening program on mechanics during running and during a single-leg squat. *J. Orthop. Sports Phys. Ther.* **2011**, *41*, 625–632. [CrossRef] [PubMed]

49. Nigg, B.M.; Emery, C.; Hiemstra, L.A. Unstable shoe construction and reduction of pain in osteoarthritis patients. *Med. Sci. Sports Exerc.* **2006**, *38*, 1701–1708. [CrossRef]
50. Noehren, B.; Hamill, J.; Davis, I. Prospective evidence for a hip etiology in patellofemoral pain. *Med. Sci. Sports Exerc.* **2013**, *45*, 1120–1124. [CrossRef]

Disclaimer/Publisher's Note: The statements, opinions and data contained in all publications are solely those of the individual author(s) and contributor(s) and not of MDPI and/or the editor(s). MDPI and/or the editor(s) disclaim responsibility for any injury to people or property resulting from any ideas, methods, instructions or products referred to in the content.

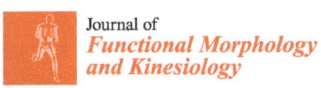

Article

Learning to Cycle: Why Is the Balance Bike More Efficient than the Bicycle with Training Wheels? The Lyapunov's Answer

Cristiana Mercê [1,2,3,4,*], Keith Davids [5], Rita Cordovil [4], David Catela [1,3,6] and Marco Branco [1,2,3,4]

1. Sport Sciences School of Rio Maior, Santarém Polytechnic University, Avenue Dr. Mário Soares No. 110, 2040-413 Rio Maior, Portugal; catela@esdrm.ipsantarem.pt (D.C.); marcobranco@esdrm.ipsantarem.pt (M.B.)
2. Physical Activity and Health—Life Quality Research Centre (CIEQV), Polytechnique University of Santarém, Complex Andaluz, Apart 279, 2001-904 Santarém, Portugal
3. Sport Physical Activity and Health Research & Innovation Center (SPRINT), Santarém Polytechnic University, Complex Andaluz, Apart 279, 2001-904 Santarém, Portugal
4. Interdisciplinary Center for the Study of Human Performance (CIPER), Faculty of Human Kinetics, University of Lisbon, Cruz Quebrada-Dafundo, 1499-002 Lisboa, Portugal; cordovil.rita@gmail.com
5. Sport & Human Performance Group, Sheffield Hallam University, Sheffield S10 2BP, UK; k.davids@shu.ac.uk
6. Quality Education—Life Quality Research Centre (CIEQV), Santarém Polytechnique University, Complex Andaluz, Apart 279, 2001-904 Santarém, Portugal
*   Correspondence: cristianamerce@esdrm.ipsantarem.pt

Citation: Mercê, C.; Davids, K.; Cordovil, R.; Catela, D.; Branco, M. Learning to Cycle: Why Is the Balance Bike More Efficient than the Bicycle with Training Wheels? The Lyapunov's Answer. *J. Funct. Morphol. Kinesiol.* **2024**, *9*, 266. https://doi.org/10.3390/jfmk9040266

Academic Editor: Pedro Miguel Forte

Received: 11 November 2024
Revised: 29 November 2024
Accepted: 5 December 2024
Published: 10 December 2024

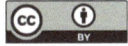

Copyright: © 2024 by the authors. Licensee MDPI, Basel, Switzerland. This article is an open access article distributed under the terms and conditions of the Creative Commons Attribution (CC BY) license (https://creativecommons.org/licenses/by/4.0/).

Abstract: Background/Objectives: Riding a bicycle is a foundational movement skill that can be acquired at an early age. The most common training bicycle has lateral training wheels (BTW). However, the balance bike (BB) has consistently been regarded as more efficient, as children require less time on this bike to successfully transition to a traditional bike (TB). The reasons for this greater efficiency remain unclear, but it is hypothesized that it is due to the immediate balancing requirements for learners. This study aimed to investigate the reasons why the BB is more efficient than the BTW for learning to cycle on a TB. Methods: We compared the variability of the child–bicycle system throughout the learning process with these two types of training bicycles and after transitioning to the TB. Data were collected during the Learning to Cycle Program, with 23 children (6.00 ± 1.2 years old) included. Participants were divided into two experimental training groups, BB (N = 12) and BTW (N = 11). The angular velocity data of the child–bicycle system were collected by four inertial measurement sensors (IMUs), located on the child's vertex and T2 and the bicycle frame and handlebar, in three time phases: (i) before practice sessions, (ii) immediately after practice sessions, and (iii) two months after practice sessions with the TB. The largest Lyapunov exponents were calculated to assess movement variability. Conclusions: Results supported the hypothesis that the BB affords greater functional variability during practice sessions compared to the BTW, affording more functionally adaptive responses in the learning transition to using a TB.

Keywords: bicycle; functional variability; nonlinear; inertial sensors; skill adaptation; postural control; learning paths; motor development; physical activity; health

1. Introduction

Riding a bicycle has recently been considered a foundational movement skill [1,2] with multiple lifetime benefits [3], which should be promoted early in development [4]. The new conceptual model proposed by Hulteen et al. [1] suggests replacing the term 'fundamental movement skills' with 'foundational movement skills', which underpins a significant conceptual adaptation to broaden the scope of skills, including specifically riding a bicycle, considered important for promoting physical activity and other positive health trajectories across a lifespan. Indeed, several studies corroborate that learning to cycle supports adherence to and the maintenance of healthy and positive trajectories, particularly due to the beneficial effects on physical health, such as improved body composition and enhanced cardiorespiratory fitness [3], and mental health, including increased socialization opportunities and the development of social skills [5,6]. For all these reasons, previous studies have considered learning to ride a bicycle an important milestone [4,7,8].

According to research, even though using a bicycle with lateral training wheels (BTW) is the most common approach to learning to cycle worldwide [9], the balance bike (BB), a bicycle without pedals nor training wheels, is the most efficient learning bicycle [4,9–13]. It has been argued that the use of the BTW is a mistake [12] which can be counterproductive [10,11,14–19]. By adding the side wheels, as an artificial method to increase stability and minimize bicycle oscillations, the child learns to pedal without directly experiencing the bicycle's instability. When training wheels are removed, the child is confronted for the first time with the instability of the bicycle and responds by organizing defensive responses, including freezing their upper limbs and trunk, impacting the imbalance of the bicycle [10,13]. On the other hand, a child using the BB from the start immediately learns to engage with instability and only has to deal with pedaling after achieving and maintaining balance. Several other studies have indicated that the balance bike (BB) is a more efficient learning tool than the bicycle with training wheels (BTW). For instance, a recent systematic review investigated the best strategies to promote efficient cycle learning [4]. Additionally, a retrospective study found that children who learn to cycle using the BB can successfully cycle independently on average 1.81 years earlier than those who use the BTW [9]. Despite the significance of these ideas [4,12,20] for learning to cycle only, one study has sought to experimentally verify the efficacy of these two training bicycles [13]. The investigation applied an intervention program (L2Cycle), comparing two groups of kindergarten and elementary school children, where one group practiced with the BTW and another with the BB. They found that the BB group learned to self-start, ride, brake, and cycle independently (i.e., all these cycling milestones performed sequentially) significantly faster than participants in the BTW group, which corroborates previous suggestions in the literature. However, the "why" question is left unresolved, with a need for research to verify possible reasons behind the greater effectiveness of the BB in learning to cycle.

Our conceptualization of the BB's learning effectiveness lies in the functionality of motor system variability for skill adaptation. Traditional approaches to interpreting movement system variability considered it 'noise' or a result of errors [21,22] to be eliminated from performance. More recently, a dynamical systems interpretation has highlighted the functionality and importance of movement variability for adapting skills [23]. That is, the same coordination task, like cycling with a training bicycle, could be performed by re-organizing multiple elements or degrees of freedom (e.g., motor units, muscles, joints, limbs, a movement axes, and planes) and a wide variety of combinations between them [24]. Functionality is assumed to be a system's ability to carry out its tasks effectively and adaptively. Movement variability, as a movement system that explores different solutions for the same task, can contribute to task functionality by affording system adaptability in facing unexpected and challenging situations [25]. The human movement system has evolved the capacity to produce several solutions for the same coordination task (e.g., locomotion), affording functional system adaptability in facing unexpected and challenging contexts, such as being able to use a traditional bicycle [21,25]. Variability during the learning process is currently considered a crucial aspect and is one of the essential elements of the recent theory of nonlinear pedagogy [23,26]. According to this theoretical framework, which is based on dynamic systems [27,28], Newell's constraints [29], and ecological dynamics [30], learning should be learner-centered rather than teacher-centered. The teacher/coach acts as a filmmaker who sets the stage for learning (i.e., manipulates various constraints) so that the main actor, the learner, can self-organize and acquire and master the new motor skill. Therefore, the teacher should introduce variability during the process, encouraging the learner to seek new and more efficient motor solutions [23,26].

Movement variability has traditionally been measured by using linear tools, like the standard deviation statistic, to quantify the amount of variability independently of their order in a data series [22]. In contrast, nonlinear methods afford analysis based on the performance process, looking for both the structure and quality of variability [31]. To analyze variability in biological systems, as in the case of a child riding a bicycle, nonlinear measurement tools can provide deeper insights in the (re)organization of movement [31]. In this sense, several nonlinear methods could be used, such as recurrence quantification analysis (RQA) [32], which evaluates the recurrence of dynamic states in time series; or, the single scale entropy could be used, which can be used as a measure of the uncertainty and irregularity of time series [33,34]. Nevertheless, considering the present study's purpose, which consists of specifically analyzing motor variability, and its specifications, including periodic data from angular velocities, the most suitable nonlinear technique consists of the largest Lyapunov exponent (LyE) [35,36]. The LyE is probably the most popular nonlinear method used to assess stability and variability [31,35]. This method is widely used in the analysis of biological systems because it offers a deeper understanding of the neuromotor control of movement. It is very sensitive to initial conditions and the divergence of trajectories in dynamic systems, providing a robust measure of system stability and variability [31,35,36]. This method reconstructs the data in a system's state phase and measures the rate at which the orbits converge or diverge. In periodic signals, the LyE value is 0, as the orbits do not converge or diverge. A positive LyE signifies that the orbits are diverging, while a negative value indicates that the orbits are converging [37]. The LyE has already proven to be a valid measure for analyzing human gait [35,36], since lower values LyE indicate rigidity in the system and an inability to adapt. In contrast, higher values indicate greater variability and adaptability, with the system being able to respond more quickly to destabilization in order to maintain system order [35,38].

Considering the gap in the literature regarding rationalizations for the greater efficiency of BBs, compared to BTWs, and the potential of using nonlinear methods to study rider–system variability, the present study sought to investigate the process of learning to cycle with either the BB or BTW. Specifically, we compared variability (by using the LyE) (i) within the same training bicycle group (BB or BTW), (ii) between bicycle groups (BB vs. BTW) at different stages of learning, and (iii), between children who did and did not learn to cycle independently. We also considered the newer theories that have highlighted the importance of variability [39] and the existing literature that points out balance exploration as the key component for the BB's efficiency [4,40]. We hypothesized that the mechanisms behind the effectiveness of the balance bike (BB) include the immediate engagement with balance and postural control, which promotes greater functional variability. This variability may allow children to explore and adapt their movements more effectively, leading to the quicker mastery of cycling skills. In this sense, we hypothesized the following: (a) the BB would afford greater functional variability, compared to the BTW, during the period of first contact with a bicycle and after training; (b) there would be no difference in variability after children learned to independently cycle on the traditional bicycle; and (c) children who did not learn to cycle independently during the program would display lower values of variability than children who did. If these hypotheses were confirmed, the findings could indicate that the greater values of variability in using the BB signal its greater efficiency in supporting children's skill adaptation in functionally using a traditional bicycle.

2. Materials and Methods

2.1. Study Design

This study was conducted during the Learning to Cycle Program (L2Cycle) intervention, a two-week bicycle camp that helped children to learn how to cycle. The program included six lessons with a BB group and a BTW group, followed by four sessions with both groups using the traditional bicycle (TB) (i.e., with pedals and without training wheels). The training environment was designed with different surfaces, slopes, and vertical obstacles, allowing children to explore actions related to the basic milestones of cycling including self-starting, maintaining balance, moving around, avoiding obstacles, and braking. Practice sessions were undertaken daily for a duration of 30 min and were conducted by physical exercise technicians with safety equipment [13]. The results regarding the effectiveness of learning to cycle between the BB and BTW, by analyzing the number of sessions required to achieve each stage of cycling, as well as independent cycling, have already been presented and discussed in a previous study (see more information in [13]). This intervention was simultaneously used to collect data on variability during the learning process using two different training bikes, which is the focus of the present study.

To analyze movements during the learning process, three evaluation phases were defined: (i) before the training program, with the training bicycle (O1), (ii) after the six training lessons, still with the training bicycle (O2), and (iii), two months after the training program, with the TB; see Figure 1. The program and the data collection procedures were approved by the Ethics Committee of the Faculty of Human Kinetics (approval number: 22/2019).

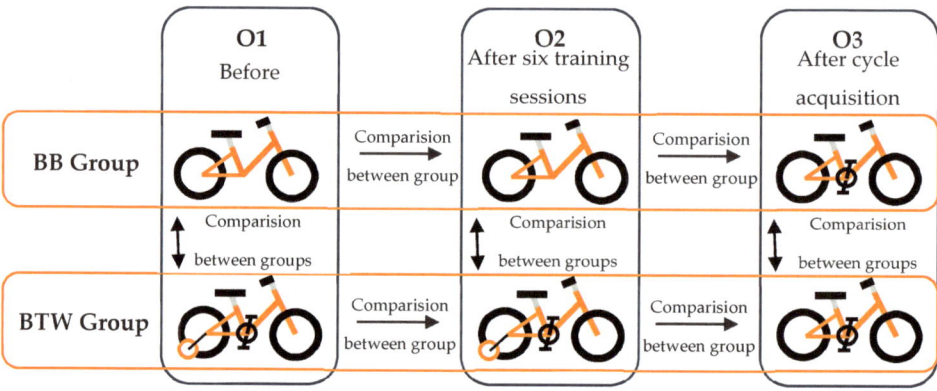

Figure 1. A presentation of the study design (2 groups × 3 moments), with the identification of the comparisons.

2.2. Participants

Twenty-three children participated in the study, aged between three and seven years (nine girls; M= 6.00; SD = 1.20 years). Random stratified samples were constituted based on sex and age. Twelve children were allocated to the BB group and eleven to the BTW group. In O1 (pre-intervention evaluation), no statistically significant differences were found between the groups regarding their weight, height, BMI, BMIs percentile, motor competence, and previous bicycle experiences (all p_s > 0.05) [13]. Participation in the study was completely voluntary and free of charge, and participants could leave the study if they wished without having to give reasons.

Before the intervention, we confirmed that none of the participants were able to cycle independently, meaning that they did not know how to ride a traditional bicycle. The ability to cycle independently prior to the intervention was an exclusion criterion. To be considered independent riders, the children needed to fulfill the following criteria: to be able to perform a self-launch (to start cycling, the researcher could only stabilize the bicycle if the child's feet could not reach the ground, due to small stature), cycle for at least 10 m, and brake safely.

All participants performed in O1 and O2. However, in O3, four children in the BB training group did not participate, with one due to health issues and three because they were not able to perform the self-launch, due to their small stature. Another four children in the BTW group did not participate in O3, with one because of their small stature and three because they could not cycle independently using the TB.

2.3. Bicycle Equipment

The bicycles used were the LittleBig Balance Bike (LittleBig, Wicklow, Ireland). This model was chosen because it can be adapted, through the rotation of its saddle, to children from 2 to 7 years old and because it allows the insertion of the pedal crank in it. The BTW group used the same LittleBig model but with the pedal crank and two lateral training wheels added. The use of the same bicycle model in the two groups also allowed us to eliminate possible variables masked by use of different bicycle models by the different groups, ruling out variations due to ergonomic issues or component friction.

2.4. Data Collection and Protocols

To ensure similarity between the groups at the beginning of the intervention, data on body composition, motor competence, and previous cycling experience were collected during the O1 evaluation. A Level II anthropometrist certified by the International Society for the Advancement of Kinanthropometry (ISAK) performed the body composition measurements, which included weight and height [41], followed by the calculation of BMI and its percentile classification according to age and sex [42]. Motor competence was assessed using the Motor Competence Assessment battery [43]. Previous cycling experience information was gathered through a brief questionnaire administered to parents or guardians [13].

To ensure that the participants were comfortable and familiar with the study procedures and equipment, a thorough familiarization process was conducted prior to the data collection [44]. This process included the following steps: (i) an introduction to the task, presented as a game; (ii) equipment familiarization, where the participants were introduced to the customized vest with the inertial measurement units (IMUs) and the equipment was presented as a superhero outfit that was going to collect some information about the game they were playing; (iii) equipment exploration, where, prior to mounting the bicycle, the children were invited to walk and run a little with the customized vest in order to get used to the feel of the equipment; (iv) safety and comfort checks, where, throughout the familiarization process, investigators conducted regular checks to ensure that the equipment was properly fitted and that the participants were comfortable.

During all moments of evaluation (O1, O2, and O3), the children were invited to ride a bicycle for five minutes, in a 10 m $\times$ 10 m area, with no further instructions or feedback from trainers (for more details, see [45]).

Considering that we wanted to calculate the variability of the child and the bicycle, four inertial measurement units (IMUs) (SparkFun 9DoF Razor, Niwot, CO, USA) were used and placed in specific locations. These specific locations were chosen to provide a comprehensive analysis of both the rider's body movements and the bicycle's dynamics, allowing for a detailed understanding of the child–bicycle system during the learning process. On the participants, one IMU was placed at the vertex point through an adjusted headband [46,47], allowing the analysis of head movements. This location was selected because head movements are crucial for understanding how the child controls their balance and spatial orientation while cycling. Another IMU was placed by the second vertebra of the thoracic column (T2) [48], through a customized vest, allowing analyses of trunk segment motions. The trunk plays a fundamental role in maintaining balance and coordinating movements during cycling. By monitoring the trunk's movements, we could assess how the child stabilized their body and adapted their posture to maintain equilibrium and control the bicycle effectively. On the bicycle, one IMU was placed in the spokes of the front wheel, providing data from the handlebar. This location was chosen because the handlebar movements were directly influenced by the child's actions and were essential for steering and maintaining the bicycle's stability. Analyzing the handlebar data helped us understand how the child manipulated the bicycle to navigate and maintain balance, which is critical for developing cycling proficiency. Another IMU was placed in the seat tube of the bicycle frame, providing motion data relating to the whole bicycle [11]. This location was selected to capture the overall dynamics of the bicycle, including its oscillations and adjustments made by the child; see Figure 2. Inertial sensors (IMUs) have been consistently shown in the previous literature to be reliable tools for capturing kinematic data [49]. These small, powerful devices allow for the quick and convenient collection of large amounts of data, enabling more ecological assessments. Winter et al. [50] highlighted their effectiveness in analyzing movement variability during cycling, demonstrating their capability in capturing kinematic data across different body segments. The excellent validity and reliability of IMUs have also been tested and proven in various other activities, such as running and walking [51,52] and jumping [53]. The sensor was calibrated according to the manufacturer's recommendations by holding the sensor in a static position for 8 s previous to each collection [54]. All collected data from the IMUs were sampled at a rate of 100 Hz, with a full scale of 4G defined for the accelerometer and 2000 deg/s for the gyroscope [45].

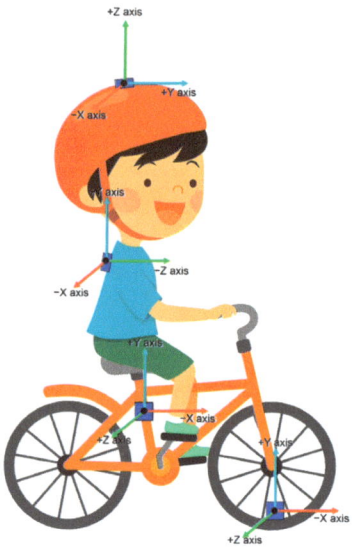

Figure 2. A graphical representation of the experimental setup with the sensor locations.

Each data collection phase was also video-recorded to identify the points in time when the child was cycling or performing other activities (e.g., stopping to rest or fall). The video was recorded with a smartphone (Samsung A71, Seoul, Republic of Korea) at 30 Hz. To synchronize the IMUs and the video, before each data collection period, the researcher lifted and dropped the bicycle's front wheel on the ground, on three consecutive occasions, with intervals of approximately five seconds between them. Before data analysis, a visual inspection was made to identify the three peaks corresponding to the three drops. The IMUs were synchronized by identifying the first acceleration peak from each drop. The video was also synchronized to the IMU data by identifying the first video frame corresponding to the first impact of the front wheel on the ground; this synchronization process allowed us to identify in the IMU data the onsets of periods of cycling and other activities previously verified in the videos [45].

2.5. Data and Statistical Treatment

Initially, all video clips were analyzed to identify the beginning and end of each data collection episode, as well as the moments when the child was not cycling (e.g., when they fell or their image exited the video frame). These were later discarded.

Data treatment was performed with a custom matlab routine. Considering that the length of a time series affects the calculation of LyE values, and following the recommendation that time-normalization to a fixed point or duration is necessary [36], all time series were cut according to the one with the lowest duration, which was fixed at three minutes. This value is within methodological recommendations established in the literature [36]. After normalization, the data were filtered using a low-pass, second-order Butterworth filter with a cutoff frequency of 10 Hz (e.g., [55,56]). Therefore, the LyE values for the angular velocity were calculated for each IMU, child, and evaluation moment. The angular velocity variable was chosen because it allows the study of postural control (e.g., [57,58]) and because the movements under analysis were mainly rotations.

For the statistical analysis of the data from the IMUs located on the children's heads and trunks, three movement planes were considered, since the movement was multiplanar. For the handlebar IMU, only the frontal and transverse planes were considered, since the handlebars did not move in the sagittal plane. For the IMU of the bicycle frame, only the frontal plane was considered since it did not move in sagittal and transversal planes.

The statistical analysis of the data was performed with the Statistical Package for Social Sciences (IBM Corp, version 26), and the statistical significance level was defined at $p < 0.05$. Descriptive statistics were used for sample characterization and for the LyE values of each IMU for each movement plane, evaluation moment, and group. The Shapiro–Wilk test was used to estimate the samples' normality of data distribution. Accordingly, paired t-tests were used to compare, within the same group, the values of each IMU, for each movement plane, between the different evaluation moments. Independent t-tests were performed to compare the same IMU, for each movement and evaluation moment, between the two training groups, BB and BTW, and between the BTW children who became independent riders and those who did not. For all significant comparisons, the effect size r was calculated [59].

3. Results

The descriptive data (average ± standard deviation) of each IMU for each movement plane, moment of evaluation (O1, O2, and O3), and group are presented in Table 1. All Lyapunov mean values were highly positive and far from zero, signifying divergent orbits or that the body and bicycle oscillations were not regular in space. These values were always higher in the BB group, except for frontal plane in the O1 and O2 moments. Per group and between movement planes, the Lyapunov standard deviations of the child and of the bicycle were small and similar, particularly very much smaller than the Lyapunov means. This finding is statistically important, considering the sample sizes. Interestingly, when the standard deviation values were analyzed, the BTW group presented higher values than the BB group for both O1 and O2, except only at the O2 point's sagittal plane. However, in O3, this tendency was inverted, and the BB group had higher standard deviation values, with the only exception of the vertex's frontal plane.

Table 1. Lyapunov descriptive statistics (M ± SD), in BB and BTW groups, for each IMU, movement plane, and evaluation moment (O1, O2, O3).

Group	IMU	Movement Plane	O1 M ± SD	O2 M ± SD	O3 M ± SD
BB	Vertex	Sagittal	58.82 ± 1.45	59.27 ± 1.03	58.50 ± 1.43
		Frontal	57.85 ± 1.14	57.72 ± 0.87	56.64 ± 1.26
		Transverse	56.51 ± 1.25	56.87 ± 1.04	55.63 ± 1.71
	T2	Sagittal	59.16 ± 1.51	58.48 ± 1.21	57.30 ± 0.99
		Frontal	56.61 ± 1.25	56.33 ± 0.77	55.39 ± 1.31
		Transverse	57.36 ± 0.80	57.16 ± 0.65	56.18 ± 1.63
	Bicycle frame	Frontal	54.32 ± 1.29	55.22 ± 0.72	55.86 ± 0.94
	Handlebar	Frontal	55.97 ± 1.08	57.33 ± 1.14	57.60 ± 1.48
		Transverse	55.84 ± 1.13	57.20 ± 1.14	57.72 ± 1.65

Table 1. *Cont.*

Group	IMU	Movement Plane	O1 M ± SD	O2 M ± SD	O3 M ± SD
BTW	Vertex	Sagittal	56.60 ± 2.13	55.39 ± 1.35	58.41 ± 1.36
		Frontal	55.18 ± 1.76	57.51 ± 1.13	56.22 ± 1.98
		Transverse	53.91 ± 1.87	54.94 ± 1.35	54.37 ± 1.45
	T2	Sagittal	56.01 ± 1.82	56.28 ± 0.98	57.58 ± 0.78
		Frontal	52.58 ± 2.16	53.43 ± 1.21	54.55 ± 1.23
		Transverse	55.02 ± 1.87	55.97 ± 1.70	55.79 ± 0.98
	Bicycle frame	Frontal	57.52 ± 1.82	58.28 ± 1.49	55.01 ± 0.47
	Handlebar	Frontal	53.39 ± 2.12	55.35 ± 2.02	57.56 ± 1.10
		Transverse	53.54 ± 2.22	55.51 ± 1.66	57.68 ± 0.67

3.1. Comparisons Between Evaluation Moments

Considering the BB group, between pre-intervention (O1) and after six training sessions (O2), there were significant increases in the variability in the following: (i) the bicycle frame for lateral rotations in the frontal plane (t(11) = −2.41; p = 0.035; r = 0.588); (ii) the handlebar for lateral rotations in the frontal plane (t(11) = −3.74; p = 0.003; r = 0.748); and (iii) left–right rotations in the transverse plane (t(11) = −2.334; p = 0.04, r = 0.576). No statistically significant changes were observed for the data from the vertex and T2 IMUs. In comparing results from after training with the BB (O2) to results from after cycling skill acquisition on the TB (O3), significant decreases occurred in the variability levels at T2 for all planes; the children reduced their velocities for flexion and extension in the sagittal plane (t(7) = 2.634; p = 0.034; r = 0.706), lateral flexions in the frontal plane (t(7) = 4.201; p = 0.004; r = 0.775), and left–right rotations in the transverse plane (t(7) = 2.467; p = 0.043, r = 0.682). No significant changes were verified for the other IMUs. The statistical outcomes are presented above in Table 2, and an illustrative schematic of all comparisons is presented in Figure 3.

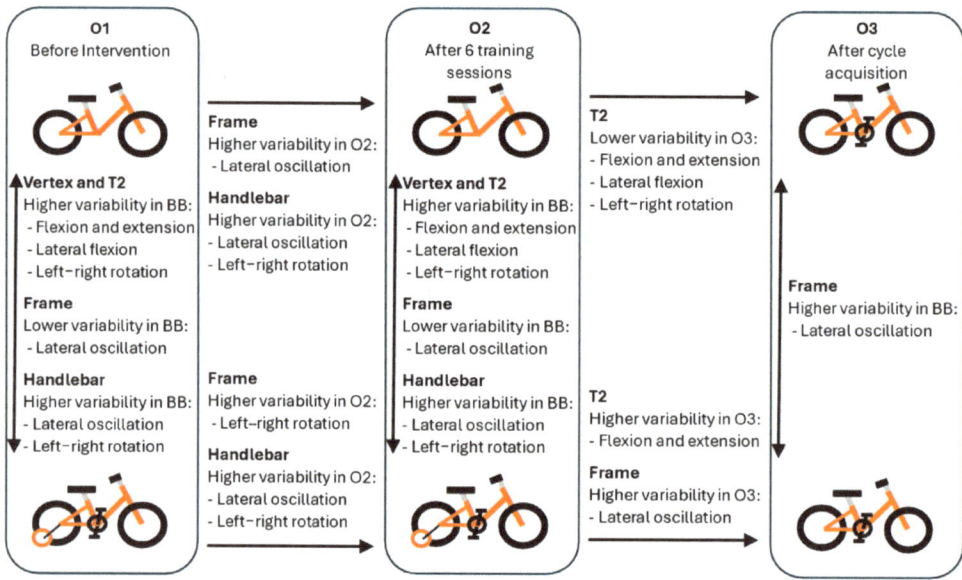

Figure 3. Abstract graph of comparisons of results between periods (O1, O2, O3) and between groups (BB, BTW).

Table 2. A table summarizing the significant differences between assessment moments within the same group.

Group	IMU	Movement Plane	O1 Versus O2 p, r, Direction Change	O2 Versus O3 p, r, Direction Change
BB	Vertex	Sagittal	ns	ns
		Frontal	ns	ns
		Transverse	ns	ns
	T2	Sagittal	ns	p = 0.034; r = 0.706; ↓
		Frontal	ns	p = 0.004; r = 0.775; ↓
		Transverse	ns	p = 0.043; r = 0.682; ↓
	Bicycle frame	Frontal	p = 0.035; r = 0.588; ↑	ns
	Handlebar	Frontal	p = 0.003; r = 0.748; ↑	ns
		Transverse	p = 0.04; r = 0.576; ↑	ns
BTW	Vertex	Sagittal	ns	ns
		Frontal	ns	ns
		Transverse	p = 0.025; r = 0.640; ↑	ns
	T2	Sagittal	ns	p = 0.020; r = 0.790; ↑
		Frontal	ns	ns
		Transverse	ns	ns
	Bicycle frame	Frontal	ns	p = 0.006; r = 0.865; ↑
	Handlebar	Frontal	p = 0.009; r = 0.713; ↑	ns
		Transverse	p = 0.012; r = 0.697; ↑	ns

Notes: ns—no statistical significance; ↑—significant increase between evaluations; ↓—significant decrease between evaluations.

Considering the BTW group, after the six training sessions, there were significant increases in the system variability in the following: (i) the vertex for left–right rotations ($t(10) = -2.636$; $p = 0.025$; $r = 0.640$); (ii) the handlebar for lateral rotations ($t(10) = -3.218$; $p = 0.009$; $r = 0.713$); and (iii) left–right rotations ($t(10) = -3.077$; $p = 0.012$; $r = 0.697$). There were no significant changes observed in the data from the T2 and bicycle frame IMUs. In comparing results from after training with the BB (O2) to results from after cycling skill acquisition on the TB (O3), significant increases in the variability for the T2 IMU were verified in the values for the velocity of the flexion and extension ($t(6) = -3.152$; $p = 0.020$; $r = 0.790$) and in the bicycle frame's velocity of lateral rotations ($t(6) = 4.219$; $p = 0.006$; $r = 0.865$); no differences were observed in the variability values for the vertex nor the handlebar (see Figure 3).

3.2. Comparisons Between Groups

The comparison between the BB and BTW groups showed significantly greater variability in the BB group during O1 and O2. This was observed for the vertex (flexion and extension, lateral oscillations, and left–right rotations), T2 (flexion and extension, lateral oscillations, and left–right rotations), and handlebar (lateral oscillations and left–right rotations). Conversely, the BTW group showed greater variability in the bicycle frame's lateral oscillations during both O1 and O2, confirming the Lyapunov mean values. The statistical results for significant differences are presented in Table 3 and Figure 3.

In O3, after acquiring cycling skills, the only difference between the groups was in the velocity of the bicycle frame's lateral oscillations, with the BB group showing greater variability.

Table 3. A table summarizing the significant differences between groups within the same assessment moments.

Groups	IMU	Movement Plane	O1	O2	O3 (in TB)
BB versus BTW	Vertex	Sagittal	$p = 0.008; r = 0.541;$ ↑	$p = 0.001; r = 0.650;$ ↑	ns
		Frontal	$p < 0.001; r = 0.689;$ ↑	$p < 0.001; r = 0.792;$ ↑	ns
		Transverse	$p = 0.001; r = 0.653;$ ↑	$p = 0.008; r = 542;$ ↑	ns
	T2	Sagittal	$p < 0.001; r = 0.771;$ ↑	$p < 0.001; r = 0.720;$ ↑	ns
		Frontal	$p < 0.001; r = 0.771;$ ↑	$p < 0.001; r = 0.833;$ ↑	ns
		Transverse	$p < 0.001; r = 0.654;$ ↑	$p = 0.034; r = 0.443;$ ↑	ns
	Bicycle frame	Frontal	$p < 0.001; r = 0.730;$ ↓	$p < 0.001; r = 0.814;$ ↓	$p = 0.048; r = 0.519;$ ↑
	Handlebar	Frontal	$p = 0.001; r = 0.630;$ ↑	$p = 0.008; r = 0.538;$ ↑	ns
		Transverse	$p = 0.005; r = 0.570;$ ↑	$p = 0.009; r = 0.530;$ ↑	ns

Notes: ns—no statistical significance; ↑—value significantly superior in BB group; ↓—value significantly inferior in BB group.

3.3. Comparisons to Children That Did Not Acquire the Skill of Cycling Independently

The L2Cycle program demonstrated an 88% success rate for achieving independent cycling on the TB. Notably, all children in the BB group successfully reached the level of independent cycling, resulting in a 100% success rate. In contrast, three children in the BTW group did not reach this level, resulting in a 75% success rate. To consider whether variability could be one of the reasons for this failure, a comparison between the performance of children in the BTW group who became independent riders and those who did not was undertaken at the first moment of evaluation, O1, and after six training lessons, in O2. In O1, there was no significant difference in the variability measures recorded by any IMU. At the beginning of training (O1), the BTW children who ended up not achieving independent cycling acted similarly to those who did. However, in O2, the independent riders had a higher level of variability in the velocity of the handlebar for lateral oscillations (t(9) = 4.411; $p = 0.002$; r = 827) and left–right rotations (t(9) = 4.191; $p = 0.002$; r = 0.813); no other statistically significant differences were observed in O2. It should be noted that children who did not acquire the level of cycling independently displayed lower mean values than the independent riders for all other measures from the IMUs and planes of movement; see Table 4.

Table 4. Lyapunov descriptive statistics of independent and non-independent riders, for each IMU, for movement planes and first (O1) and second (O2) periods.

BTW Group	IMU	Movement Plane	O1 M ± SD	O2 M ± SD
Independent Riders of BTW group	Vertex	Sagittal	56.72 ± 2.41	57.83 ± 1.18
		Frontal	55.08 ± 1.96	55.25 ± 1.30
		Transverse	54.07 ± 1.92	55.51 ± 1.43
	T2	Sagittal	56.14 ± 1.27	56.38 ± 1.07
		Frontal	52.48 ± 2.4	53.57 ± 1.37
		Transverse	55.04 ± 2.12	56.21 ± 1.65
	Bicycle frame	Frontal	57.43 ± 1.90	58.40 ± 1.66
	Handlebar	Frontal	53.96 ± 2.00	56.32 ± 1.12
		Transverse	54.18 ± 2.04	56.30 ± 0.98

Table 4. Cont.

BTW Group	IMU	Movement Plane	O1 M ± SD	O2 M ± SD
Non-Independent Riders of BTW group	Vertex	Sagittal	56.28 ± 1.43	56.65 ± 0.26
		Frontal	55.43 ± 1.39	54.09 ± 1.31
		Transverse	53.49 ± 2.05	55.08 ± 1.29
	T2	Sagittal	55.65 ± 1.00	56.02 ± 0.80
		Frontal	52.84 ± 1.70	53.05 ± 0.69
		Transverse	54.98 ± 1.37	55.30 ± 1.99
	Bicycle frame	Frontal	57.78 ± 1.92	57.97 ± 1.03
	Handlebar	Frontal	51.86 ± 1.93	52.74 ± 1.45
		Transverse	51.83 ± 2.04	53.41 ± 1.16

4. Discussion

Despite the widespread use of the BTW, several previous studies suggest that the BB may be more effective in facilitating the transition to the TB. However, the reasons behind this greater effectiveness remain unclear, with the assumption that it may be linked to their inherent exploration of balance. In the present study, we sought to analyze the movement variability that emerged from participants during the process of learning to cycle, at different evaluation times, using the BB or the BTW training cycles, as well as after the cycling skill acquisition with the traditional bicycle (TB). We hypothesized that the BB would provide greater functional variability, which, in turn, could favor skill adaptation and more effective learning outcomes. The greatest exponent of LyE, as a nonlinear measure of movement variability, did emerge as a sensitive system parameter, increasing in value after six training sessions in both groups, recorded at several points on the body and the bicycle, with differing movement planes. Since the LyE measure was calculated through the variable of the angular velocity, its increased variability implied greater and faster variations in rotations, which could represent the bicycle's and children's postural oscillations. The implication is that, after training, the children were adapting their postural regulation and exploring more (and faster). This performance characteristic was reflected in increases in the velocity of the left–right rotations of the head on the BTW. In controlling the bicycle, movement variability as a skill adaptation was reflected in increases in the velocities of the handlebar's lateral oscillations and left–right rotations in both groups and in the velocity of the bicycle frame's lateral oscillations in the BB group. These increments in movement variability measures could reflect the children's search of, exploration of, and adaptation to a more freely movable instrument for locomotion, the bicycle. Also, it is interesting to note that not only were patterns of increased movement variability common to both groups but also were their variations. While between O1 and O2 the BB children increased their exploration of the bicycle frame's control, the BTW children did not. The BB group also displayed increases in the variability of head segment rotations. The use of the BTW when learning to cycle presents similarities with the use of baby walkers in the process of learning to walk. Infants/children sit on the walker/bicycle and just need to walk/pedal without having to worry about balance control or lateral oscillations. Although the use of baby walkers is still not consensual [60], some studies have argued that they delay the child's movement development with respect to walking [61,62]. Other studies have not confirmed a developmental delay in using walkers but have instead identified kinematic changes in gait patterns [63]. It could be argued that artificial support for movement systems' postural regulation and stability during locomotion and transport, which both aids provide, when walking or cycling may not provide the necessary task constraints for a child to self-organize and adapt their movement skills for achieving a new task or locomotion pattern.

When analyzing different stages of the learning process, comparing the end of the practice period with the learning bicycles (i.e., BB or BTW, O2) to the end of the period of practice with the TB (O3), it was observed that the variability pattern differed among the two groups; while the BB children reduced their levels of variability in the trunk velocity (represented by data from the T2 IMU) in all movement planes, the BTW group participants increased their variability in the velocity of the trunk flexion and extension and in the velocity of the bicycle's lateral oscillations (represented by data from the bicycle frame IMU). In the last observation phase, O3, the BTW children could not use their training wheels (like infants leaving a baby walker), so their center of gravity was no longer stable. Consequently, they were forced to explore how to regulate the postural control of their trunk, as well as controlling the bicycle.

As hypothesized, when comparing the movement variability of postural control between the two learning bikes, the BB provided greater postural variability in the child–bicycle system from the point of initial contact, in O1, as well as after practice, in O2. The BB group displayed greater variability in all movement planes for the head (represented by data from the vertex IMU) and for the trunk, as well as in all planes for the steering wheel. By not having any artificial support (i.e., the absence of the training wheels), it was more difficult to keep the BB balanced, even when feet were in contact with the ground, than to keep the BTW balanced. This is because, even when there are no feet in contact with the ground, the BTW bicycle does not fall and has small lateral oscillations. Besides this difference in task constraint, to ride the BB, the children had to self-propel with their feet on the ground. These relations of the children with the BB could result in the emergence of what has been termed a 'neutral' affordance landscape, supporting agency in exploring multiple BB cycle patterns, e.g., walking, running, hopping, and others [45,64]. Not long after the first contact with the BB, a child could simply push and maintain balance with the BB by gliding [45]. The BB supported the exploration of a greater variety of cycle patterns, leading the children to explore greater spatiotemporal variability in several segments and movement planes, which was reflected by the higher LyE values. The only exception was in the velocity of the bicycle frame's lateral rotations, in which the BTW children displayed greater system variability compared to the BB group. This is a result that may not have been expected since the lateral wheels limited the amplitude of the bicycle's lateral oscillations. However, even with lateral wheels, in tight curves or at higher speeds, the experimenters observed that the centrifugal force pushed the children's trunk to move laterally, lifting one of the training wheels off the ground, resulting in a fall or an abrupt return of the wheel to the ground. This rapid oscillation produced by mechanical factors may have led to a higher LyE value, thus justifying this unexpected observation.

In comparing the measures of movement variability in the TB between both groups, only one statistically significant difference was found, with the BB group participants displaying higher variability in the velocity of the bicycle frame's lateral rotations. Generally, these results show that the same foundational motor developmental capacities, in this case, the ability to cycle, can be achieved along different pathways, by using different training bicycles like the BB or BTW [9]. This observation is in line with what Waddington defined as the equifinality principle [65]. Interestingly, when analyzing movement variability in the two groups across all observations, in O1 and O2, the BB participants displayed significantly higher LyE values with lower standard deviations for all points and planes, except in the T2-O2-sagittal plane. But, this tendency was inverted in O3, when the BB children continued to display higher LyE mean values (with the only statistically significant difference being observed for bicycle frame's rotation). Higher standard deviation values were observed for all points in time and movements, except in the vertex's frontal plane. Despite having reduced the variability of their oscillation velocity when they transferred to the TB, between O2 and O3, the BB participants continued to display higher mean values of variability, especially in O3, when even higher standard deviation values were observed in this group. Considering that the standard deviation of LyE is a variability measure of variability itself, and that the BB participants showed greater success in learning to cycle than the BTW group, these findings imply that variability seems to have been used in a functional way as a performance solution and not as a problem.

These data corroborate the idea of Bernstein [66] that learning to coordinate complex actions, like riding a bicycle, is acquired by unfreezing, controlling, and mastering degrees of freedom (DOF), i.e., motor units, muscles, joints, limbs, movement axes, and planes. More recently, Berthouze and Lungarella [67] proposed an update to these ideas, verifying that the acquisition of coordination results from dynamic alternations between freezing and freeing DOFs, also arguing that the movement system needs to be perturbed to trigger these freezing and freeing mechanisms. Our hypothesis is that the functional properties of the BB may have the necessary structural level of perturbation to trigger the child–BB system for the emergence of diverse self-organized cycle patterns. However, this might require a complexification of the child's postural variability, as was observed in the head and trunk IMUs' values, in order to be attuned with the emergence of a greater BB functional variability, as expressed in bicycle frame and handlebar IMUs' values.

Previous studies in movement science using LyE measures have reported that higher values have been associated with greater movement system variability and flexibility in responding more quickly to perturbations in order to better control balance [35,38]. Indeed, children from the BB group adapted more easily to the TB, being able to self-launch, ride for 10 m, and brake significantly more quickly than participants in the BTW group [13]. In contrast, the BTW participants needed more time to adapt and three of them were not able to cycle independently after practicing with that bike. As already noted by Burt et al. [10], when children training with a BB transit to a TB, they tend to reveal defensive responses with an increasing stiffness in the trunk and arms, which tends to impact their capacity to balance on the bicycle and, consequently, their ability to cycle independently. The lower-level variability afforded by training with the BTW did not propitiate the children with enough opportunities to achieve greater postural flexibility on the bike. In response, they ended up freezing their movement system's DOF, which is typical in those in the early learning stage according to Bernstein [66].

The present findings are aligned with previous research on motor skill acquisition, particularly studies focusing on the development of balance and coordination in children. For instance, research on the acquisition of gross motor skills, such as running and jumping, has shown that variability in practice can enhance motor learning by promoting adaptability and variability in motor performance [68]. Similarly, studies on fine motor skills, such as handwriting and object manipulation, have demonstrated that diverse practice conditions can lead to more adaptive skill acquisition [69]. These parallels suggest that the principles of motor variability and adaptive learning observed in our study with balance bikes (BB) are consistent with broader motor learning theories.

This hypothesis was confirmed by the significantly lower levels of movement variability displayed by the non-riders in our study, especially in all movement planes analyzed at the BTW handlebar. The non-riders displayed lower mean values for movement variability measures than the independent riders in all analyzed segments (IMUs) and in all motion planes; see Table 2.

4.1. Pratical Aplications

The present results contribute to shedding more light on the reasons why the BB proves to be more efficient in learning to cycle compared to the more traditional BTW approach. The inherent exploration of balance and the provision of greater motor variability during the learning process are potential catalysts. These results, as well as those of previous studies which show that it is possible to learn to cycle independently through a BB from the age of three [9,13], have practical applications for both school and family contexts. Kindergarten teachers, primary school teachers, physical education teachers, coaches, parents, and family members who want to encourage children to learn to cycle independently at a young age should make a BB available to their children as early as possible [70], e.g., as soon as they have acquired independent walking skills. Providing this equipment in a school context contributes not only to learning to cycle but also to increasing motor skills, developing coordination skills such as balance and spatial orientation, and [20,40], not least, providing moments of sharing and fun between peers, contributing to the development of relational skills [71].

4.2. Strengths, Limitations, and Considerations for Future Studies

The results of this study highlight that higher levels of movement system variability may be one of the important reasons for greater efficiency in learning to cycle when using a BB. Indeed, this finding also provides insights about the most efficient motor learning strategy for learning to cycle, based on allowing learners to explore movement system variability. In studies of learning to cycle using different learning bikes, the LyE has presented itself as a useful nonlinear measure which is a reliable tool for studying human gait [35,36]. Here, we demonstrated its use for studying learning behaviors in cycling, reinforcing the utility and versatility of the LyE.

The small sample size of the present study may limit the generalizability of the findings. Despite the effort and methodological rigor in controlling several possibly confounding variables (e.g., body composition and motor competence), it was not possible to control others that may also have had some influence on learning, such as physical fitness levels or socio-economic factors. Future research needs to verify the current findings with a larger sample size, controlling more possible confounding variables and perhaps using a longer learning phase.

Balance ability in children can be influenced by intrinsic constraints such as age, motor competence, and prior experience. Research indicates that balance performance improves with age, as older children typically exhibit better postural control and stability due to more advanced neuromuscular development [72]. Higher motor competence is associated with better balance abilities, as children with greater motor skills can more effectively manage their body's movements and maintain stability [73]. Prior experience with activities that challenge balance can also enhance a child's ability to control their posture and respond to balance-related tasks [74]. Given these potential influences, it was crucial to evaluate these variables at the beginning of our intervention. Our assessments confirmed that there were no significant differences between the two groups in terms of age, motor competence, or prior cycling experience at the start of the study. This homogeneity reinforces the internal validity of our study, ensuring that the observed effects could be attributed to the intervention itself rather than pre-existing differences between the groups. Additionally, a child's height can be considered an individual constraint and may affect their ability to learn how to ride a bike. Depending on the bike's features, particularly the height of the seat from the ground, shorter children might not be able to sit with their feet comfortably touching the ground. This affects their ability to self-launch on the bike without assistance. This issue was observed in the current study, with the youngest children, aged three, representing a limitation of the study. It is recommended that future studies consider the suitability of bicycle dimensions for their sample and that bicycle manufacturers adjust their designs to better accommodate younger children.

Furthermore, there are several other nonlinear methodologies that could provide complementary insights into the coordination of movements, such as recurrence quantification analysis (RQA) [32], single scale entropy [34], and refined composite multiscale dispersion entropy (RCMDE) [33]. To gain a deeper understanding of the processes coordinating actions when learning to cycle, further investigations could be designed using and combining these nonlinear techniques. Incorporating these advanced methodologies can enhance our understanding of motor behavior and its underlying mechanisms, particularly in the context of motor development [75,76].

5. Conclusions

Our results revealed that using the BB allowed for the greater postural variability of the child–bicycle system formed during learning, compared to using the BTW. The BB technology allowed children to use it to explore skill adaptation, facilitating a faster to the TB. Movement system variability, viewed in more traditional theories as error or noise, needs to be re-evaluated as a part of a system's adaptive dynamics, supporting the capacity to adapt to the environment and learn more efficiently. The variability captured by the LyE technique may reflect the freezing and freeing of DOFs, which afford the emergence of synergies between a child and bicycle, supporting the acquisition of the foundational motor skill of riding a bicycle.

The results of this study also provide empirical support, verifying the choice of the balance bike as an adequate instrument for learning to cycle autonomously. The data suggest that policy makers, cycling federations, coaches, educators, and parents should choose the BB over the BTW for children to learn to cycle.

Author Contributions: Methodology, formal analysis, resources: C.M., R.C., D.C. and M.B.; software: M.B.; validation, data curation: C.M. and M.B.; investigation: C.M.; writing—original draft preparation: C.M.; conceptualization, writing—review and editing, visualization: C.M., K.D., R.C., D.C. and M.B.; project administration: C.M.; funding acquisition: C.M. and D.C. All authors have read and agreed to the published version of the manuscript.

Funding: The work of C.M., R.C., and M.B. was partially supported with a grant from FCT, UIDB/00447/2020 CIPER, Interdisciplinary Center for the Study of Human Performance (unit 447). The work of C.M., D.C., and M.B. was partially supported by a grant from Fundacão para a Ciência e a Tecnologia (FCT) (UIDP/04748/2020 and UIDB/04748/2020—CIEQV-Life Quality Research Center) and by the SPRINT, Sport Physical Activity and Health Research & Innovation Center, Polytechnic University of Santarém.

Institutional Review Board Statement: This study was conducted according to the guidelines of the Declaration of Helsinki and approved by Ethics Committee of the Faculty of Human Kinetics, University of Lisbon, number 22/2019.

Informed Consent Statement: Informed consent was obtained from all guardians of the participants involved in this study, as well as the consent of all participants.

Data Availability Statement: Data availability is possible upon request and with the approval of an institutional ethics committee.

Acknowledgments: The authors would like to thank the Association of Early Childhood Education Professionals (APEI), both schools, and all the families and children who participated in this study.

Conflicts of Interest: The authors declare no conflicts of interest.

References

1. Hulteen, R.M.; Morgan, P.J.; Barnett, L.M.; Stodden, D.F.; Lubans, D.R. Development of Foundational Movement Skills: A Conceptual Model for Physical Activity Across the Lifespan. *Sports Med.* **2018**, *48*, 1533–1540. [CrossRef] [PubMed]
2. Kavanagh, J.A.; Issartel, J.; Moran, K. Quantifying cycling as a foundational movement skill in early childhood. *J. Sci. Med. Sport* **2020**, *23*, 171–175. [CrossRef] [PubMed]
3. Ramírez-Vélez, R.; García-Hermoso, A.; Agostinis-Sobrinho, C.; Mota, J.; Santos, R.; Correa-Bautista, J.E.; Amaya-Tambo, D.C.; Villa-González, E. Cycling to School and Body Composition, Physical Fitness, and Metabolic Syndrome in Children and Adolescents. *J. Pediatr.* **2017**, *188*, 57–63. [CrossRef] [PubMed]
4. Mercê, C.; Pereira, J.V.; Branco, M.; Catela, D.; Cordovil, R. Training programmes to learn how to ride a bicycle independently for children and youths: A systematic review. *Phys. Educ. Sport Pedagog.* **2021**, *28*, 530–545. [CrossRef]
5. Karabaic, L. Putting the Fun Before the Wonk: Using Bike Fun to Diversify Bike Ridership. 2016. Available online: http://archives.pdx.edu/ds/psu/18207 (accessed on 12 September 2024).
6. O'Brien, E.; Pickering, T.; Asmar, R.; Myers, M.; Parati, G.; Staessen, J.; Mengden, T.; Imai, Y.; Waeber, B.; Palatini, P.; et al. Working Group on Blood Pressure Monitoring of the European Society of Hypertension International Protocol for validation of blood pressure measuring devices in adults. *Blood Press. Monit.* **2002**, *7*, 3–17. [CrossRef]
7. Zeuwts, L.; Deconinck, F.; Vansteenkiste, P.; Cardon, G.; Lenoir, M. Understanding the development of bicycling skills in children: A systematic review. *Saf. Sci.* **2020**, *123*, 104562. [CrossRef]
8. Zeuwts, L.; Ducheyne, F.; Vansteenkiste, P.; D'Hondt, E.; Cardon, G.; Lenoir, M. Associations between cycling skill, general motor competence and body mass index in 9-year-old children. *Ergonomics* **2015**, *58*, 160–171. [CrossRef]
9. Mercê, C.; Branco, M.; Catela, D.; Lopes, F.; Cordovil, R. Learning to Cycle: From Training Wheels to Balance Bike. *Int. J. Environ. Res. Public Health* **2022**, *19*, 1814. [CrossRef]
10. Burt, T.L.; Porretta, D.P.; Klein, R.E. Use of Adapted Bicycles on the Learning of Conventional Cycling by Children with Mental Retardation. *Educ. Train. Dev. Disabil.* **2007**, *42*, 364–379.

11. Cain, S.M.; Ulrich, D.A.; Perkins, N.C. Using Measured Bicycle Kinematics to Quantify Increased Skill as a Rider Learns to Ride a Bicycle. In Proceedings of the ASME 2012 5th Annual Dynamic Systems and Control Conference Joint with the JSME 2012 11th Motion and Vibration Conference, Fort Lauderdale, FL, USA, 17–19 October 2012; pp. 195–199.
12. Ballantine, R.; Grant, R. *The Ultimate Bicycle Book*; Dorling Kindersley: London, UK, 1992.
13. Mercê, C.; Davids, K.; Catela, D.; Branco, M.; Correia, V.; Cordovil, R. Learning to cycle: A constraint-led intervention programme using different cycling task constraints. *Phys. Educ. Sport Pedagog.* 2023, 1–14. [CrossRef]
14. Newell, K.M.; Mcdonald, P.V. Learning to Coordinate Redundant Biomechanical Degrees of Freedom. In *Interlimb Coordination: Neural, Dynamical, and Cognitive Constraints*; Swinnen, S., Massion, J., Heuer, H., Casaer, P., Eds.; Academic Press: London, UK, 1994.
15. Temple, V.A.; Purves, P.L.; Misovic, R.; Lewis, C.J.; DeBoer, C. Barriers and Facilitators for Generalizing Cycling Skills Learned at Camp to Home. *Adapt. Phys. Act. Q.* 2016, 33, 48–65. [CrossRef]
16. Hauck, J.; Jeong, I.; Esposito, P.; MacDonald, M.; Hornyak, J.; Argento, A.; Ulrich, D.A. Benefits of Learning to Ride a Two-Wheeled Bicycle for Adolescents with Down Syndrome and Autism Spectrum Disorder. *PALAESTRA* 2017, 31, 35.
17. MacDonald, M.; Esposito, P.; Hauck, J.; Jeong, I.; Hornyak, J.; Argento, A.; Ulrich, D.A. Bicycle Training for Youth with Down Syndrome and Autism Spectrum Disorders. *Focus Autism Other Dev. Disabil.* 2012, 27, 12–21. [CrossRef]
18. Hawks, Z.; Constantino, J.N.; Weichselbaum, C.; Marrus, N. Accelerating Motor Skill Acquisition for Bicycle Riding in Children with ASD: A Pilot Study. *J. Autism Dev. Disord.* 2020, 50, 342–348. [CrossRef] [PubMed]
19. Ulrich, D.A.; Burghardt, A.R.; Lloyd, M.; Tiernan, C.; Hornyak, J.E. Physical activity benefits of learning to ride a two-wheel bicycle for children with Down syndrome: A randomized trial. *Phys. Ther.* 2011, 91, 1463–1477. [CrossRef] [PubMed]
20. Shim, A.L.; Norman, S. Incorporating Pedal-less Bicycles into a Pre-K through Third-grade Curriculum to Improve Stability in Children. *J. Phys. Educ. Recreat. Danc.* 2015, 86, 50–51. [CrossRef]
21. van Emmerik, R.E.A.; van Wegen, E.E.H. On the Functional Aspects of Variability in Postural Control. *Exerc. Sport Sci. Rev.* 2002, 30, 177–183. [CrossRef]
22. Stergiou, N.; Harbourne, R.T.; Cavanaugh, J.T. Optimal Movement Variability: A New Theoretical Perspective for Neurologic Physical Therapy. *J. Neurol. Phys. Ther.* 2006, 30, 120–129. [CrossRef]
23. Chow, J.Y.; Davids, K.; Button, C.; Renshaw, I. *Nonlinear Pedagogy in Skill Acquisition: An Introduction*, 2nd ed.; Routledge: New York, NY, USA, 2022; pp. 1–159.
24. Latash, M.L.; Scholz, J.P.; Schöner, G. Motor control strategies revealed in the structure of motor variability. *Exerc. Sport Sci. Rev.* 2002, 30, 26–31. [CrossRef]
25. Davids, K.; Button, C.; Bennett, S. *Dynamics of Skill Acquisition: A Constraints-Led Approach*; Human Kinetics: Champaign, IL, USA, 2008; pp. 1–28.
26. Correia, V.; Carvalho, J.; Araújo, D.; Pereira, E.; Davids, K. Principles of nonlinear pedagogy in sport practice. *Phys. Educ. Sport Pedagog.* 2019, 24, 117–132. [CrossRef]
27. Kelso, J.A.S. *Dynamic Patterns: The Self-Organization of Brain and Behavior*; MIT Press: Cambridge, MA, USA, 1995; pp. 1–28; 334p.
28. Kelso, S. Coordination Dynamics. In *Encyclopedia of Complexity and Systems Science*; Meyers, R.A., Ed.; Springer: New York, NY, USA, 2009; pp. 1537–1564.
29. Newell, K.M. Constraints on the development of coordination. In *Motor Development in Children: Aspects of Coordination and Control*; Wade, M.G., Whiting, H.T.A., Eds.; Martinus Nijhoff: Dordrecht, The Netherlands, 1986; pp. 341–360.
30. Button, C.; Seifert, L.; Chow, J.Y.; Araujo, D.; Davids, K. *Dynamics of Skill Acquisition: An Ecological Dynamics Approach*; Human Kinetics Publishers: Champaign, IL, USA, 2020.
31. da Costa, C.S.; Batistão, M.V.; Rocha, N.A. Quality and structure of variability in children during motor development: A systematic review. *Res. Dev. Disabil.* 2013, 34, 2810–2830. [CrossRef] [PubMed]
32. Webber, C.L.; Marwan, N. (Eds.) *Recurrence Quantification Analysis: Theory and Best Practices*; Springer: Cham, Switzerland, 2015.
33. Azami, H.; Rostaghi, M.; Abásolo, D.; Escudero, J. Refined Composite Multiscale Dispersion Entropy and its Application to Biomedical Signals. *IEEE Trans. Biomed. Eng.* 2017, 64, 2872–2879. [CrossRef] [PubMed]
34. Yentes, J.M.; Raffalt, P.C. Entropy Analysis in Gait Research: Methodological Considerations and Recommendations. *Ann. Biomed. Eng.* 2021, 49, 979–990. [CrossRef] [PubMed]
35. Kędziorek, J.; Błażkiewicz, M. Nonlinear Measures to Evaluate Upright Postural Stability: A Systematic Review. *Entropy* 2020, 22, 1357. [CrossRef]
36. Mehdizadeh, S. The largest Lyapunov exponent of gait in young and elderly individuals: A systematic review. *Gait Posture* 2018, 60, 241–250. [CrossRef]
37. Harbourne, R.T.; Stergiou, N. Nonlinear analysis of the development of sitting postural control. *Dev. Psychobiol.* 2003, 42, 368–377. [CrossRef]
38. Smith, B.A.; Stergiou, N.; Ulrich, B.D. Lyapunov exponent and surrogation analysis of patterns of variability: Profiles in new walkers with and without down syndrome. *Mot. Control* 2010, 14, 126–142. [CrossRef]
39. Chow, J.Y.; Davids, K.; Button, C.; Shuttleworth, R.; Renshaw, I.; Araújo, D. The role of nonlinear pedagogy in physical education. *Rev. Educ. Res.* 2007, 77, 251–278. [CrossRef]
40. Becker, A.; Jenny, S.E. No Need for Training Wheels: Ideas for Including Balance Bikes in Elementary Physical Education. *J. Phys. Educ. Recreat. Danc.* 2017, 88, 14–21. [CrossRef]

41. Norton, K. Standards for Anthropometry Assessment. In *Kinanthropometry and Exercise Physiology*; Routledge: London, UK, 2018; pp. 68–137.
42. WHO. WHO Child Growth Standards based on length/height, weight and age. *Acta Paediatr. Suppl.* **2006**, *450*, 76–85. [CrossRef]
43. Luz, C.; Rodrigues, L.P.; Almeida, G.; Cordovil, R. Development and validation of a model of motor competence in children and adolescents. *J. Sci. Med. Sport* **2016**, *19*, 568–572. [CrossRef] [PubMed]
44. Whiteley, A.M.; Whiteley, J. The familiarization study in qualitative research: From theory to practice. *Qual. Res. J.* **2006**, *6*, 69–85. [CrossRef]
45. Mercê, C.; Cordovil, R.; Catela, D.; Galdino, F.; Bernardino, M.; Altenburg, M.; António, G.; Brígida, N.; Branco, M. Learning to Cycle: Is Velocity a Control Parameter for Children's Cycle Patterns on the Balance Bike? *Children* **2022**, *9*, 1937. [CrossRef] [PubMed]
46. Shurtleff, T.L.; Engsberg, J.R. Changes in Trunk and Head Stability in Children with Cerebral Palsy after Hippotherapy: A Pilot Study. *Phys. Occup. Ther. Pediatr.* **2010**, *30*, 150–163. [CrossRef] [PubMed]
47. Wolter, N.E.; Gordon, K.A.; Campos, J.L.; Vilchez Madrigal, L.D.; Pothier, D.D.; Hughes, C.O.; Papsin, B.C.; Cushing, S.L. BalanCI: Head-Referenced Cochlear Implant Stimulation Improves Balance in Children with Bilateral Cochleovestibular Loss. *Audiol. Neurotol.* **2020**, *25*, 60–71. [CrossRef]
48. Li, Y.; Koldenhoven, R.M.; Liu, T.; Venuti, C.E. Age-related gait development in children with autism spectrum disorder. *Gait Posture* **2021**, *84*, 260–266. [CrossRef]
49. Camomilla, V.; Bergamini, E.; Fantozzi, S.; Vannozzi, G. Trends Supporting the In-Field Use of Wearable Inertial Sensors for Sport Performance Evaluation: A Systematic Review. *Sensors* **2018**, *18*, 873. [CrossRef]
50. Winter, L.; Bellenger, C.; Grimshaw, P.; Crowther, R.G. Analysis of Movement Variability in Cycling: An Exploratory Study. *Sensors* **2023**, *23*, 4972. [CrossRef]
51. Zeng, Z.; Liu, Y.; Hu, X.; Tang, M.; Wang, L. Validity and Reliability of Inertial Measurement Units on Lower Extremity Kinematics During Running: A Systematic Review and Meta-Analysis. *Sports Med.-Open* **2022**, *8*, 86. [CrossRef]
52. Kobsar, D.; Charlton, J.M.; Tse, C.T.F.; Esculier, J.-F.; Graffos, A.; Krowchuk, N.M.; Thatcher, D.; Hunt, M.A. Validity and reliability of wearable inertial sensors in healthy adult walking: A systematic review and meta-analysis. *J. NeuroEng. Rehabil.* **2020**, *17*, 62. [CrossRef]
53. Clemente, F.; Badicu, G.; Hasan, U.; Akyildiz, Z.; Pino Ortega, J.; Silva, R.; Rico-González, M. Validity and reliability of inertial measurement units (IMUs) for jump height estimations: A systematic review. *Hum. Mov.* **2021**, *23*, 1–20. [CrossRef]
54. 9DoF Razor IMU M0 Hookup Guide. Available online: https://learn.sparkfun.com/tutorials/9dof-razor-imu-m0-hookup-guide/all (accessed on 26 November 2024).
55. Stins, J.F.; Michielsen, M.E.; Roerdink, M.; Beek, P.J. Sway regularity reflects attentional involvement in postural control: Effects of expertise, vision and cognition. *Gait Posture* **2009**, *30*, 106–109. [CrossRef]
56. Donker, S.F.; Ledebt, A.; Roerdink, M.; Savelsbergh, G.J.P.; Beek, P.J. Children with cerebral palsy exhibit greater and more regular postural sway than typically developing children. *Exp. Brain Res.* **2008**, *184*, 363–370. [CrossRef] [PubMed]
57. Budini, K.; Richards, J.; Cole, T.; Levine, D.; Trede, R.; George, L.S.; Selfe, J. An exploration of the use of Inertial Measurement Units in the assessment of dynamic postural control of the knee and the effect of bracing and taping. *Physiother. Pract. Res.* **2018**, *39*, 91–98. [CrossRef]
58. Allum, J.H.; Carpenter, M.G. A speedy solution for balance and gait analysis: Angular velocity measured at the centre of body mass. *Curr. Opin. Neurol.* **2005**, *18*, 15–21. [CrossRef]
59. Field, A. *Discovering Statistics Using IBM SPSS Statistics*; SAGE Publications: Thousand Oaks, CA, USA, 2013.
60. Badihian, S.; Adihian, N.; Yaghini, O. The Effect of Baby Walker on Child Development: A Systematic Review. *Iran. J. Child Neurol.* **2017**, *11*, 1–6. [PubMed]
61. Siegel, A.C.; Burton, R.V. Effects of baby walkers on motor and mental development in human infants. *J. Dev. Behav. Pediatr.* **1999**, *20*, 355–361. [CrossRef]
62. Garrett, M.; McElroy, A.M.; Staines, A. Locomotor milestones and babywalkers: Cross sectional study. *BMJ* **2002**, *324*, 1494. [CrossRef]
63. Chagas, P.S.C.; Fonseca, S.T.; Santos, T.R.T.; Souza, T.R.; Megale, L.; Silva, P.L.; Mancini, M.C. Effects of baby walker use on the development of gait by typically developing toddlers. *Gait Posture* **2020**, *76*, 231–237. [CrossRef]
64. Withagen, R.; de Poel, H.J.; Araújo, D.; Pepping, G.-J. Affordances can invite behavior: Reconsidering the relationship between affordances and agency. *New Ideas Psychol.* **2012**, *30*, 250–258. [CrossRef]
65. Waddington, C.H. *The Strategy of the Genes*; A Discussion of Some Aspects of Theoretical Biology; Allen & Unwin: London, UK, 1957; p. ix. 262p.
66. Bernstein, N.A. *The Co-Ordination and Regulation of Movements*, 1st ed.; Pergamon Press: Oxford, NY, USA, 1967; p. xii. 196p.
67. Berthouze, L.; Lungarella, M. Motor Skill Acquisition Under Environmental Perturbations: On the Necessity of Alternate Freezing and Freeing of Degrees of Freedom. *Adapt. Behav.* **2004**, *12*, 47–64. [CrossRef]
68. Leech, K.A.; Roemmich, R.T.; Gordon, J.; Reisman, D.S.; Cherry-Allen, K.M. Updates in Motor Learning: Implications for Physical Therapist Practice and Education. *Phys. Ther.* **2021**, *102*, pzab250. [CrossRef]
69. Kafri, M.; Atun-Einy, O. From Motor Learning Theory to Practice: A Scoping Review of Conceptual Frameworks for Applying Knowledge in Motor Learning to Physical Therapist Practice. *Phys. Ther.* **2019**, *99*, 1628–1643. [CrossRef]

70. Mercê, C.; Branco, M.; Catela, D.; Lopes, F.; Rodrigues, L.P.; Cordovil, R. Learning to Cycle: Are Physical Activity and Birth Order Related to the Age of Learning How to Ride a Bicycle? *Children* **2021**, *8*, 487. [CrossRef]
71. Schoen, S.A.; Ferrari, V.; Valdez, A. It's Not Just about Bicycle Riding: Sensory-Motor, Social and Emotional Benefits for Children with and without Developmental Disabilities. *Children* **2022**, *9*, 1224. [CrossRef]
72. Schedler, S.; Tenelsen, F.; Wich, L.; Muehlbauer, T. Effects of balance training on balance performance in youth: Role of training difficulty. *BMC Sports Sci. Med. Rehabil.* **2020**, *12*, 71. [CrossRef] [PubMed]
73. Blodgett, J.M.; Cooper, R.; Pinto Pereira, S.M.; Hamer, M. Stability of Balance Performance from Childhood to Midlife. *Pediatrics* **2022**, *150*, e2021055861. [CrossRef] [PubMed]
74. Liu, R.; Yang, J.; Xi, F.; Xu, Z. Relationship between static and dynamic balance in 4-to-5-year-old preschoolers: A cross-sectional study. *BMC Pediatr.* **2024**, *24*, 295. [CrossRef]
75. Moreno, F.J.; Caballero, C.; Barbado, D. Editorial: The role of movement variability in motor control and learning, analysis methods and practical applications. *Front. Psychol.* **2023**, *14*, 1260878. [CrossRef]
76. Getchell, N.; Schott, N.; Brian, A. Motor Development Research: Designs, Analyses, and Future Directions. *J. Mot. Learn. Dev.* **2020**, *8*, 410–437. [CrossRef]

Disclaimer/Publisher's Note: The statements, opinions and data contained in all publications are solely those of the individual author(s) and contributor(s) and not of MDPI and/or the editor(s). MDPI and/or the editor(s) disclaim responsibility for any injury to people or property resulting from any ideas, methods, instructions or products referred to in the content.

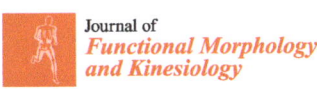

Article

Design of a Freely Accessible Web Application (Instrument for the Measurement of Balance in Primary Education, IMEP) for the Assessment of Static and Dynamic Balance in Children Aged 6–9 Years Based on Force Platforms

Julio Martín-Ruiz [1], Ignacio Tamarit-Grancha [2], Carlos Cordente-Martínez [3], Raúl Santamaría-Fernández [4], Concepción Ros Ros [5] and Laura Ruiz-Sanchis [5,*]

1. Department of Health and Functional Assessment, Catholic University of Valencia, 46900 Valencia, Spain; julio.martin@ucv.es
2. Department of Physical Preparation and Conditioning, Catholic University of Valencia, 46900 Valencia, Spain; ignacio.tamarit@ucv.es
3. Department of Sports, Polytechnic University of Madrid, 28040 Madrid, Spain; carlos.cordente@upm.es
4. Faculty of Sciences of Physical Activity and Sports, Catholic University of Valencia, 46900 Valencia, Spain; rasanfer@mail.ucv.es
5. Department of Sports Management and Physical Activity, Catholic University of Valencia, 46900 Valencia, Spain; concepcion.ros@ucv.es
* Correspondence: laura.ruiz@ucv.es; Tel.: +34-963637412

Abstract: Background: The proper development of balance is essential in the acquisition of a correct physical condition, as well as in the evolutionary follow-up at early ages, and its periodic evaluation is very relevant in the educational environment. **Objectives**: The objective of this research was to design an accessible web application for static and dynamic balance assessment, based on a force platform and motion analysis software. **Methods:** The Single leg balance test (SLB), Tandem balance test (TBT), and Y balance test (YBT) were performed on a sample of 75 children aged 6 to 9 years. **Results**: The results show that static balance is more complex at an older age, greater standing height, and with eyes closed ($p < 0.001$). Regarding the center of pressure (COP), its variability was greater in girls owing to a lower Total Force (TF) at the time of the test ($p < 0.05$). Parallel observation with the Kinovea software has made it possible to elaborate a scale from 1 to 10 points for integration into an open-access web application (IMEP) to assess static and dynamic balance. **Conclusions:** The creation of an ad hoc application for primary school teachers and students has been possible by using validated devices obtaining a rating scale, which facilitate the monitoring of students' functional evolution and offers the possibility of scheduling physical education sessions with a preventive approach as well as a focus on improving physical condition.

Keywords: motion analysis; physical activity; educational application; balance; primary education

1. Introduction

Balance is fundamental to the development of motor skills, body schemas, and tonic functions [1]. It is the basis of coordination and spatial–temporal control, always represented by an initial imbalance until the end of rebalance, particularly in sports movements [2–4]. The interaction of its variables, the base of sustenance, center of mass (COM) [5], and changing the center of pressure (COP) at each joint [6] is basic for an efficient and precise motor sequence. A balanced action [7] is defined by cooperation between the central nervous system as a regulator and the musculoskeletal system as the executor.

Balance control is primordial at early ages; up to three years of age, it allows the first tasks of displacement, position maintenance, and dynamic balance [8]. Between 4 and 5 years of age, there is no established relationship between static and dynamic balance [9] (ability to stand upright with or without movement, respectively) because of the maturation of brain areas related to motor control. This relationship is slightly better in girls, without being significant [10,11]. At eight and nine years of age, some studies relate children's development to improved self-concept and self-efficacy [12] when the movement is clearer and more oriented, owing to the plasticity of the nervous system that leads to a great gestural improvement, highlighting the oculo-segmental, a qualitative change in the activities of balance and general coordination [13], which makes this age group the most suitable for static balance work [14]. From the age of 9 years, anatomical growth results in a motor imbalance that improves with adequate and continuous physical exercise [15] and reaches its peak at approximately 23 years of age [16].

The role of Physical Education teachers in consolidating this achievement is fundamental from the age of six years, guaranteeing greater motor richness with the application of different skills: physical–motor, socio-motor, and perceptual–motor [17]. Its systematic and structured work [18] provides benefits when prolonged for more than one month [19]. The use of interactive balance tools such as the MABC-2 Battery can aid in the early detection of coordination disorders [20]; thus, the integration of these types of resources in the classroom with an adequate evaluation and interpretation of data [16] is of added value and great support to the teaching staff.

Traditionally, balance assessment consists of measuring the time it takes to maintain a position, minimizing visual stimuli, as it depends on the functions of the vestibular and proprioceptive (somatosensory) systems [21–23]. Measurement techniques are complex and, being proprioceptive in nature, take the physiological mechanisms, influencing factors, and location of the variable within the system as a reference. The complex interactions between these elements make it difficult to analyze and measure their specific functions and characteristics [24]. Most current techniques assess the integrity and function of proprioceptive components with measurements along afferent and efferent pathways, the result of musculoskeletal activation, or a combination of the two [25].

The static tests include unipodal tests, such as the flamingo test [26], with its variant with eyes closed [27], and the bipodal ones, such as the tandem or Romberg's test, which includes hands at the side and eyes closed [24]. In unipodal dynamics, the equilibrium test in T [28], the well-known Y balance test (YBT), and the Star Excursion Balance Test (SEBT) [29,30] are widely used in recovery protocols, with work suggesting the integration of other movement models [31]. In the case of bipodal tests, the Gesell balance test can be used [16], or tandem walking, which is also used in special populations [32]. In general, the differences between tests usually boil down to the placement of body segments and the execution time [33,34].

For accurate assessment, isolating dependent variables with direct measurements from medical applications, such as the Biodex Balance System [35], force platforms [36], pressure analysis, or the use of the baropodometer [5], is ideal for measuring symmetry, moment of force, COM and COP projection, plantar support, barycenter, or stabilometry in a static position [37]. However, in the educational field, this type of instrumentation is inaccessible owing to the cost and student ratio. Alternative tools, mainly mobile applications, have been designed to calculate the balance with increasing accuracy [38,39], taking advantage of the fact that, by default, these devices include an accelerometer but offer only one form of balance, are not open source, and are not globally accessible. A shortage of open and collective resources that measure the precision of validated instruments and can be integrated into the specific contents of the curriculum has been detected [40].

For these reasons, the objective of this research was to develop an objective and accessible tool that allows teachers and students between six and nine years of age to assess static and dynamic balance. This would allow obtaining an accurate measurement of different types of balance with different applications: school for teachers and students and personal monitoring adjusted to individual characteristics, with the incentive of being open and having a comparative reference with other cases of the same educational cycle.

2. Materials and Methods

2.1. Experimental Approach to the Problem

To develop an objective and accessible tool that allows Physical Education professionals to evaluate balance in children aged 6–9 years, a cross-sectional study was carried out using quantitative biomechanical tests and field evaluations with movement analysis instruments.

Five primary schools participated in this study and provided authorization. Informed consent was obtained from the parents/legal guardians of all participants. The timetable for measuring the tests agreed with the Physical Education teachers of each center. The study was designed in accordance with the Declaration of Helsinki to guarantee the fundamental rights of research on human subjects and was approved by the Ethics Committee of the Catholic University of Valencia (reference number: UCV/2015-2016/049).

2.2. Participants

The sample was selected based on the accessibility of the participating schools and was therefore non-probabilistic by convenience. The inclusion criteria were as follows: being a student from the 1st to 3rd year of Primary Education (6 to 9 years old), not suffering from any lower limb injury, and voluntary participation of the Physical Education teacher in the research. The reasons for exclusion were limited to non-compliance with the age of the study. The descriptive data for the sample are shown in Table 1.

Table 1. Characteristics of the students participating in the study (mean ± standard deviation).

		Global	Female	Male
N		75	44	31
Age		7.27 ± 0.74	7.23 ± 0.71	7.32 ± 0.79
Weight (kg)		27.25 ± 7.37	25.91 ± 5.93	29.16 ± 8.79
High (m)		1.28 ± 0.06	1.27 ± 0.05	1.29 ± 0.08
BMI		16.59 ± 3.64	16.1 ± 3.2	17.29 ± 4.14
Dominant foot	Right	68 (90.67%)	42 (95.45%)	26 (83.87%)
Non dominant foot	Left	6 (8%)	2 (4.55%)	4 (12.9%)
Foot Size		32.95 ± 2.14	32.48 ± 1.66	33.63 ± 2.56
Leg length		67.45 ± 4.62	67.28 ± 4.5	67.69 ± 4.85

Note: BMI = Body mass index. SD = Standard deviation.

2.3. Procedure

Informed consent was obtained (guardians/parents), and anthropometric measurements of weight (Seca 750, Hamburg, Germany) and height (Seca 213, Hamburg, Germany) were measured by a qualified professional (ISAK-I).

Leg length: With the knee extended, the talus (ankle) and greater trochanter of the femur (hip) were located, and the distance between the two was measured with a metallic tape measure. Next, the laterality of the lower extremities was identified using an accurate chopstick test [41].

Finally, self-adhesive markers were placed on the following bony landmarks: (1) acromion: starting from the distal third of the clavicle, the thumb was slid to its end point, and the marker was placed on the most prominent edge on the glenoid surface of the humerus; (2) navel: in the anterior frontal plane, the marker was placed in the hollow located in the abdomen; and (3) the external border of the greater trochanter of the femur, starting from the sagittal plane, and the most prominent lateral bony border was located. The thumb was placed, and the subject was asked to perform hip flexion to detect the pivot point [42] and (4) L3 lumbar vertebra: from the posterior frontal plane, in a standing position, both hands were placed on the edges of the pelvis located at the L4 lumbar vertebra by palpation, and one vertebra ascended and was located at L3.

To proceed with the measurement, the space was adapted in such a way that the portable force platform (Kistler, Model 9260AA, Winterthur, Switzerland) was placed in the center and with four cameras (GoPro Hero, Model 3+ Silver, San Mateo, CA, USA): one front (displacement of the umbilicus), one rear (of L3), and two lateral (variation of the greater trochanter and acromion) located at a distance of 2 m from the central point of the platform (150 × 250 mm) and at a height of 0.7 m. Finally, a camera perpendicular to the subject (Panasonic, Model HC-V130, Osaka, Japan) in HD (17 Mbps/VBR) with 1920 × 1080 px resolution for subsequent analysis using the Kinovea software (Kinovea, v2023.1, Bordeaux, France) and two 1m red marks visible from all cameras as a reference for this software (Figure 1).

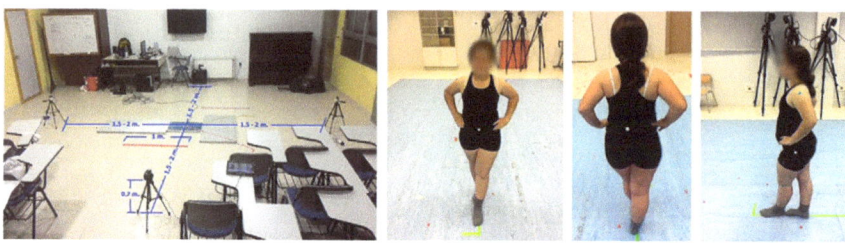

Figure 1. Adequacy of the measurement environment and joint markers. Note: (**Left**) Study environment; (**Center-left**): frontal marker, umbilicus; (**Center-right**): dorsal marker, lumbar L3; (**Right**): lateral markers, acromion, and greater trochanter.

A single measurement session was performed without prior standardized warm-up to avoid conditioning the tone of muscle activation during the test. They were shown the procedure of each test and were familiarized with each test for five minutes before performing the actual measurement and were able to ask the questions they needed. A total of 3 tests were performed with a total of 14 different balance positions: 4 unipodal support (single-leg balance, SLB) of 16 s with eyes open (2) and closed (2); 4 tandem balance test (tandem balance test, TBT) of 16 s, with eyes open (2) and closed (2); and 3 dynamic balance of 5 s (Y balance test, YBT), in the frontal (2), posteromedial (2), and posterolateral (2) directions [43]. In the cases of the SLB and TBT, they were always started with the right leg.

The objective of the SLB is to maintain balance with one leg on the reference marks placed on the platform [34], with the subject immobile with hands on the waist, repeating the test if there is support from both feet.

In TBT, the load differences in the lower extremities in the standing position were evaluated [44]. It is performed by touching the toe of the rear foot to the heel of the front foot and the hands on the waist. If a change in foot landing occurred, the test was repeated.

Finally, the YBT modified the SEBT, which is a valid and reliable tool for assessing unipodal dynamic balance [45]. Movements were performed in three different directions (frontal, posteromedial, and posterolateral), maintaining the position for 1 s without losing support, looking for symmetry on both sides of the body through the distances reached using the following formula [46]:

$$YBT = \text{distance in frontal direction} + \text{distance in posteromedial direction} + \text{distance in posterolateral direction} / (\text{leg length} \times 3) \times 10$$

The execution of each test is illustrated in Figure 2.

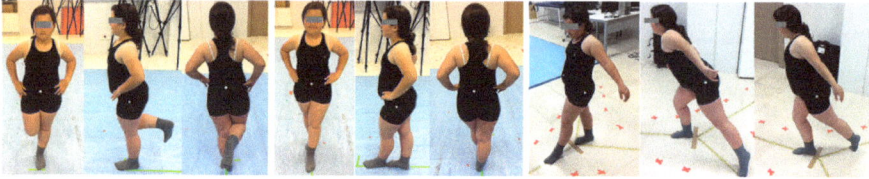

Figure 2. Representation of the balance tests used. Note: (**Left**): Single-leg test; (**Center**): tandem balance test; (**Right**): Y balance test.

Data from the force platform were collected using the Bioware software (Kistler, v5.3.0.7, Winterthur, Switzerland) and exported as a .txt extension file, and signal processing was performed using MATLAB (2024b) (Mathworks Inc., Natick, MA, USA). The signal was digitally cleaned with a 10–50HZ bandpass filter to collect only the useful signals. The Root Mean Square (RMS) was then performed, and the data were segmented as follows: from Test 1 to Test 8 (SLB and TBT test), the first 3 and last 3 s of the 16 total were removed to avoid peaks at the start setting and fatigue at the end of the test. From records 9 to 14 (YBT), the initial 4 s corresponding to the performance of each movement was used. In all cases, the force and COP data along the X-, Y-, and Z-axes were collected.

Similarly, with the Kinovea software (no possibility of synchronization with the platform), the variations in the movement of each of the tests were collected with the cameras in centimeters (1920 × 1080 px minimum resolution). Each video was labeled to distinguish the number of attempts (from 1 to 14); whether it was a frontal or lateral camera, considering the joint markers, the cm of deviation in each case were noted to relate them statistically and establish a correct rating scale in the design of the web application designed ad hoc, as shown in Figure 3.

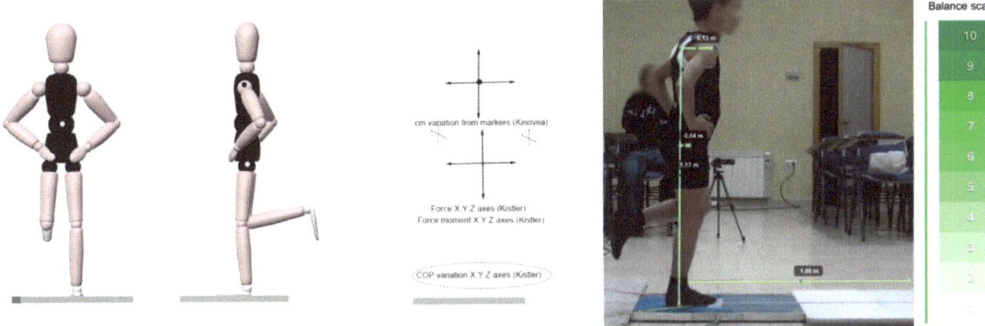

Figure 3. Study workflow. Note: (**Left**): Performance of the balance tests; (**Center-left**): registration of variables; (**Center-right**): analysis with the Kinovea software; (**Right**): conversion to the equilibrium rating scale.

2.4. Web Application Design

A responsive web application (with functionality on mobile devices) was designed for use by teachers and students of Physical Education in primary education. The name ascribed to it was the Instrument for the Measurement of Balance in Primary Education (IMEP). It is hosted in the subdomain imep.giepafs.net/IMEP/, dependent on the main domain giepafs.net and its access is free.

The programming was performed on a Linux server, CentOS v.7.9.2009 (Core), in the PHP language (PHP, v8.1.29., Greenland), and MariaDB (MariaDb, v. 10.5.26., Tampere, Finland).

It starts with a panel in which one can choose the balancing test to be performed. Once selected, there is an area in which to enter the user data; a nickname or pseudonym is preferred for data protection. In each field, the cm of deviation of the test is indicated, and at the end, a score of between 1 and 10 points is obtained, based on the research carried out on the forces platform (the value 0 was avoided as it is carried out for educational contexts). If each participant has several records and returns to the home page, you can see all the results by choosing the nickname, at which time the attempts and results of all the tests will be displayed (Figure 4).

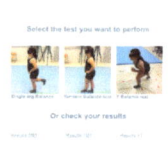
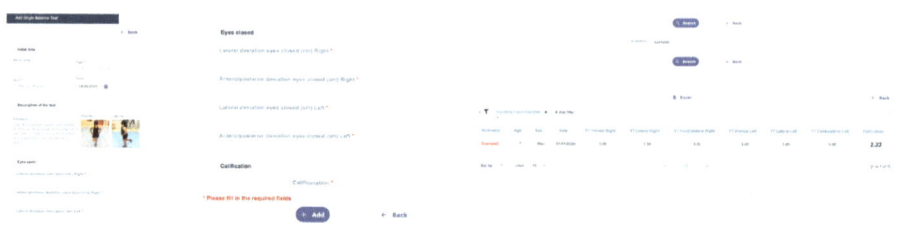

Figure 4. Sequence of use of the IMEP web application. Note: (**Left**): Application input interface; (**Center**): example of SLB test (two images); (**Right**): individual results search engine; * = mandatory answer.

2.5. Statistical Analysis

2.5.1. Descriptive Analysis

The data were described as means and standard deviations, as well as medians and interquartile ranges for continuous quantitative variables. For qualitative variables, proportions and 95% confidence intervals were determined.

2.5.2. Logistic Regression Models

To determine the causes of test complexity, YBT score, and changes in balance and movement, mixed-effects regression models were performed with the packages lme4 [47] v.1.1-30 and lmerTest [48] v.3.1-3, according to the protocol of Zuur and Ieno [49]. First, the error structure of the data was determined by fitting the beyond optimal model, which included the factors of interest in each case, along with test-related factors (test type, eyes open or closed, and dominance in the supporting foot), age, sex, and foot number.

Second, the random structure of the model was fitted using the participant ID, and coefficients were estimated using the REML method. Finally, a simplified optimal model was reported by estimating the coefficients using the REML method. To interpret the model, the coefficients and the results of the ANOVA were calculated using the car package [50] v.3.1.0. For significant categorical factors, post hoc comparisons were performed using the emmeans package [51] v.1.7.5.

All nested models were compared using the corrected Akaike information criterion (AICc) calculated using the MuMIn package [52] v.1.46.0. In all cases, the assumptions of the linear models were checked by visually inspecting the residuals and performing the Shapiro–Wilk (normality) and Levene (homoscedasticity) tests, as well as with the v.0.10.3 package [53]. The models were fitted with the package lme4 [47] v.1.1-30.

2.5.3. Calculation of Scales

To obtain a score on a scale of 1 to 10 for each test (SLB, TBT, and YTest), the following procedure was followed:

2.6. Notation

In the following mathematical demonstration, a test is defined as a set of static or dynamic balance exercises. Thus, in the present study, there were three tests: SLB, TBT, and YTest, each of which was composed of four exercises.

2.6.1. Reference Point Motion Calculation

In each exercise of a given test, displacement was measured at three reference points: the acromion, umbilicus, and trochanter. The Pythagorean theorem was used on the X- and Y-axes. Subsequently, three displacements were added to obtain the movement of a given exercise.

$$mvtu\ mbilicus. = \sqrt{despl.X^2umb. + despl.Y^2umb.}$$

In the case of the YBT, the score is calculated in the usual way:

YBT = distance in frontal direction + distance in posteromedial direction + distance in posterolateral direction/(leg length) × 10

2.6.2. Total Movement and Gross Score Calculation

The movements of each exercise were summed to obtain the total movement of the test, which was used as a reference for the raw score of the test. Because a higher amount of movement indicates a lower performance, the value of the total movement is inverted. To conduct this, the total movement is subtracted from a constant (*cte*), thus ensuring that the resulting values are positive. The value of *cte* is determined for each test by attending to the range of variation in the amount of total motion.

$$Raw\ score = (mvt\ umb\ a + mvt\ umb\ b + mvt\ umb\ c + mvt\ umb\ d) + cte$$

In the case of the YBT, the scores are added together to obtain the raw score. In this case, a greater movement implies a better performance; so, there is no need to reverse the value. Since this score has a logarithmic scale, it is transformed, and a constant is subtracted, cte:

$$Raw\ score = log(YBT\ a + YBT\ b + YBT\ c + YBT\ d + YBT\ e + YBT\ f - cte)$$

2.6.3. Adjustment of the Raw Score by Demographic Variables

To adjust the raw scores for demographic variables (sex, foot size, and age), a linear regression model was fitted to generate a correction factor for each participant. This was applied to the raw scores, as follows:

$$Adjusted\ score = Raw\ score - 0.5 \cdot FC$$

where FC is the correction factor obtained from the linear regression model. It is multiplied by 0.5 to smooth its impact on the adjusted score.

2.6.4. Rescaling to the Scale of 1 to 10

The adjusted score was rescaled to a range from 1 to 10 to obtain the final test score. This rescaling varied according to the test type.

$$Adjusted\ score = \frac{Adjusted\ score - min(Adjusted\ score)}{max(Adjusted\ score) - min(Adjusted\ score)} \cdot 9 - 1$$

In all analyses, the following was used: $\alpha = 0.05$.

The analyses were performed using R [54] v.4.2.2. Data tables were read with the openxlsx package [55] v.4.2.5 (for xlsx files) and/or haven [56] v. (for sav files). The graphics were constructed with ggplot2 [57] v.3.5.1 ggpubr [58] v.0.4.0, and other functions integrated in the mentioned packages.

3. Results

3.1. Analysis of the Complexity of Each Test

An equation was designed to determine the complexity of the exercise based on the beyond optimal model.

$$Complexity \sim FootSupport + Age + TestType \times (Foot\_Size + Sex) +$$
$$EyesOpen \times Foot\_Size$$
$$(1\ |\ ID)$$

After fitting it to a gamma distribution with logarithmic linkage, the model presents a good fit of the residuals, complying with linearity, normality, homoscedasticity, and absence of outliers. Table 2 shows the six significant effects after the application of a type III ANOVA.

Table 2. Evaluation of the balance test complexity.

Variable	χ^2	Df	p-Valor
(Intercept)	5.402	1	0.02 *
Standing foot	0.578	1	0.447
Age	78.617	1	7.5×10^{-19} ***
Type of test	44.931	2	1.8×10^{-10} ***
Foot size	12.605	1	0.00038 ***
Sex	0.479	1	0.489
Open eyes	4.492	1	0.034 *
Type of test: Foot size	29.247	2	4.5×10^{-7} ***
Type of test: Sex	4.6	2	0.1
Foot Size: Open eyes	2.984	1	0.084

Note: * = $p < 0.05$. *** = $p < 0.001$.

As it can be seen, a greater age, foot size, and performing the test with eyes closed (in SLB and TBT) significantly conditioned the complexity, increasing the score of this variable by 1.3 ± 0.05 (Figure 5).

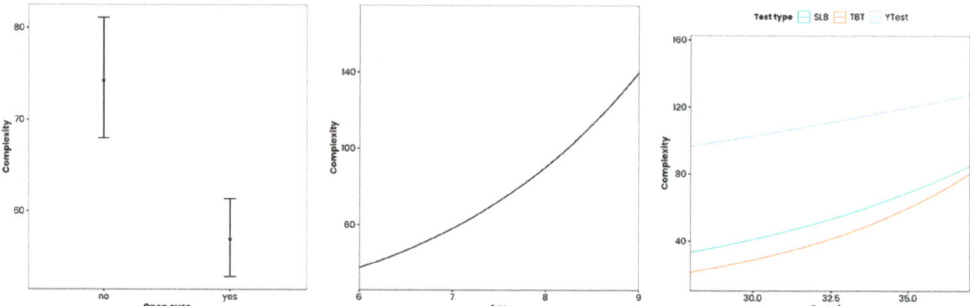

Figure 5. Variation in the complexity score as a function of eye opening, age, and standing size. Note: SLB = Single-leg balance. TBT = Tandem balance test.

3.2. Effect of Leg Length on YBT

In the case of YBT, we used the beyond optimal model to calculate whether the leg length influenced the results using the following equation:

$$\text{Complexity} \sim \text{FootSupport} + \text{Age} + \text{TestType} \times (\text{Foot\_Size} + \text{Sex}) + \text{EyesOpen} * \text{Foot\_Size}$$
$$(1 \mid \text{ID})$$

Table 3 shows with a type II ANOVA that the scores are higher for anterior movement, lower for posterolateral movement, and intermediate for posteromedial movement.

Table 3. Effect of the type of movement performed on YBT.

YBT	Emmean (95%)	Contrast	Estimate	t Ratio	p Value
Anterior	18.57 ± 0.23 [18.11–19.03]	Anterior–Posterolateral	2.27 ± 0.22	10.45	0.0 ***
Posterolateral	16.3 ± 0.23 [15.84–16.76]	Anterior–Posteromedial	1.09 ± 0.22	5.04	2.2×10^{-6} ***
Posteromedial	17.47 ± 0.23 [17.01–17.93]	Posterolateral–Posteromedial	-1.18 ± 0.22	−5.41	3.4×10^{-7} ***

Note: *** = $p < 0.001$.

3.3. Relationship Between Equilibrium and COP Modification

In addition, by applying the beyond optimal model, it was determined that the best structure for equilibrium is:

Balance ~ TestType + FootSupport + Eyes Open + FT + MT + COP_A + Foot_Size + Sex + FT + MT + COP_A + Sex + FT + MT + COP_A + Sex + Foot_Size + Sex + Sex +FT + MT + Sex + COP_A + Sex

Age + TestType: SizeFoot + TestType: Sex + EyesOpen:Size_Foot + EyesOpen:Sex + FT:Sex + MT + COP_A:Sex

Age affected balance, with older participants showing a better balance than younger participants ($p < 0.001$). The type of test affected the balance according to the foot size. The greater the number, the greater the static balance with eyes open (SLB and TBT) ($p < 0.01$) as well as sex, showing better results in girls in the case of SLB and TLB and neutral in YBT (Table 4).

Table 4. Balance ratio according to foot size and sex.

Sexo	Test	Emmean	Contrast	Estimate	t Ratio	p Value
Female	SLB	158.89 ± 9.55 [141.21–178.78]	SLB/TBT	0.78 ± 0.07	−2.82	0.014 *
Female	TBT	202.54 ± 13.53 [177.65–230.92]	SLB/YTest	1.07 ± 0.1	0.77	0.724
Female	YTest	147.93 ± 10.09 [129.4–169.11]	TBT/YTest	1.37 ± 0.14	3.06	0.006 **
Male	SLB	118.96 ± 8.65 [103.13–137.21]	SLB/TBT	0.91 ± 0.09	−0.87	0.662
Male	TBT	130.04 ± 10 [111.82–151.21]	SLB/YTest	0.8 ± 0.09	−1.99	0.116
Male	YTest	148.68 ± 12.21 [126.56–174.68]	TBT/YTest	0.87 ± 0.1	−1.13	0.497

Note: * = $p < 0.05$. ** = $p < 0.01$.

In the case of the center of pressure (COP), the greater the variation, the higher the girls' score in equilibrium, whereas the opposite phenomenon occurred in the case of boys, who improved their score when the COP was reduced (Figure 6).

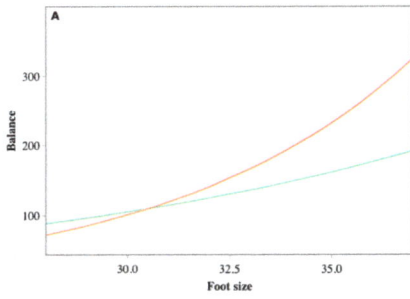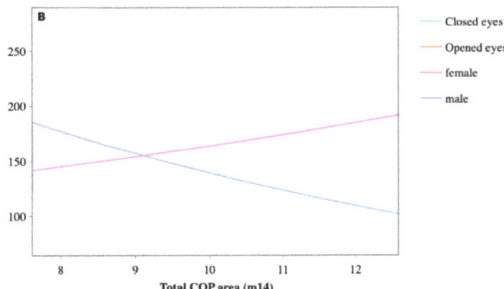

Figure 6. Variation in the balance score with eyes open or closed (**A**) and POP by sex (**B**).

3.4. Relationship Between Complexity and POP Modification

As in the previous case, through the beyond optimal model, it was determined that the best structure to establish the complexity was:

Complexity ~ TypeTest + FootSupport + Eyes open +FT + MT + COP_A + Foot_Size + Sex + Age + TestType: FootSize + TestType:Sex + FT:Foot_Size + MT:Sex + CO:A:Sex

Age was a determinant in assessing complexity, increased the older they get ($p < 0.001$), TBT, and foot size ($p < 0.001$), especially in girls (Table 5).

Table 5. Complexity by gender and type of test.

Sex	Test	Emmean	Contrast	Estimate	t Ratio	p Value
Female	SLB	63.56 ± 3.07 [57.82–69.88]	SLB/TBT	1.07 ± 0.07	1.01	0.570
Female	TBT	59.28 ± 3.28 [53.18–66.09]	SLB/YTest	0.58 ± 0.04	−7.47	8.5×10^{-13} ***
Female	YTest	109.76 ± 5.65 [99.21–121.43]	TBT/YTest	0.54 ± 0.05	−7.36	1.4×10^{-12} ***
Male	SLB	55.71 ± 3.43 [49.37–62.87]	SLB/TBT	1.36 ± 0.11	3.74	5.6×10^{-4} ***
Male	TBT	40.96 ± 2.76 [35.89–46.75]	SLB/YTest	0.54 ± 0.05	−7.07	9.2×10^{-12} ***
Male	YTest	102.41 ± 6.22 [90.9–115.38]	TBT/YTest	0.4 ± 0.04	−9.69	3.2×10^{-13} ***

Note: *** = $p < 0.001$.

The application of force is fundamental for describing the complexity related to the foot size. It decreased with the increase in the force in each axis and with the increase in the foot size (Table 6).

Table 6. Complexity according to applied force and foot size.

Foot Size	TF	Emmean	Contrast	Estimate	t Ratio	p Value
32	229.1	65.75 ± 2.13 [61.69–70.07]	TF 229.12/TF 265.59	1.07 ± 0.02	3.41	0.002 **
32	265.6	61.69 ± 1.73 [58.4–65.18]	TF 229.12/TF 318.31	1.17 ± 0.05	3.41	0.002 **
32	318.3	56.27 ± 2.27 [51.99–60.91]	TF 265.59/TF 318.31	1.10 ± 0.03	3.41	0.002 **
33	229.1	74.03 ± 2.47 [69.34–79.03]	TF 229.12/TF 265.59	1.05 ± 0.02	3.16	0.005 **
33	265.6	70.30 ± 1.79 [66.88–73.91]	TF 229.12/TF 318.31	1.13 ± 0.05	3.16	0.005 **
33	318.3	65.25 ± 1.99 [61.46–69.27]	TF 265.59/TF 318.31	1.08 ± 0.03	3.16	0.005 **
34	229.1	83.35 ± 3.21 [77.29–89.89]	TF 229.12/TF 265.59	1.04 ± 0.02	2.55	0.030 *
34	265.6	80.12 ± 2.30 [75.72–84.77]	TF 229.12/TF 318.31	1.10 ± 0.04	2.55	0.030 *
34	318.3	75.66 ± 2.05 [71.75–79.79]	TF 265.59/TF 318.31	1.06 ± 0.02	2.55	0.030 *

Note: TF = Total force. * = $p < 0.05$. ** = $p < 0.01$.

Finally, the COP area is an element that affects the complexity score, with an unequal relationship between sexes. In boys, the greater the area, the lower the balance score, while in girls, the complexity was independent of the variation in COP (Figure 7).

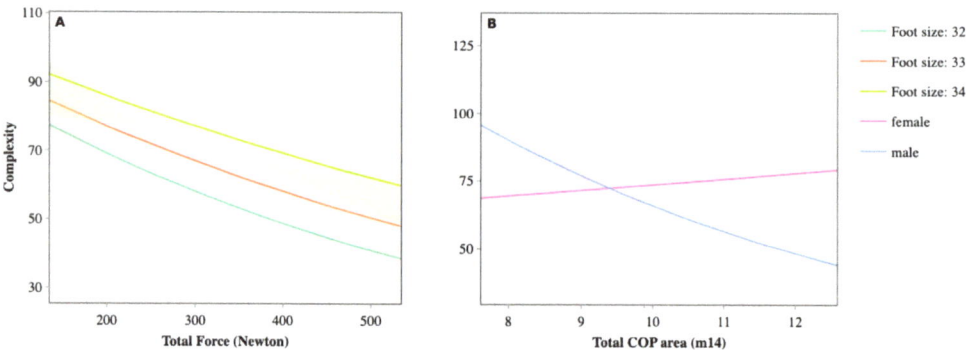

Figure 7. Variation in the complexity score as a function of total strength (A), COP, and sex (B).

3.5. Design of Scoring Scales

After performing the total motion study in the SLB test, the maximum value of motion recorded was 347.53. With this, it is decided to apply *cte* = 350 to invert the scale and obtain the raw score. In the case of the TBT, the maximum value was 288.80 and its value *cte* = 300. Finally, in the YBT, a maximum value of 84 was obtained, with a value *cte* = 80.

Raw score SLB $= -(mvt\ exercise\ a + mvt\ exercise\ b + mvt\ exercise\ c + mvt\ exercise\ d) + 350$

$$Raw\ score\ TBT = -(mvt\ exercise\ a + mvt\ exercise\ b + mvt\ exercise\ c + mvt\ exercise\ d) + 300$$

$$Raw\ score\ YTB = log(YBT\ a + YBT\ b + YBT\ c + YBT\ d + YBT\ e + yby\ f - 80)$$

The linear model to determine the variation in the raw score from sex, age, and foot size resulted in the following formulas, from which the correction factor, FC, was obtained:

$$SLB\ FC = 1053.32 + 6.03 \cdot (Sex == male) - 53.41 \cdot Age - 12.46 \cdot Foot\ size$$

$$TBT\ FC = 1009.87 + 10.96 \cdot (Sex == male) - 54.58 \cdot Age - 11.90 \cdot Foot\ size$$

$$YBT\ FC = 1.61 + 0.11 \cdot (Sex == male) + 0.05 \cdot Age - 0.04 \cdot Foot\ size$$

By applying the correction factor to the raw scores obtained for the population studied, it was determined that the range of these adjusted scores is, in the case of the SLB, from −72 to 230; for the TBT, from −54 to 206; and finally, for the YBT, from −175 to 526. Figure 8 shows the raw score obtained from the total amount of movement and adjusted and rescaled values on YBT.

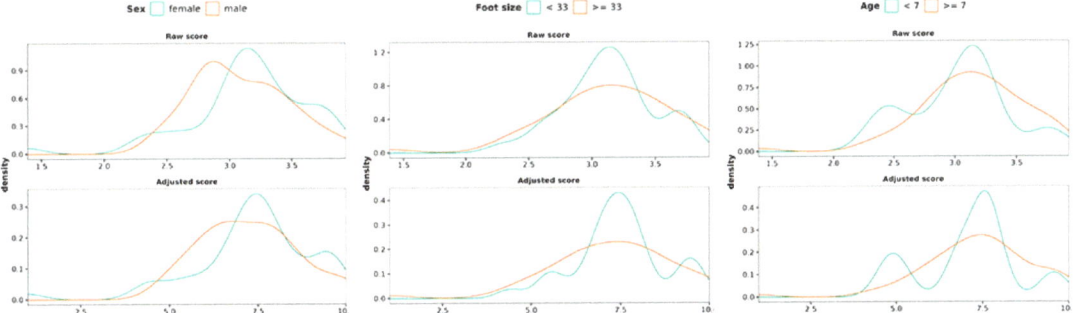

Figure 8. Raw score for the total amount of movement, together with adjusted and rescaled values for sex (**left**), foot size (**center**), and age (**right**).

4. Discussion

The objective of this study was to design a free application for the assessment of static and dynamic balance using a force platform for children between 6 and 9 years of age. The use of mobile applications to monitor fitness indicators has become widespread, providing immediate information on different variables to users with few instructions, even in gamified form [59], for various purposes [60].

As indicated by Kabir et al. [61], the current reliability of these applications is very low, and the accuracy of the data received is essential for their correct interpretation and subsequent decision-making [62]. It is important that they are intuitive, simple, and allow quick understanding [63] based on validated instruments to favor the programming of conditioning work [64].

Balance is fundamental in the perceptual–motor phase, since, in addition to the work on the vestibular system, it integrates determining social functions in preadolescence. Moreover, it is part of all general motor patterns of both basic and more sophisticated techniques, helping the correct location in space in a prominent manner when visual tasks are added [65]. Therefore, it is important to identify whether there is an adequate level of development statically or dynamically, and to observe possible anomalies or dysfunctions in relation to the age of measurement [66], and in this case, the difference in performance competence can be a useful indicator.

A greater complexity was found in the tests performed with closed eyes (SLB and TBT), with a greater height and standing height, possibly due to a greater COM height (Table 3).

In the case of YBT, beyond the complexity, joint mobility is relevant. A greater posteromedial and posterolateral mobility are linked to a greater strength in the lower extremities in 7-year-old children [67]. In this study, it was added to this information that the subject profile with a greater leg length facilitates a better balance in the anterior direction and less in the posterolateral direction.

In the case of the COP, in girls, a greater variation means a better score in the balance variable, as opposed to boys, with less fluctuation due to the difference in the base of support (foot size). Furthermore, it can be affirmed that, in the case of girls, with a lower application of force, they increase the global complexity by having a greater variability in the COP, unlike the boys, whose greater total force decreases this variable for the achievement of balance. Therefore, it can be deduced that a greater movement in girls is the reason for a higher score, unlike in boys (Figure 7).

In addition to evaluating the level of static or dynamic balance and the degree of complexity, these tests are useful for identifying ankle instability by the level of applied force and the detection of a lower participation in physical activities, with possible negative consequences for their health [68]; therefore, they are an excellent reference for Physical Education teachers in the selection of tasks to be developed. The greater or lesser total strength identified in relation to the variation in the COP opens a line of preventive work [69] that would allow correcting the variations that occur, with a greater assistance in the case of girls.

In this line, the observational tool Kinovea, used in similar work with children [70], captured the interrelation between interaxial forces and postural control, allowing for the establishment of a scale of easy interpretation after a sequence of four phases: (1) calculation of movement at reference points, (2) calculation of total movement and raw score, (3) score adjustment attending to demographics, and (4) rescaling to a scale with a score from 1 (greatest imbalance) to 10 (greatest balance), with which to differentiate the level of development by age and sex [71] (unpublished data). These procedures are in line with other studies that have used conventional cameras for kinematic calculations of balance [72] and are similar to those proposed in the Berg scale [73], except that these and other similar designs were intended for special populations without differentiating the specific characteristics of children [59].

This study has several limitations. It should be noted that the age range was small, and the measurement of such young people can be complex. The application requires bridging software to be used to change position (Kinovea, MyLab, or the mobile device's measurement level widget). Finally, it is necessary to apply it in school courses to determine its accessibility and applicability in the educational environment, which would be facilitated by the conversion of the responsive web application into a native mobile app for the two most used operating systems. In any case, it allows the measurement of several tests (dynamic and static) to collect periodic monitoring by keeping data from several dates and to compare, by age, the perceptual–motor evolution of the children.

5. Conclusions

After this investigation, it can be affirmed that static balance is more complex with a greater age, greater standing height, and keeping the eyes closed without significant changes. For dynamic balance, the highest score was associated with anterior mobility and leg length.

With respect to the COP, its variability is greater in girls than in boys, who present less complexity when maintaining balance due to a greater total force at the time of the test.

Finally, the objectivity of the data collected on the force platform, together with the observation with Kinovea, allows the elaboration of an easily interpretable scoring scale, whose environment is an open-access web application (IMEP) to objectify static and dynamic balance tests.

Author Contributions: Conceptualization, J.M.-R. and L.R.-S.; Methodology, J.M.-R., C.R.R. and L.R.-S.; Software, J.M.-R.; Investigation, I.T.-G., C.R.R. and R.S.-F.; Resources, C.C.-M.; Data curation, L.R.-S.; Writing—original draft preparation, J.M.-R.; Writing—review and editing, J.M.-R. and L.R.-S.; Visualization, R.S.-F.; Supervision, I.T.-G. All authors have read and agreed to the published version of the manuscript.

Funding: This research received no external funding.

Institutional Review Board Statement: The study was conducted in accordance with the Declaration of Helsinki and approved by the Ethics Committee of the Catholic University of Valencia (protocol code UCV/2015-16/49) for studies involving humans.

Informed Consent Statement: Informed consent was obtained from all the subjects involved in the study. Written informed consent was obtained from the patients for the publication of this paper.

Data Availability Statement: The datasets used and analyzed during the current study are available from the corresponding author upon reasonable request due to privacy and ethical restrictions.

Acknowledgments: We would like to thank all centers, teachers, and students who made this work possible for their participation.

Conflicts of Interest: The authors declare no conflicts of interest. The funders had no role in the design of the study; in the collection, analyses, or interpretation of data; in the writing of the manuscript; or in the decision to publish the results.

Abbreviations

COM = Centre of mass; COP = Centre of pressure; SLB = Single leg balance test; TBT = Tandem balance test; YBT = Y balance test; SEBT = Star excursion balance test; TF = Total force; IMEP = Instrumento para la Medición del Equilibrio en Primaria.

References

1. Cañizares, J.; Carbonero, C. *Coordinación y Equilibrio en el Niño: Su Desarrollo en la Edad Escolar*; Editorial Wanceulen: Seville, Spain, 2016.
2. Griffin, L. Neuromuscular Training and Injury Prevention in Sports. *Clin. Orthop. Relat. Res.* **2003**, *409*, 53–60. [CrossRef] [PubMed]
3. Mitrousis, I.; Bourdas, D.I.; Kounalakis, S.; Bekris, E.; Mitrotasios, M.; Kostopoulos, N.; Ktistakis, I.E.; Zacharakis, E. The Effect of a Balance Training Program on the Balance and Technical Skills of Adolescent Soccer Players. *J. Sports Sci. Med.* **2023**, *22*, 645–657. [CrossRef] [PubMed]
4. Kounalakis, S.; Karagiannis, A.; Kostoulas, I. Balance Training and Shooting Performance: The Role of Load and the Unstable Surface. *J. Funct. Morphol. Kinesiol.* **2024**, *9*, 17. [CrossRef] [PubMed]
5. Redín, M.I. *Biomecánica y Bases Neuromusculares de la Actividad Física y el Deporte*; Editorial Médica Panamericana: Madrid, Spain, 2008.
6. Muehlbauer, T.; Besemer, C.; Wehrle, A.; Gollhofer, A.; Granacher, U. Relationship between Strength, Power and Balance Performance in Seniors. *Gerontology* **2012**, *58*, 504–512. [CrossRef] [PubMed]
7. Häfelinger, U.; Schuba, V. *La Coordinación y el Entrenamiento Propioceptivo (Bicolor)*, 1st ed.; Paidotribo: Badalona, Spain, 2019.
8. Bueno Moral, M.; Valle Díaz, F.; Vega Marcos, R. *Los Contenidos Perceptivo-Motrices, Las Habilidades Motrices y la Coordinación*; Virtual Sport Publicaciones: Madrid, Spain, 2011.
9. Liu, R.; Yang, J.; Xi, F.; Xu, Z. Relationship between static and dynamic balance in 4-to-5-year-old preschoolers: A cross-sectional study. *BMC Pediatr.* **2024**, *24*, 295. [CrossRef]
10. Sirard, J.R.; Pate, R.R. Physical Activity Assessment in Children and Adolescents. *Sports Med.* **2001**, *31*, 439–454. [CrossRef]
11. García-Liñeira, J.; Leirós-Rodríguez, R.; Romo-Pérez, V.; García-Soidán, J.L. Static and dynamic postural control assessment in schoolchildren: Reliability and reference values of the Modified Flamingo Test and Bar Test. *J. Bodyw. Mov. Ther.* **2023**, *36*, 14–19. [CrossRef]
12. Vedul-Kjelsås, V.; Sigmundsson, H.; Stensdotter, A.K.; Haga, M. The relationship between motor competence, physical fitness and self-perception in children. *Child Care Health Dev.* **2012**, *38*, 394–402. [CrossRef]
13. Bucco-dos Santos, L.; Zubiaur-González, M. Desarrollo de las habilidades motoras fundamentales en función del sexo y del índice de masa corporal en escolares. *Cuad. De Psicol. Del Deporte* **2013**, *13*, 63–72. [CrossRef]
14. Schedler, S.; Brock, K.; Fleischhauer, F.; Kiss, R.; Muehlbauer, T. Effects of Balance Training on Balance Performance in Youth: Are There Age Differences? *Res. Q. Exerc. Sport.* **2020**, *91*, 405–414. [CrossRef]
15. Valero, A.T. *Desarrollo Cognitivo y Motor*; Síntesis: Madrid, Spain, 2016.
16. Cabedo i Sanromá, J.; Roca i Balasch, J. Evolución del equilibrio estático y dinámico desde los 4 hasta los 74 años—INEFC. Apunts. *Educ. Física Y Deportes* **2008**, *2*, 15–25.
17. Castañer Balsells, M.; Camerino Foguet, O. *Manifestaciones Básicas de la Motricidad*; Edicions de la Universitat de Lleida: Lleida, Spain, 2016.

18. Kojić, F.; Arsenijević, R.; Grujić, G.; Toskić, L.; Šimenko, J. Effects of Structured Physical Activity on Motor Fitness in Preschool Children. *Children* **2024**, *11*, 433. [CrossRef] [PubMed]
19. Martín-Ruiz, J.; da Vinha Ricieri, D.; Ruiz-Sanchis, L. Improvement of balance in a 7-year-old child through a six-week learning programme. *J. Hum. Sport Exerc.* **2018**, *13*, 205–217.
20. Eddy, L.H.; Preston, N.; Boom, S.; Davison, J.; Brooks, R.; Bingham, D.D.; Mon-Williams, M.; Hill, L.J.B. The validity and reliability of school-based fundamental movement skills screening to identify children with motor difficulties. *PLoS ONE* **2024**, *19*, e0297412. [CrossRef]
21. Vuillerme, N.; Danion, F.; Marin, L.; Boyadjian, A.; Prieur, J.M.; Weise, I.; Nougier, V. The effect of expertise in gymnastics on postural control. *Neurosci. Lett.* **2001**, *303*, 83–86. [CrossRef]
22. Guimaraes-Ribeiro, D.; Hernández-Suárez, M.; Rodríguez-Ruiz, D.; García-Manso, J.M. Efecto del entrenamiento sistemático de gimnasia rítmica sobre el control postural de niñas adolescentes. *Rev. Andal. De Med. Del Deporte* **2015**, *8*, 54–60. [CrossRef]
23. Golomer, E.; Dupui, P.; Monod, H. The effects of maturation on self-induced dynamic body sway frequencies of girls performing acrobatics or classical dance. *Eur. J. Appl. Physiol.* **1997**, *76*, 140–144. [CrossRef]
24. Riemann, B.L.; Guskiewicz, K.M.; Shields, E.W. Relationship between Clinical and Forceplate Measures of Postural Stability. *J. Sport. Rehabil.* **1999**, *8*, 71–82. [CrossRef]
25. Walicka-Cupryś, K.; Przygoda, Ł.; Czenczek, E.; Truszczyńska, A.; Drzał-Grabiec, J.; Zbigniew, T.; Tarnowski, A. Balance assessment in hearing-impaired children. *Res. Dev. Disabil.* **2014**, *35*, 2728–2734. [CrossRef]
26. Graybiel, A.; Fregly, A.R. A New Quantitative Ataxia Test Battery: APPENDIX A. Postural Equilibrium Tests and Clinical-Type Ataxia Tests: Apparatus, Administration, and Scoring Procedures. *Acta Oto-Laryngol.* **1966**, *61*, 292–312. [CrossRef]
27. Ricotti, L. Static and dynamic balance in young athletes. *J. Hum. Sport Exerc.* **2011**, *6*, 616–628. [CrossRef]
28. Villa, C. Coordinación y equilibrio: Base para la educación física en primaria. *Rev. Digit. Innovación Y Exp. Educ.* **2010**, *37*, 1–11.
29. Faigenbaum, A.D.; Myer, G.D.; Fernandez, I.P.; Carrasco, E.G.; Bates, N.; Farrell, A.; Ratamess, N.A.; Kang, J. Feasibility and reliability of dynamic postural control measures in children in first through fifth grades. *Int. J. Sports Phys. Ther.* **2014**, *9*, 140–148. [PubMed]
30. Faigenbaum, A.D.; Bagley, J.; Boise, S.; Farrell, A.; Bates, N.; Myer, G.D. Dynamic Balance in Children: Performance Comparison Between Two Testing Devices. *Athl. Train. Sports Health Care* **2015**, *7*, 160–164. [CrossRef]
31. Eriksrud, O.; Federolf, P.; Sæland, F.; Litsos, S.; Cabri, J. Reliability and Validity of the Hand Reach Star Excursion Balance Test. *J. Funct. Morphol. Kinesiol.* **2017**, *2*, 28. [CrossRef]
32. Göktürk Usta, A.; Armutlu, K. Comparison of different methods used in balance evaluation in children with diparetic cerebral palsy. *Neurol. Res.* **2024**, *46*, 49–53. [CrossRef]
33. Sheehan, D.P.; Katz, L. The effects of a daily, 6-week exergaming curriculum on balance in fourth grade children. *J. Sport Health Sci.* **2013**, *2*, 131–137. [CrossRef]
34. Guzmán, L.A.; González, F.V.; Jorquera, I.A.; Oyaneder, H.F.; Campoverde, M.S.; Bornand, C.M. Diferencias en equilibrio estático y dinámico entre niños de primero básico de colegios municipales y particulares subvencionados. *Rev. Cienc. De La Act. Física* **2014**, *15*, 17–23.
35. Dabbs, N.C.; Sauls, N.M.; Zayer, A.; Chander, H. Balance Performance in Collegiate Athletes: A Comparison of Balance Error Scoring System Measures. *J. Funct. Morphol. Kinesiol.* **2017**, *2*, 26. [CrossRef]
36. Villalobos-Samaniego, C.; Rivera-Sosa, J.M.; Ramos-Jimenez, A.; Cervantes-Borunda, M.S.; Lopez-Alonzo, S.J.; Hernandez-Torres, R.P. Métodos de evaluación del equilibrio estático y dinámico en niños de 8 a 12 años (Evaluation methods of static and dynamic balance in children aged 8 to 12 years old). *Retos* **2020**, *37*, 793–801. [CrossRef]
37. Saito, A.K.; Navarro, M.; Silva, M.F.; Arie, E.K.; Peccin, M.S. Oscilação do centro de pressão plantar de atletas e não atletas com e sem entorse de tornozelo. *Rev. Bras. De Ortop.* **2016**, *51*, 437–443. [CrossRef]
38. Shafi, H.; Awan, W.A.; Olsen, S.; Siddiqi, F.A.; Tassadaq, N.; Rashid, U.; Niazi, I.K. Assessing Gait & Balance in Adults with Mild Balance Impairment: G&B App Reliability and Validity. *Sensors* **2023**, *23*, 9718. [CrossRef] [PubMed]
39. Balsalobre-Fernández, C.; Bishop, C.; Beltrán-Garrido, J.V.; Cecilia-Gallego, P.; Cuenca-Amigó, A.; Romero-Rodríguez, D.; Madruga-Parera, M. The validity and reliability of a novel app for the measurement of change of direction performance. *J. Sports Sci.* **2019**, *37*, 2420–2424. [CrossRef]
40. Saucedo-Araujo, R.G.; Huertas-Delgado, F.J.; Barranco-Ruiz, Y.M.; Perez-Lopez, I.J.; Aznar-Lain, S.; Chillon, P.; Herrador-Colmenero, M. Testing the Mystic School Mobile Application to Promote Active Commuting to School in Spanish Adolescents: The PACO Study. *Children* **2022**, *9*, 1997. [CrossRef]
41. Mayolas, M. Un nuevo test de valoración de la lateralidad para los profesionales de la Educación Física—INEFC. *Apunts. Educ. Física Y Deportes* **2003**, *71*, 14–22.
42. Tixa, S. *Atlas de Anatomía Palpatoria. Tomo 2. Miembro Inferior*; Elsevier Health Sciences: Philadelphia, PA, USA, 2024.
43. Pérez, F.V.; Vicén, J.A. Efectos de Power Balance® en el equilibrio estático y dinámico en sujetos físicamente activos. *Apunts.Med. De L'esport* **2011**, *46*, 109–115. [CrossRef]
44. Jaworska, M.; Tuzim, T.; Starczyńska, M.; Wilk-Frańczuk, M.; Pedrycz, A. Assessment of the effects of rehabilitation on balance impairment in patients after ischemic stroke according to selected tests and scales. *Pol. Hyperb. Res.* **2015**, *51*, 55–63. [CrossRef]
45. Gribble, P.A.; Hertel, J.; Plisky, P. Using the Star Excursion Balance Test to assess dynamic postural-control deficits and outcomes in lower extremity injury: A literature and systematic review. *J. Athl. Train.* **2012**, *47*, 339–357. [CrossRef]

46. Rabello, L.M.; Macedo, C.d.S.G.; Oliveira MRd Fregueto, J.H.; Camargo, M.Z.; Lopes, L.D.; Shigaki, L.; Gobbi, C.; Gil, A.W.; Kamuza, C.; Silva, R.A., Jr. Relationship between functional tests and force platform measurements in athletes' balance. *Rev. Bras. De Med. Do Esporte* **2014**, *20*, 219–222. [CrossRef]
47. Bates, D.; Mächler, M.; Bolker, B.; Walker, S. Fitting linear mixed-effects models using lme4. *J. Stat. Softw.* **2015**, *67*, 1–48. [CrossRef]
48. Kuznetsova, A.; Brockhoff, P.B.; Christensen, R.H. lmerTest package: Tests in linear mixed effects models. *J. Stat. Softw.* **2017**, *82*, 1–26. [CrossRef]
49. Zuur, A.F.; Ieno, E.N.; Freckleton, R. A protocol for conducting and presenting results of regression-type analyses. *Methods Ecol. Evol.* **2016**, *7*, 636–645. [CrossRef]
50. Fox, J.; Weisberg, S. *An R Companion to Applied Regression*; Sage Publications: Thousand Oaks, CA, 2018.
51. Lenth, R.; Singmann, H.; Love, J.; Buerkner, P.; Herve, M. Emmeans: Estimated Marginal Means, Aka Least-Squares Means (Version 1.3. 4). Emmeans Estim.Marg.Means Aka Least-Sq.Means. 2019. Available online: https://CRAN.R-project.org/package=emmeans (accessed on 20 July 2024).
52. Barton, K. MuMIn: Multi-Model Inference. 2009. Available online: http://r-forge.r-project.org/projects/mumin/ (accessed on 20 July 2024).
53. Lüdecke, D.; Ben-Shachar, M.S.; Patil, I.; Waggoner, P.; Makowski, D. Performance: An R package for assessment, comparison and testing of statistical models. *J. Open Source Softw.* **2021**, *6*, 3139. [CrossRef]
54. R Core Team. *R: A Language and Environment for Statistical Computing, R Foundation for Statistical Computing*; R Foundation for Statistical Computing: Vienna, Austria, 2022.
55. Schauberger, P.; Walker, A.; Braglia, L. Openxlsx: Read, Write and Edit Xlsx Files. *R Package Version* 2020, 4. Available online: https://cran.r-project.org/web/packages/openxlsx/openxlsx.pdf (accessed on 20 July 2024).
56. Wickham, H.; Miller, E. Haven: Import and Export "SPSS", "Stata" and "SAS" Files. 2019. Available online: https://cran.r-project.org/package=haven (accessed on 1 June 2020).
57. Wickham, H. *ggplot2: Elegant Graphics for Data Analysis*; Springer: New York, NY, USA, 2009; Preprint at 2016.
58. Kassambara, A. Ggpubr:"ggplot2" Based Publication Ready Plots. *R Package Version 0.4.0.* 2020. Available online: https://rpkgs.datanovia.com/ggpubr/ (accessed on 20 July 2024).
59. Cash, J.J.; Velozo, C.A.; Bowden, M.G.; Seamon, B.A. The Functional Balance Ability Measure: A Measure of Balance Across the Spectrum of Functional Mobility in Persons Post-Stroke. *Arch. Rehabil. Res. Clin. Transl.* **2023**, *5*, 100296. [CrossRef] [PubMed]
60. Metzendorf, M.; Wieland, L.S.; Richter, B. Mobile health (m-health) smartphone interventions for adolescents and adults with overweight or obesity. *Cochrane Database Syst. Rev.* **2024**, *2*, CD013591.
61. Kabir, M.A.; Samad, S.; Ahmed, F.; Naher, S.; Featherston, J.; Laird, C.; Ahmed, S. Mobile Apps for Wound Assessment and Monitoring: Limitations, Advancements and Opportunities. *J. Med. Syst.* **2024**, *48*, 80. [CrossRef]
62. Bucher, S.L.; Young, A.; Dolan, M.; Padmanaban, G.P.; Chandnani, K.; Purkayastha, S. The NeoRoo mobile app: Initial design and prototyping of an Android-based digital health tool to support Kangaroo Mother Care in low/middle-income countries (LMICs). *PLOS Digit Health* **2023**, *2*, e0000216. [CrossRef]
63. Kim, G.S.; Kim, L.; Baek, S.; Shim, M.; Lee, S.; Kim, J.M.; Yoon, J.Y.; Choi, J.; Choi, J.-P. Three cycles of mobile app design to improve HIV self-management: A development and evaluation study. *Digit Health* **2024**, *10*, 20552076241249294. [CrossRef]
64. Gómez-Hernández, M.; Ferre, X.; Moral, C.; Villalba-Mora, E. Design Guidelines of Mobile Apps for Older Adults: Systematic Review and Thematic Analysis. *JMIR Mhealth Uhealth* **2023**, *11*, e43186. [CrossRef]
65. Yin, R.; Zhu, G.; Liu, A.; Wang, M.; Li, L.; Dai, S. The impact of additional visual tasks in physical exercise on balance ability among 9–10-year-old children: The mediating effect of visual acuity. *Front. Public Health* **2023**, *11*, 1270947. [CrossRef]
66. Nagy, Á.V.; Wilhelm, M.; Domokos, M.; Győri, F.; Berki, T. Assessment Tools Measuring Fundamental Movement Skills of Primary School Children: A Narrative Review in Methodological Perspective. *Sports* **2023**, *11*, 178. [CrossRef] [PubMed]
67. Ituen, O.A.; Duysens, J.; Ferguson, G.; Smits-Engelsman, B. The strength of balance: Strength and dynamic balance in children with and without hypermobility. *PLoS ONE* **2024**, *19*, e0302218. [CrossRef] [PubMed]
68. Suphasubtrakul, T.; Lekskulchai, R.; Jalayondeja, C. Balance, strength and physical activity after ankle sprain: Comparison between children with chronic ankle instability and copers. *Phys. Ther. Sport* **2024**, *65*, 49–53. [CrossRef] [PubMed]
69. Cleworth, T.; Tondat, A.; Goomer, K.; Kalra, M.; Laing, A.C. Effects of flooring on static and dynamic balance in young and older adults. *Gait Posture* **2024**, *107*, 42–48. [CrossRef] [PubMed]
70. Ferreiro-Pérez, M.; Abuín-Porras, V.; Martín-Casas, P.; Ortiz-Gutiérrez, R.M. Postural Control and Sensory Processing in Preschool Children with Autistic Spectrum Disorder: A Cross-Sectional Study. *Children* **2024**, *11*, 303. [CrossRef]
71. Rusu, L.; Marin, M.I.; Geambesa, M.M.; Rusu, M.R. Monitoring the Role of Physical Activity in Children with Flat Feet by Assessing Subtalar Flexibility and Plantar Arch Index. *Children* **2022**, *9*, 427. [CrossRef]
72. Eveleigh, K.J.; Deluzio, K.J.; Scott, S.H.; Laende, E.K. Principal component analysis of whole-body kinematics using markerless motion capture during static balance tasks. *J. Biomech.* **2023**, *152*, 111556. [CrossRef]
73. Miranda, N.; Tiu, T.K. *Berg Balance Testing*; StatPearls Publishing: Treasure Island, FL, USA, 2024.

Disclaimer/Publisher's Note: The statements, opinions and data contained in all publications are solely those of the individual author(s) and contributor(s) and not of MDPI and/or the editor(s). MDPI and/or the editor(s) disclaim responsibility for any injury to people or property resulting from any ideas, methods, instructions or products referred to in the content.

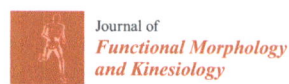

Article

Insights on the Selection of the Coefficient of Variation to Assess Speed Fluctuation in Swimming

Mafalda P. Pinto [1,2], Daniel A. Marinho [1,2], Henrique P. Neiva [1,2], Tiago M. Barbosa [3,4] and Jorge E. Morais [3,4,*]

1. Department of Sport Sciences, University of Beira Interior, 6201-001 Covilhã, Portugal; marinho.d@gmail.com (D.A.M.); henriquepn@gmail.com (H.P.N.)
2. Research Centre in Sports, Health and Human Development (CIDESD), 6201-001 Covilhã, Portugal
3. Department of Sport Sciences, Instituto Politécnico de Bragança, 5300-253 Bragança, Portugal; barbosa@ipb.pt
4. Research Centre for Active Living and Wellbeing (LiveWell), Instituto Politécnico de Bragança, 5300-253 Bragança, Portugal
* Correspondence: morais.jorgestrela@ipb.pt

Abstract: The aim of this study was to compare swimming speed and speed fluctuations in front crawl between swimmers of different performance levels using discrete variables against statistical parametric mapping (SPM). The sample was composed of 34 male swimmers divided into three groups: (i) group #1—recreational swimmers; (ii) group #2—competitive swimmers aged 12 to 14 years; (iii) group #3—competitive swimmers aged 15 to 17 years. Swimming speed and speed fluctuations (calculated based on four different conditions) were used as discrete variables. Using these discrete variables, ANOVA one-way was used to verify differences between groups, and Bonferroni post-hoc correction for pairwise comparison whenever suitable. SPM (with similar statistical tests) was used to analyze the swimming speed and fluctuation as a continuous variable. Overall, both statistical approaches revealed significant differences ($p < 0.001$) in swimming speed and speed fluctuations. However, as discrete variables (in four different conditions), the speed fluctuation was not able to detect significant differences between groups #2 and #3. Conversely, SPM was more sensitive and did yield significant differences between these two groups. Therefore, researchers and coaches should be aware that the speed fluctuation as a discrete variable may not identify differences in swimming speed fluctuations when the average value between groups is marginal. On the other hand, SPM was more sensitive in analyzing all groups.

Keywords: statistical parametric mapping; continuous analysis; comparison; swimmers; performance

Citation: Pinto, M.P.; Marinho, D.A.; Neiva, H.P.; Barbosa, T.M.; Morais, J.E. Insights on the Selection of the Coefficient of Variation to Assess Speed Fluctuation in Swimming. J. Funct. Morphol. Kinesiol. 2024, 9, 129. https://doi.org/10.3390/jfmk9030129

Academic Editor: Peter Hofmann

Received: 21 June 2024
Revised: 18 July 2024
Accepted: 23 July 2024
Published: 25 July 2024

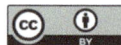

Copyright: © 2024 by the authors. Licensee MDPI, Basel, Switzerland. This article is an open access article distributed under the terms and conditions of the Creative Commons Attribution (CC BY) license (https://creativecommons.org/licenses/by/4.0/).

1. Introduction

Swimming is characterized as being a periodic acceleration/deceleration sport [1,2]. Thus, researchers and coaches put a lot of focus on understanding the balance between thrust (acceleration) and drag (deceleration) [3,4]. From this interaction between thrust and drag, several fluctuations in swimming speed can be observed [5,6]. These fluctuations within a swim stroke cycle are usually measured by a discrete variable called the intra-cyclic variation of the horizontal velocity of the center of mass, which is a feasible way to examine the swimmers' overall mechanics [7]. This variable is also called "speed fluctuation" and can be calculated based on: (i) the coefficient of variation (one standard deviation/mean × 100)—dv1; (ii) the difference between maximal and minimum instantaneous swimming speed—dv2; (iii) the ratio of the mean swimming speed/difference between the maximal and minimum instantaneous swimming speed—dv3; (iv) the ratio of the minimum and maximum swimming speeds/intracycle mean swimming speed—dv4 [8].

Both the swimming speed and speed fluctuation (this latter one irrespective of the way of calculation) are used as discrete variables, i.e., with no time dimension to understand the swimmers' stroke kinematics [9–11]. In the case of swimming speed, several research groups with expertise in swimming use the average swimming speed during the intermediate section of the swimming pool [9,12,13]. Afterwards, the speed fluctuation variable (irrespective of the way) is calculated. The literature reports speed fluctuation as an indicator of swimming efficiency [7,14,15]. Indeed, the overall trend is that smaller values of speed fluctuation are related to the fastest swimming speeds [16,17]. Because it is a variable that is simple to calculate and interpret, coaches and practitioners can easily give insights to their swimmers.

Recently, a study raised the fact that some issues could emerge when using speed fluctuation as the coefficient of variation [18]. Overall, the authors argued that researchers and coaches should take care when using the coefficient of variation as an indicator of the front crawl intra-cycle speed fluctuation since it is likely biased by the mean swimming speed. Moreover, it was suggested that analysis of the swimming speed as a continuous variable (with a time dimension) and comparing different swimming levels could bring greater practical relevance. Indeed, it was reported that using continuous analysis procedures (i.e., with a time dimension), such as statistical parametric mapping (SPM) can give deeper insights into hypothetical differences in these speed fluctuations [19,20]. This statistical method exploits the use of random field theory to perform topological inference by directly mapping the conventional Gaussian distribution onto smooth n-dimensional data [21]. By using SPM for time series data, the statistical result is still a time series (e.g., a time series of t-values) and allows for better interpretation of data [22]. SPM application is increasing in sports sciences, contributing to more detailed movement analyses in biomechanical and performance contexts [23–25]. In the case of swimming, for instance, it was used to investigate differences between elite and sub-elite adult swimmers in the 100 m breaststroke [20] and to identify differences within the front-crawl stroke cycle between age-group swimmers of both sexes [26]. Additionally, we could not find any information about research that used all these discrete ways of calculating speed fluctuations and comparing the outputs with a time dimension procedure such as SPM.

Therefore, the aim of this study was to compare swimming speeds in front crawl between swimmers of different performance levels using discrete variables against SPM. Based on discrete variables, both the swimming speed and speed fluctuation (calculated based on four different conditions) were compared. Based on SPM, the swimming speed was analyzed as a continuous variable, and thus all fluctuations within the stroke cycle were considered. It was hypothesized that SPM would be more sensitive in detecting differences in speed fluctuation with the add-on of identifying where in the stroke cycle such differences would occur.

2. Materials and Methods

2.1. Sample

The sample was composed of 34 male swimmers divided into three groups: #1—recreational swimmers (N = 14); #2—competitive swimmers aged 12 to 14 years (N = 10); #3—competitive swimmers aged 15 to 17 years (N = 10). Part of this sample was retrieved from the study by Morais and co-workers [12]. Their demographics are presented in Table 1. The oldest group (#1—recreational swimmers) presented the greatest body mass, height, and arm span, followed by group #3 (competitive aged 15 to 17 years), and group #2 (competitive aged 12 to 14 years), respectively. The performance level (World Aquatic Points—WAPS) of competitive swimmers was calculated based on the 100 m freestyle short-course event. They were recruited from a national team that regularly participated in regional, national, and international competitions. The sample (groups #2 and #3) included age-group national record holders, age-group national champions, and other swimmers who enrolled in national talent identification programs (Tier 3 athletes) [27]. They trained six to nine times a week. At the time of data collection, they were in peak form at the end of the second macro-cycle. As for the recreational swimmers, these were classified as Tier #1 athletes [27]. Inclusion criteria were that the swimmers should be front-crawl experts and have no limitations (e.g., no injuries in the past 6 months) that would prevent them from performing at their best. An informed consent was obtained by the coaches and/or parents and the swimmers themselves to participate in this study. All procedures followed the Declaration of Helsinki regarding human research. The Polytechnic Ethic Committee also approved the study design (N. ° 72/2022).

Table 1. Descriptive statistics (mean ± one standard deviation—SD) of the swimmers' demographics by group.

	Mean ± SD		
	Group #1 (N = 14)	Group #2 (N = 10)	Group #3 (N = 10)
Age [years]	20.07 ± 1.93	13.20 ± 0.79	16.39 ± 0.69
Body mass [kg]	73.87 ± 8.00	57.30 ± 8.20	70.38 ± 5.97
Height [cm]	179.48 ± 6.54	169.95 ± 8.78	177.30 ± 5.60
Arm span [cm]	183.86 ± 8.06	174.05 ± 10.08	183.60 ± 10.01
WAPS [100 m freestyle]	-	357.90 ± 47.69	578.40 ± 57.49

WAPS—World Aquatic Points.

2.2. Swimming Speed and Speed Fluctuation

Swimmers were invited to perform three all-out 25 m trials, with a push-off start, with a 10-min interval to ensure full recovery. The best trial (i.e., the one with the fastest swimming speed) was used for analysis. Swimmers were instructed to perform non-breathing strokes during such a distance to avoid changes in coordination or technique [28]. Three consecutive stroke cycles between the 10th and 20th meters were analyzed. This was done to avoid any advantage of the wall push-off. The average of the three-stroke cycles was used for analysis.

The string of a mechanical apparatus (SpeedRT, ApLab, Rome, Italy) was attached to the swimmers' waist [29]. The speedometer calculated the displacement and speed of the swimmers (f = 100 Hz). Afterwards, the speed–time series were imported into signal processing software (AcqKnowledge v.3.9.0, Biopac Systems, Santa Barbara, CA, USA). The signal was handled with a Butterworth 4th order low-pass filter (cut-off: 5 Hz) based on the analysis of the residual error vs. cut-off frequency output [30]. A video camera GoPro (Hero 7, San Mateo, CA, USA) filmed the swimmers in the sagittal plane to identify the hand's water entry and exit. This was synchronized with the mechanical device. The beginning and end of each stroke cycle were set by the consecutive entry of the right hand into the water. A swim stroke cycle is composed of the following phases: (i) entry and catch; (ii) downsweep; (iii) insweep; (iv) upsweep, and; (v) exit and recovery [31]. The swimming speed (m/s) was retrieved from the software and the speed fluctuations were calculated as aforementioned (i.e., dv1, dv2, dv3, and dv4).

2.3. Statistical Analysis

The mean plus one standard deviation (SD) was computed as descriptive statistics. The ANOVA one-way was used to measure differences between groups (α = 0.05). The effect size index (eta square—η^2) was computed and interpreted as: without effect if $0 < \eta^2 \leq 0.04$; minimum if $0.04 < \eta^2 \leq 0.25$; moderate if $0.25 < \eta^2 \leq 0.64$; strong if $\eta^2 > 0.64$ [32]. The Bonferroni post-hoc correction was used to verify pairwise differences ($p < 0.017$). Cohen's d estimated the standardized effect sizes and deemed as: trivial if $0 \leq d < 0.20$; small if $0.20 \leq d < 0.60$; moderate if $0.60 \leq d < 1.20$; large if $1.20 \leq d < 2.00$; very large if $2.00 \leq d < 4.00$; nearly distinct if $d \geq 4.00$ [33].

SPM ANOVA one-way was used to verify the differences between groups (α = 0.05) [21]. SPM Bonferroni post-hoc correction was used to verify differences between pairwise ($p < 0.017$). Before such analysis, each stroke cycle was normalized to its duration on R software (version 2024.04.02). The normalization procedure implies creating a near-identical copy of each signal segment that is resampled to a normalized length of 100% [34]. In this case, all swim stroke cycles were stretched/compressed to the same length. Consequently, each normalized curve consisted of 101 points, irrespective of how many points each original curve contained. This is a procedure commonly used in human gait that allows comparison across different gait cycles, subjects, and conditions due to the inherent variability in human gait [35]. The same rationale is applied to swimming. By normalizing the stroke cycles, coaches can identify differences within the swim stroke. SPM analyses were implemented using the open source spm1d code on Matlab (v.M0.1, www.spm1d.org).

3. Results

Table 2 presents the descriptive data related to swimming speed and speed fluctuation by group. Swimmers in group #3 were the fastest, in group #2 the second fastest, and in group #1 the slowest. As for speed fluctuation, this was greater in group #1, followed by group #3, and group #2, respectively (all conditions). Regarding the swimming speed, the ANOVA one-way yielded significant differences between groups (F = 75.01, $p < 0.001$, η^2 = 0.83). Bonferroni post-hoc correction revealed significant differences between group #1 and groups #2 ($p < 0.001$, d = 3.60) and #3 ($p < 0.001$, d = 4.38), but not between group #2 and #3 (Table 2). As for speed fluctuation (all conditions), these presented similar findings. That is, significant differences between groups were noted ($p < 0.001$) (Table 2). The pairwise comparison also revealed significant differences between group #1 and groups #2 and #3, but not between groups #2 and #3 (Table 1).

Table 2. Descriptive statistics (mean ± one standard deviation—SD) of the participants' swimming speed and speed fluctuation (dv) as being the coefficient of variation (CV). The one-way ANOVA and pairwise comparison is also presented.

	Mean ± SD			ANOVA One-Way		Post-Hoc Comparison		
	Group #1	Group #2	Group #3	F-Ratio (p)	η^2	#1 vs. #2	#1 vs. #3	#2 vs. #3
Speed [m/s] [a,b]	1.17 ± 0.15	1.56 ± 0.03	1.67 ± 0.06	75.01 ($p < 0.001$)	0.83	$p < 0.001$; d = 3.60	$p < 0.001$; d = 4.38	-
dv1 [%] [a,b]	23.90 ± 5.06	7.33 ± 2.11	7.69 ± 1.37	88.04 ($p < 0.001$)	0.85	$p < 0.001$; d = 4.27	$p < 0.001$; d = 4.37	-
dv2 [m/s]	0.96 ± 0.21	0.39 ± 0.11	0.45 ± 0.06	54.42 ($p < 0.001$)	0.78	$p < 0.001$; d = 3.40	$p < 0.001$; d = 3.30	-
dv3 [a.u.]	1.27 ± 0.28	4.25 ± 1.34	3.79 ± 0.53	49.47 ($p < 0.001$)	0.76	$p < 0.001$; d = 3.08	$p < 0.001$; d = 5.95	-
dv4 [a.u.]	0.36 ± 0.09	0.50 ± 0.04	0.45 ± 0.02	17.40 ($p < 0.001$)	0.53	$p < 0.001$; d = 2.01	$p = 0.001$; d = 1.38	-

dv1—speed fluctuation based on the coefficient of variation; dv2—speed fluctuation based on the difference between maximal and minimum instantaneous speed; dv3—speed fluctuation based on the ratio of the mean speed/difference between the maximal and minimum instantaneous speed; dv4—speed fluctuation based on the ratio of the minimum and maximum speeds/intracycle mean speed; η^2—effect size index; a—significant differences ($p < 0.001$) between group #1 and #2; b—significant differences ($p < 0.001$) between group #1 and #3; d—Cohen's d (effect size index).

Figure 1 depicts the swimming speed curve differences by SPM (Panel A). There was a significant difference (F = 12.016, $p < 0.001$) between the three groups mainly over the entire stroke cycle. SPM post-hoc comparison between group #1 and #2 (Panel B) revealed significant differences mainly over the entire stroke cycle. Non-significant differences were only noted between ~16% and ~29% (end of the downsweep and insweep of the right hand), and between ~68% and ~82% (end of the downsweep and beginning of the upsweep of the left hand). The comparison between the group #1 and #3 trend (Panel C) was similar (i.e., differences over the entire stroke cycle), except between ~73% and ~80% (insweep and beginning of the upsweep of the left hand). Contrary to what was observed with the dv as a discrete variable, the post-hoc correction through SPM was able to detect significant differences between group #2 and #3 (Panel D). These were noted between ~17% and ~27% (end of the downsweep phase and insweep of the right hand), and between ~44% and ~51% (end of the downsweep phase of the right hand).

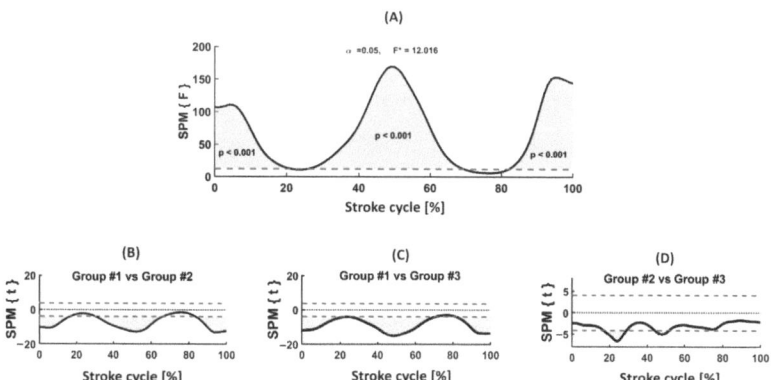

Figure 1. (A) ANOVA one-way of swimming speed by SPM between the three groups, and the corresponding post-hoc analysis (B)—group #1 vs. #2; (C)—group #1 vs. #3; (D)—group #2 vs. #3). (F)—variance statistic for statistical parametric mapping. SPM {t}—post-hoc statistic for statistical parametric mapping. Grey areas indicate significant differences. In panels (B–D) these areas correspond to $p < 0.017$. The dotted black line indicates the null hypothesis. Dash red lines represent the 95% confidence intervals (95 CI).

4. Discussion

The aim of this study was to compare swimming speeds in front crawl between swimmers of different performance levels using discrete variables against SPM. The main findings indicate that, by analyzing discrete variables, i.e., average swimming speed and speed fluctuation (calculated based on four different conditions), significant differences between groups were noted (Table 2). However, post-hoc comparisons indicated a non-significant difference between groups #2 and #3 (similar values of speed fluctuation considering the four conditions of calculation) (Table 2). SPM was revealed to be a more sensitive analysis of the speed–time curve as a continuous time-series. Contrary to discrete variables analysis, SPM detected significant differences between groups #2 and #3 in the post-hoc correction (Figure 1, Panel D).

Speed fluctuation (calculated based on the aforementioned four different conditions, but particularly based on the coefficient of variation) has been considered a good proxy of the intra-cyclic variation of the horizontal speed of the center of mass within a stroke cycle, and thus a mechanical efficiency indicator [7]. Among the swimming community, this is deemed to be a feasible and straightforward procedure to analyze the swimmers' overall stroke kinematics. Moreover, several practical advantages for researchers and coaches can be listed: (i) identification of key moments in different phases of the cycle; collection of relevant details; (ii) easily interpretable data for coaches and practitioners, and; (iii) a straightforward way of setting the swimmer's competitive level [7]. At least in front crawl, it was shown that the fastest or most highly skilled swimmers have smaller speed fluctuations (particularly calculated as the coefficient of variation and reporting to the average of the stroke cycle) than their slower or less skilled counterparts [9,10,16]. It must be mentioned that such smaller speed fluctuations might not be significant [9]. Nonetheless, this confirms that speed fluctuation can be useful in discriminating against the best or poorest swimmers and delivering important insights to coaches.

Notwithstanding, and as mentioned previously, concerns were raised about the use of speed fluctuation (calculated as being the coefficient of variation) because this reports the average of what happens within the stroke cycle [18]. Indeed, authors who aimed to compare the swimming speed and speed fluctuation in front crawl between competitive swimmers of different age-groups reported contradictory findings [12]. Even though significant differences were noted in swimming speed between groups, speed fluctuation revealed non-significant differences. Conversely, the same comparison selecting SPM did yield significant differences in the speed fluctuation at a given moment of the stroke cycle [12]. Thus, it seems that whenever marginal differences are noted by the speed fluctuation (in such cases as being the coefficient of variation), classical statistics using discrete values are not sensitive enough to identify hypothetical differences. On the other hand, in the present study, classical statistics detected significant differences between groups (ANOVA) by both the swimming speed and speed fluctuation. One can speculate that this occurred because performance-level group #1 presented both a substantially slower swimming speed and larger speed fluctuation. But pairwise comparison revealed only significant differences between group #1 and groups #2 and #3. Once again, classical statistics did not detect significant differences between the fastest groups (#2 and #3) in swimming speed and speed fluctuation.

In another study that compared swimmers of different performance levels, the authors noted that the poorest performance level group was significantly slower than the intermediate and fastest groups (the intermediate and fastest groups were not significantly different) [10]. However, regarding speed fluctuation, this was only significantly different between the slowest and intermediate groups with the fastest group (the slowest and intermediate groups were not significantly different) [10]. This shows that there are studies where significant differences in swimming speed were noted, but this did not happen in speed fluctuation [9,36]. This allows us to indicate that the fastest swimmers may present smaller speed fluctuations than their slower counterparts, but a cause–effect phenomenon may not happen (i.e., small speed fluctuation leads to the fastest swimming speeds). It argued that despite speed fluctuation being a gross propulsive efficiency proxy (for the same hydrodynamic drag condition), swimmers can adopt different mechanical strategies that will affect such gross swimming efficiency [37]. Aiming to better understand this swimming speed–speed fluctuation relationship, Pinto et al. [38] measured these variables in a stroke-by-stroke analysis. These authors noted that non-significant relationships were verified between the swimming speed and speed fluctuations. Moreover, this relationship (despite being non-significant) was not always inverse, i.e., small speed fluctuations did not always lead to the fastest swimming speeds [38]. This highlights the rationale indicating that this variable may not be a cause of a given behavior, but a consequence [37].

Notwithstanding, SPM being, a continuous time-series analysis, was more sensitive to the speed fluctuations enabling the detection of differences within the stroke cycle and pinpointing where these happened. Therefore, one can suggest that for those who aim to identify differences in speed fluctuations (where the average values are close), a continuous time-series analysis seems to be the best approach at least in comparison to classical statistics that use discrete variables. Researchers aimed to compare swimming speed and speed fluctuations at different competitive levels of young swimmers of both sexes as a discrete variable and based on SPM [26]. The main outcomes were that, overall, non-significant differences were noted between performance levels in boys, and between boys and girls of the same performance level. Significant differences were noted in girls between the two fastest performance levels and the slowest one. Which, curiously, was where the greatest absolute difference was noted [26]. Data from the present study revealed a similar trend where differences in the speed fluctuation between the two competitive groups (fastest ones) were only noted through SPM. Once again, classical statistics were able to detect differences between group #1 (recreational swimmers with the poorest performances) and the two remaining groups (competitive swimmers with the best performances). This indicates that the speed fluctuation, irrespective of the way of calculation, can only be compared based on discrete values (through classical statistics) when the groups do not present very close or similar values. For instance, in a study by Lopes and co-workers [39], the authors aimed to detect differences between two sections of the swimming pool (10–15 m vs.

15–20 m) in a set of variables related to stroke kinematics including the speed fluctuation (calculated as being the coefficient of variation). They noted significant differences in the speed fluctuation between sections (10–15 m: speed fluctuation = 33.82 ± 15.22%; 15–20 m: speed fluctuation = 25.59 ± 13.15%; $p = 0.005$; $d = 0.58$). Referring again to the study of Figueiredo et al. [10] it was noted that significant differences were only verified between groups that had the greatest difference. Once again, it was not possible to detect differences between groups that had close values of speed fluctuation through discrete variables. These findings corroborate our previous statement, where differences in speed fluctuation (based on discrete values) can only be detected when the average values are not close or similar. Otherwise, when the discrete values are close or similar, the continuous analysis approach (such as SPM) seems to be the most appropriate way of detecting hypothetical differences as shown in other studies [12].

In summary, continuous speed–time analysis by SPM analysis revealed itself to be more sensitive than the speed fluctuation (calculated based on four different conditions) when examining speed fluctuations. This procedure also has the advantage of identifying where within the stroke cycle such differences occur. At least in competitive swimming, the speed fluctuation as a discrete variable was not able to detect differences between performance groups where the average value was similar. Researchers and coaches should be aware that when the speed fluctuation values are similar between different groups, skill levels or tiers, it may not be possible to detect differences based on discrete variables. As a main limitation, it can be considered the sample size. An a priori power analysis was performed using G*Power [40]. A total of 66 participants were required to detect a large effect size ($f^2 = 0.40$) with 80% power ($\alpha = 0.05$) for an "ANOVA: Fixed effects, omnibus, one-way" statistical test. Therefore, researchers could aim to better understand this speed fluctuation phenomenon in different competitive levels and female swimmers as it is of paramount importance for coaches and practitioners. It is also suggested that larger sample sizes be used to understand if the outcomes are like those presented in this study.

5. Conclusions

Swimming speed and speed fluctuation (calculated based on four different conditions), as discrete variables, revealed an overall significant difference between groups. However, pairwise comparison did not identify significant differences between the two fastest groups. Conversely, SPM (a continuous time-series procedure, i.e., with a time dimension) did identify significant differences between such groups. This indicates that SPM is a more sensitive approach to the analysis of swimming speed fluctuations, particularly when the differences between these are marginal.

Author Contributions: Conceptualization, D.A.M., T.M.B. and J.E.M.; methodology, M.P.P., H.P.N. and J.E.M.; formal analysis, M.P.P. and J.E.M.; data curation, M.P.P.; writing—original draft preparation, M.P.P.; writing—review and editing, D.A.M., H.P.N., T.M.B. and J.E.M.; supervision, D.A.M., H.P.N. and J.E.M. All authors have read and agreed to the published version of the manuscript.

Funding: This research was funded by FCT—the Portuguese Foundation for Science and Technology, grant number UIDB/DTP/04045/2020.

Institutional Review Board Statement: All procedures were in accordance with the Declaration of Helsinki regarding human research. The Polytechnic Ethic Committee also approved the study design (N.º 72/2022).

Informed Consent Statement: Informed consent was obtained by the coaches and/or parents and the swimmers themselves to participate in this study.

Data Availability Statement: The data presented in this study are available on request from the corresponding author. The data are not publicly available due to privacy or ethical restrictions.

Conflicts of Interest: The authors declare no conflicts of interest.

References

1. Toussaint, H. Biomechanics of Drag and Propulsion in Front Crawl Swimming. In *World Book of Swimming: From Science to Performance*; Nova Science Publishers, Inc.: New York, NY, USA, 2011; pp. 3–20.
2. Ganzevles, S.P.; Beek, P.J.; Daanen, H.A.; Coolen, B.M.; Truijens, M.J. Differences in Swimming Smoothness between Elite and Non-Elite Swimmers. *Sports Biomech.* 2019, 22, 675–688. [CrossRef] [PubMed]
3. Gatta, G.; Cortesi, M.; Zamparo, P. The Relationship between Power Generated by Thrust and Power to Overcome Drag in Elite Short Distance Swimmers. *PLoS ONE* 2016, 11, e0162387. [CrossRef] [PubMed]
4. Narita, K.; Nakashima, M.; Takagi, H. Developing a Methodology for Estimating the Drag in Front-Crawl Swimming at Various Velocities. *J. Biomech.* 2017, 54, 123–128. [CrossRef]
5. Psycharakis, S.G.; Naemi, R.; Connaboy, C.; McCabe, C.; Sanders, R.H. Three-Dimensional Analysis of Intracycle Velocity Fluctuations in Frontcrawl Swimming. *Scand. J. Med. Sci. Sports* 2010, 20, 128–135. [CrossRef] [PubMed]
6. Gourgoulis, V.; Boli, A.; Aggeloussis, N.; Toubekis, A.; Antoniou, P.; Kasimatis, P.; Vezos, N.; Michalopoulou, M.; Kambas, A.; Mavromatis, G. The Effect of Leg Kick on Sprint Front Crawl Swimming. *J. Sports Sci.* 2014, 32, 278–289. [CrossRef] [PubMed]
7. Barbosa, T.M.; Bragada, J.A.; Reis, V.M.; Marinho, D.A.; Carvalho, C.; Silva, A.J. Energetics and Biomechanics as Determining Factors of Swimming Performance: Updating the State of the Art. *J. Sci. Med. Sport* 2010, 13, 262–269. [CrossRef] [PubMed]
8. Fernandes, A.; Afonso, J.; Noronha, F.; Mezêncio, B.; Vilas-Boas, J.P.; Fernandes, R.J. Intracycle Velocity Variation in Swimming: A Systematic Scoping Review. *Bioengineering* 2023, 10, 308. [CrossRef] [PubMed]
9. Silva, A.F.; Figueiredo, P.; Ribeiro, J.; Alves, F.; Vilas-Boas, J.P.; Seifert, L.; Fernandes, R.J. Integrated Analysis of Young Swimmers' Sprint Performance. *Motor Control* 2019, 23, 354–364. [CrossRef]
10. Figueiredo, P.; Silva, A.; Sampaio, A.; Vilas-Boas, J.P.; Fernandes, R.J. Front Crawl Sprint Performance: A Cluster Analysis of Biomechanics, Energetics, Coordinative, and Anthropometric Determinants in Young Swimmers. *Motor Control* 2016, 20, 209–221. [CrossRef] [PubMed]
11. Correia, R.A.; Feitosa, W.G.; Figueiredo, P.; Papoti, M.; Castro, F.A.S. The 400-m Front Crawl Test: Energetic and 3D Kinematical Analyses. *Int. J. Sports Med.* 2020, 41, 21–26. [CrossRef] [PubMed]
12. Morais, J.E.; Barbosa, T.M.; Lopes, T.; Moriyama, S.-I.; Marinho, D.A. Comparison of Swimming Velocity between Age-Group Swimmers through Discrete Variables and Continuous Variables by Statistical Parametric Mapping. *Sports Biomech.* 2023, 1–12. [CrossRef] [PubMed]
13. Strzala, M.; Stanula, A.; Krezalek, P.; Ostrowski, A.; Kaca, M.; Glab, G. Influence Of Morphology And Strength On Front Crawl Swimming Speed In Junior And Youth Age Group Swimmers. *J. Strength Cond. Res.* 2017, 33, 2836–2845. [CrossRef] [PubMed]
14. Figueiredo, P.; Kjendlie, P.L.; Vilas-Boas, J.P.; Fernandes, R.J. Intracycle Velocity Variation of the Body Centre of Mass in Front Crawl. *Int. J. Sports Med.* 2012, 33, 285–290. [CrossRef] [PubMed]
15. Seifert, L.; Toussaint, H.M.; Alberty, M.; Schnitzler, C.; Chollet, D. Arm Coordination, Power, and Swim Efficiency in National and Regional Front Crawl Swimmers. *Hum. Mov. Sci.* 2010, 29, 426–439. [CrossRef] [PubMed]
16. Matsuda, Y.; Yamada, Y.; Ikuta, Y.; Nomura, T.; Oda, S. Intracyclic Velocity Variation and Arm Coordination for Different Skilled Swimmers in the Front Crawl. *J. Hum. Kinet.* 2014, 44, 67–74. [CrossRef] [PubMed]
17. Morais, J.E.; Barbosa, T.M.; Neiva, H.P.; Marques, M.C.; Marinho, D.A. Young Swimmers' Classification Based on Performance and Biomechanical Determinants: Determining Similarities Through Cluster Analysis. *Motor Control* 2022, 26, 396–411. [CrossRef] [PubMed]
18. Gonjo, T.; Fernandes, R.J.; Vilas-Boas, J.P.; Sanders, R. Is the Use of Coefficient of Variation a Valid Way to Assess the Swimming Intra-Cycle Velocity Fluctuation? *J. Sci. Med. Sport* 2023, 26, 328–334. [CrossRef] [PubMed]
19. Gourgoulis, V.; Nikodelis, T. Comparison of the Arm-Stroke Kinematics between Maximal and Sub-Maximal Breaststroke Swimming Using Discrete Data and Time Series Analysis. *J. Biomech.* 2022, 142, 111255. [CrossRef]
20. Gonjo, T.; Olstad, B.H. Differences between Elite and Sub-Elite Swimmers in a 100 m Breaststroke: A New Race Analysis Approach with Time-Series Velocity Data. *Sports Biomech.* 2021, 22, 1722–1733. [CrossRef] [PubMed]
21. Pataky, T. Generalized N-Dimensional Biomechanical Field Analysis Using Statistical Parametric Mapping. *J. Biomech.* 2010, 43, 1976–1982. [CrossRef] [PubMed]
22. Serrien, B.; Goossens, M.; Baeyens, J.-P. Statistical Parametric Mapping of Biomechanical One-Dimensional Data with Bayesian Inference. *Int. Biomech.* 2019, 6, 9–18. [CrossRef] [PubMed]
23. Bertozzi, F.; Porcelli, S.; Marzorati, M.; Pilotto, A.M.; Galli, M.; Sforza, C.; Zago, M. Whole-Body Kinematics during a Simulated Sprint in Flat-Water Kayakers. *Eur. J. Sport Sci.* 2022, 22, 817–825. [CrossRef] [PubMed]
24. Warmenhoven, J.; Harrison, A.; Robinson, M.A.; Vanrenterghem, J.; Bargary, N.; Smith, R.; Cobley, S.; Draper, C.; Donnelly, C.; Pataky, T. A Force Profile Analysis Comparison between Functional Data Analysis, Statistical Parametric Mapping and Statistical Non-Parametric Mapping in on-Water Single Sculling. *J. Sci. Med. Sport* 2018, 21, 1100–1105. [CrossRef] [PubMed]
25. Bini, R. Influence of Saddle Height in 3D Knee Loads Commuter Cyclists: A Statistical Parametric Mapping Analysis. *J. Sports Sci.* 2021, 39, 275–288. [CrossRef] [PubMed]
26. Morais, J.E.; Marinho, D.A.; Cobley, S.; Barbosa, T.M. Identifying Differences in Swimming Speed Fluctuation in Age-Group Swimmers by Statistical Parametric Mapping: A Biomechanical Assessment for Performance Development. *J. Sports Sci. Med.* 2023, 22, 358–366. [CrossRef] [PubMed]

27. McKay, A.; Stellingwerff, T.; Smith, E.; Martin, D.; Mujika, I.; Goosey-Tolfrey, V.; Sheppard, J.; Burke, L. Defining Training and Performance Caliber: A Participant Classification Framework. *Int. J. Sports Physiol. Perform.* **2022**, *17*, 317–331. [CrossRef]
28. McCabe, C.B.; Sanders, R.H.; Psycharakis, S.G. Upper Limb Kinematic Differences between Breathing and Non-Breathing Conditions in Front Crawl Sprint Swimming. *J. Biomech.* **2015**, *48*, 3995–4001. [CrossRef] [PubMed]
29. Morouço, P.; Lima, A.B.; Semblano, P.; Fernandes, D.; Gonçalves, P.; Sousa, F.; Fernandes, R.; Barbosa, T.M.; Velhote, M.; Vilas-Boas, J.P. Validation of a Cable Speedometer for Butterfly Evaluation. *Rev. Port. Ciências Desporto* **2006**, *6*, 236–239.
30. Winter, D.A. *Biomechanics and Motor Control of Human Movement*; John Wiley & Sons: Hoboken, NJ, USA, 2009; ISBN 0-470-39818-3.
31. Maglischo, E.W. *Swimming Fastest*; Human Kinetics: Champaign, IL, USA, 2003; ISBN 0-7360-3180-4.
32. Ferguson, C.J. An Effect Size Primer: A Guide for Clinicians and Researchers. *Prof. Psychol. Res. Pract.* **2009**, *40*, 532–538. [CrossRef]
33. Hopkins, W. A Scale of Magnitudes for Effect Statistics. A New View of Statistics. 2002. Available online: http://sportsci.org/resource/stats/effectmag.html (accessed on 10 January 2024).
34. Helwig, N.E.; Hong, S.; Hsiao-Wecksler, E.T.; Polk, J.D. Methods to Temporally Align Gait Cycle Data. *J. Biomech.* **2011**, *44*, 561–566. [CrossRef] [PubMed]
35. Pinzone, O.; Schwartz, M.H.; Baker, R. Comprehensive Non-Dimensional Normalization of Gait Data. *Gait Posture* **2016**, *44*, 68–73. [CrossRef] [PubMed]
36. Morais, J.E.; Saavedra, J.M.; Costa, M.J.; Silva, A.J.; Marinho, D.A.; Barbosa, T.M. Tracking Young Talented Swimmers: Follow-up of Performance and Its Biomechanical Determinant Factors. *Acta Bioeng. Biomech.* **2013**, *15*, 129–138. [CrossRef] [PubMed]
37. Fernandes, A.; Mezêncio, B.; Soares, S.; Duarte Carvalho, D.; Silva, A.; Vilas-Boas, J.P.; Fernandes, R.J. Intra-and Inter-Cycle Velocity Variations in Sprint Front Crawl Swimming. *Sports Biomech.* **2022**, 1–14. [CrossRef] [PubMed]
38. Pinto, M.P.; Marinho, D.A.; Neiva, H.P.; Morais, J.E. Relationship between Swimming Speed, Intra-Cycle Variation of Horizontal Speed, and Froude Efficiency during Consecutive Stroke Cycles in Adolescent Swimmers. *PeerJ* **2023**, *11*, e16019. [CrossRef] [PubMed]
39. Lopes, T.J.; Sampaio, T.; Oliveira, J.P.; Pinto, M.P.; Marinho, D.A.; Morais, J.E. Using Wearables to Monitor Swimmers' Propulsive Force to Get Real-Time Feedback and Understand Its Relationship to Swimming Velocity. *Appl. Sci.* **2023**, *13*, 4027. [CrossRef]
40. Faul, F.; Erdfelder, E.; Buchner, A.; Lang, A.G. Statistical Power Analyses Using G*Power 3.1: Tests for Correlation and Regression Analyses. *Behav. Res. Methods* **2009**, *41*, 1149–1160. [CrossRef]

Disclaimer/Publisher's Note: The statements, opinions and data contained in all publications are solely those of the individual author(s) and contributor(s) and not of MDPI and/or the editor(s). MDPI and/or the editor(s) disclaim responsibility for any injury to people or property resulting from any ideas, methods, instructions or products referred to in the content.

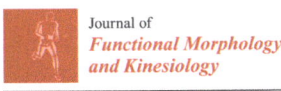

Article

Anthropometric and Somatotype Profile of Elite Finn Class Sailors

Luka Pezelj [1,*], Boris Milavić [2,*] and Mirjana Milić [2]

[1] Faculty of Maritime Studies, University of Split, 21000 Split, Croatia
[2] Faculty of Kinesiology, University of Split, 21000 Split, Croatia; mirjana.milic@kifst.hr
* Correspondence: luka.pezelj@pfst.hr (L.P.); boris.milavic@kifst.hr (B.M.);
  Tel.: +385-95-539-7714 (L.P.); +385-95-818-5328 (B.M.)

Abstract: Determining the reference base of anthropometric parameters on a sample of elite athletes is one of the foundations of further research and forming a clearer picture of each sport and sports discipline. In this study, the aim was to describe the anthropometric and somatotype profiles of elite Finn class sailors and to determine the differences in the measured parameters between sailors at different levels of general competitive success. The subject sample included 57 Finn class sailors who competed at the open Finn European Championship. A set of 25 anthropometric variables were applied. The sailors were divided into three groups according to their level of general competitive success using World Sailing Rankings. Finn sailors had higher average values in almost all morphological characteristics when compared to the sailors in other Olympic classes. Considering the average values of somatotype categories, we determined that Finn sailors fit the *endomorphic mesomorph* somatotype category (3.94 ± 1.19 − 5.50 ± 1.19 − 1.63 ± 0.74). Significant differences were observed between more-successful, medium, and less-successful sailors in the variables of *age, body mass, muscle mass, arm muscle mass,* and *endomorphy rating*. These results indicate the possibility of selection processes and/or adaptation to sailing occurring in the Finn class. The anthropometric characteristics of Finn sailors compared to sailors in Olympic classes further "support" the Finn class being called the "heavy dinghy" male class. This study on anthropometric parameters, determined via a sample of top Finn sailors, may be of great help to coaches and young sailors when deciding on the selection of an adult sailing class.

Keywords: dinghy sailing; elite athletes; Finn class; fitness testing; morphological characteristics; Olympic sailing; sailing; somatotype

Citation: Pezelj, L.; Milavić, B.; Milić, M. Anthropometric and Somatotype Profile of Elite Finn Class Sailors. *J. Funct. Morphol. Kinesiol.* **2024**, *9*, 121. https://doi.org/10.3390/jfmk9030121

Academic Editor: Pedro Miguel Forte

Received: 29 April 2024
Revised: 2 July 2024
Accepted: 3 July 2024
Published: 5 July 2024

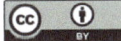

Copyright: © 2024 by the authors. Licensee MDPI, Basel, Switzerland. This article is an open access article distributed under the terms and conditions of the Creative Commons Attribution (CC BY) license (https://creativecommons.org/licenses/by/4.0/).

1. Introduction

Determining the reference base of anthropometric parameters on a sample of elite athletes is one of the foundations of further research and forming a clearer picture of each sport and sports discipline. Somatotype, the quantification of the present shape and composition of the human body calculated from the values of anthropometric parameters, provides an additional dimension that is useful in understanding and interpreting the anthropometric profile of elite athletes. It is expressed as representing relative fatness as an endomorphy rating, musculoskeletal robustness as a mesomorphy rating, and relative linearity of a physique as an ectomorphy rating [1]. Relations of amount and relations of muscle and fat mass according to a somatotype rating report a high positive correlation between endomorphy and percentage of body fat, a low positive correlation between mesomorphy and fat free weight, and a low know negative correlation between ectomorphy and percentage of body fat and fat-free weight [2,3].

Reference bases should be up to date as anthropometric characteristics are constantly evolving as a response to changes in the sporting and external environment [4]. Reference bases for anthropometric parameters and the somatotype on a sample of elite athletes have been determined for numerous sports [5–10], as well as the impact of some anthropometric characteristic [5,8,11–15] and somatotype ratings on competitive success [7,8,12,14,16]. Higher lean mass does appear to benefit sprint athletes [5] and sprint cross-country skiers [13], lower values of body mass index and percentage of body fat benefit elite mountain bikers [8], and the performance of the sailors in the Laser class, among other parameters, are determined by height and sitting height [11]. Results from somatotype rating research present significantly lower values for the endomorphic component in more-successful mountain bikers [8] and windsurfers [12].

Sailing is a sport in which athletes have the opportunity to compete in many sailing classes. The most competitive, i.e., the most "sportlike", sailing classes are those included in the Olympic program, the so-called Olympic classes. The Finn class was the longest-serving Olympic class as it had been included in the Olympic program from 1952 to Tokyo 2020, and the adjective accompanying its name (heavy-weight dinghy) suggests that it is a class intended for the "biggest" of sailors.

The selection of a sailing class that allows a sailor to use his or her potential to the fullest is one of the most important steps in every sailor's sports career. One of the criteria for the selection of a sailing class is the compatibility of the anthropometric profile of the sailor with the technical specifications and other specificities of sailing in each sailing class. Coaches and athletes are familiar with some anthropometric parameters from their experience and mutual exchange of data; however, scientific studies with standardized measurements and valid data are substantially lacking. There are papers which do not even focus their research on anthropometric parameters but still offer useful data on the anthropometric parameters of stature and body mass for sailors in some sailing classes [17–26]; however, more detailed studies, including a greater number of anthropometric parameters and (or) somatotype, are considerably less common.

This study aimed to describe the anthropometric and somatotype profile of elite former Olympic Finn class sailors and to determine the differences in the measured parameters between sailors at different levels of general competitive success.

2. Materials and Methods

2.1. Participants

The subject sample included 57 elite Olympic Finn class sailors who competed at the Open Finn European Championship (FEC), held 9–17 May 2015, in Split, Croatia. The FEC is an open type of competition; thus, apart from the European sailors, it also included the best-ranked world sailors, among which were Olympic, world, and continental medal-winners. The competition included 70 sailors; therefore, the 57 sailors who participated in the study represent 81% of the total number of participants in the competition.

All sailors participated in the study voluntarily. The study was approved by the Scientific Committee of the Faculty of Kinesiology in Split, was conducted with the support of the Executive Committee of the International Finn Association, and met the requirements of the Declaration of Helsinki (1964) and the ethical standards in sports and exercise research.

2.2. Measures

A set of anthropometric variables measured by anthropometric measuring tools was applied—stature, sitting height, biepicondylar humerus width, biepicondylar femur width, upper arm girth (flexed and tensed), calf girth, triceps skinfold, subscapular skinfold, supraspinale skinfold, and medial calf skinfold—from which we subsequently calculated body mass index, sum of skinfolds, and somatotype following the Heat–Carter method [1]. Cut-off values for the endomorphy rating were set from 0.5 to 16, for the mesomorphy rating from 0.5 to 12, and for the ectomorphy rating from 0.5 to 9 [27].

All measurements were conducted following the International Society for the Advancement of Kinanthropometry (ISAK) protocol [28] on the dominant side of the body, as suggested in the original instructions for using the Heath–Carter method for somatotype calculation [1]. Moreover, the subjects were measured by using the Tanita BC-418

(Tanita Corp., Tokyo, Japan) device, which uses a constant current source with a high frequency current (50 kHz, 90 µA), following the recommendations given by Kyle et al. [29]. The method of bioelectric impedance was used to determine the results of the following morphological measures: *body mass, fat range, muscle mass, trunk muscle mass, arms muscle mass, legs muscle mass, fat mass, trunk fat mass, arms fat mass,* and *legs fat mass*. The subjects took the BIA measurement barefoot and only in dry underwear. All jewelry, watches, or any other pieces of clothing were taken off. The GMON software was used to conduct measurements where the "body type" value was set for all subjects to "sports mode" and the "clothing weight" value was set to 0.0 kg.

Considering that sailing experience can be an important factor of success in sailing, in addition to the previously mentioned sets of variables, we also applied the *age* variable.

2.3. Procedures

This study was designed as a single cross-sectional study.

The same morphologically expert measurer conducted all the measurements in the week before the competition in the morning hours before the first training session. Every measurement per sailor was conducted in a maximum time of 30 min.

The sailors were divided into three groups according to their level of general competitive success: more successful (1), medium (2), and less successful (3). We determined the general success criterion via their ranking in the World Sailing Rankings (WSR). The WSR is formed by collecting the points from the six most successful competitions for each sailor in the 12 months from the publishing of the table. For this study, the WSR table for the Finn class published on 27 April 2015—the last one before the FEC started—was used. The group of sailors with a higher level of general success (1) included the subjects ranked among the first 20 sailors according to the WSR; the group of sailors with a medium level of general success (2) included the subjects ranked from the 20th to the 40th place of the WSR; and the group of sailors with a lower level of general success (3) included the subjects ranked lower than the 41st place of the WSR.

2.4. Statistical Analysis

Methods of data analysis included the calculation of basic statistical indicators—mean, standard deviation, minimum result, maximum result—and the determination of the measures of sensitivity of result distribution: skewness, kurtosis, maximum distance between relative cumulative theoretical frequency (normal), and relative cumulative empirical frequency (obtained by measuring). The results of the Kolmogorov–Smirnov test of the observed variables indicate that neither of the variables exceeds the cut-off value of the Kolmogorov–Smirnov test, which is 0.18 for the observed sample. These findings indicate that the variables do not deviate significantly from the normal distribution, and all variables are suitable for further parametric statistical analysis. The differences between groups of sailors were determined via one-way analysis of variance (ANOVA). Further, post hoc analyses of differences between the groups of Finn sailors were made using Fisher's LSD test. To determine effect size of the differences found, squared eta (η^2) coefficients were calculated and interpreted according to the criterion of Gamst et al. (2008) [30].

Data analysis was performed by using the STATISTICA software package (ver. 14.00).

3. Results

Table 1 presents descriptive indicators of all the measured variables: arithmetic mean, standard deviation, median, and minimum and maximum result. We conducted the analysis of sensitivity based on coefficients of asymmetry and peakedness of distribution, whereas we used the Kolmogorov–Smirnov test to test the normality of distribution.

Coefficients of asymmetry for the variables *legs fat mass, subscapular skinfold,* and *medial calf skinfold* indicate a slightly positive asymmetry, whereas the *calf girth* variable has a slight negative skew. Coefficients of peakedness indicate a somewhat lower sensitivity of the *legs fat mass* and *calf girth* variables.

Table 1. Descriptive statistics of anthropometric and somatotype variables of Finn sailors (N = 57).

Variables	Mean ± SD	M	Min	Max	Skew	Kurt	MaxD
Age (yrs)	25.54 ± 4.64	24.96	17.95	41.07	0.90	1.04	0.08
Stature (m)	1.88 ± 0.05	1.87	1.76	2.00	0.35	0.21	0.09
Sitting height (m)	0.98 ± 0.03	0.98	0.89	1.05	−0.53	0.98	0.07
Body mass (kg)	95.17 ± 5.03	95.40	76.30	106.80	−0.85	3.00	0.10
Body mass index (kg/m^2)	27.07 ± 1.76	27.13	23.17	31.71	0.09	0.13	0.06
Fat range (%)	14.29 ± 3.60	14.20	6.50	20.90	−0.26	−0.56	0.09
Muscle mass (kg)	77.73 ± 4.24	77.90	64.10	90.60	−0.07	1.93	0.07
Trunk muscle mass (kg)	41.67 ± 2.81	41.30	34.00	49.60	0.37	0.83	0.11
Arms muscle mass (kg)	10.14 ± 0.72	10.20	8.50	11.50	−0.10	−0.42	0.07
Legs muscle mass (kg)	25.91 ± 1.34	25.80	21.50	30.10	−0.12	2.33	0.09
Fat mass (kg)	13.62 ± 3.72	13.60	5.70	21.30	−0.09	−0.52	0.06
Trunk fat mass (kg)	7.40 ± 2.53	7.50	1.70	11.90	−0.29	−0.50	0.08
Arms fat mass (kg)	1.51 ± 0.39	1.40	0.80	2.80	0.74	1.54	0.12
Legs fat mass (kg)	4.79 ± 1.22	4.70	2.60	10.20	1.40	5.61	0.09
Biepicondilar humerus width (cm)	7.22 ± 0.40	7.15	6.35	8.15	0.12	−0.37	0.08
Biepicondilar femur width (cm)	9.92 ± 0.57	9.90	8.75	11.40	0.52	0.49	0.08
Upper arm girth flexed and tensed (cm)	38.53 ± 2.13	38.70	32.05	42.85	−0.54	0.37	0.07
Calf girth (cm)	41.06 ± 3.32	41.55	28.20	46.35	−1.62	3.94	0.12
Sum of skinfolds (mm)	57.41 ± 19.14	54.65	24.40	109.75	0.75	0.43	0.10
Triceps skinfold (mm)	12.38 ± 3.92	12.10	5.80	24.05	0.76	1.00	0.10
Subscapular skinfold (mm)	16.58 ± 5.83	15.00	9.20	36.20	1.28	1.62	0.12
Supraspinale skinfold (mm)	16.03 ± 8.88	13.70	5.00	42.20	0.93	0.34	0.13
Medial calf skinfold (mm)	12.42 ± 5.74	11.30	4.40	31.30	1.14	1.25	0.13
Endomorphy rating	3.94 ± 1.19	3.91	1.67	6.73	0.26	−0.51	0.07
Mesomorphy rating	5.50 ± 1.19	5.54	2.10	7.87	−0.42	0.21	0.06
Ectomorphy rating	1.63 ± 0.74	1.52	0.43	3.66	0.79	0.29	0.10

Notes: SD—standard deviation; M—median; Min—minimum result; Max—maximum result; Skew—skewness; Kurt—kurtosis; MaxD—maximum distance between relative cumulative theoretical frequency (normal) and relative cumulative empirical frequency obtained by measuring. The limit value of the KS test for N = 57 is 0.18.

Table 2 presents the descriptive parameters (arithmetic means and standard deviations) results of the univariate analysis of differences (ANOVA) (coefficient of analysis of variance and significance of differences) and the results of the post hoc analysis of differences conducted via the Fisher's LSD test (significance of differences).

Table 2. Analysis of variance (ANOVA) and post hoc analysis between groups of Finn sailors according to their different levels of general success.

Variables	LEVEL OF SUCCESS			ANOVA		Post-hoc LSD Test (between Groups)		
	Higher (N = 13)	Medium (N = 13)	Lower (N = 31)	F	p=	p = *		
	Mean ± SD	Mean ± SD	Mean ± SD			1–2	1–3	2–3
Age (yrs)	28.74 ± 5.30	27.48 ± 4.39	23.38 ± 3.21	10.07	**0.000**	0.43	**0.000**	**0.003**
Stature (m)	1.89 ± 0.04	1.88 ± 0.05	1.87 ± 0.06	0.53	0.59	0.63	0.31	0.66
Sitting height (m)	0.99 ± 0.03	0.98 ± 0.02	0.98 ± 0.03	0.49	0.61	0.78	0.36	0.55
Body mass (kg)	96.73 ± 3.86	97.49 ± 2.41	93.54 ± 5.73	4.02	**0.02**	0.69	**0.049**	**0.02**
Body mass index (kg/m^2)	27.18 ± 1.62	27.67 ± 1.17	26.77 ± 1.99	1.23	0.30	0.48	0.49	0.13
Fat range (%)	13.85 ± 3.04	15.48 ± 2.54	13.98 ± 4.15	0.91	0.41	0.26	0.91	0.22
Muscle mass (kg)	79.43 ± 2.91	78.59 ± 2.83	76.65 ± 4.92	2.44	0.10	0.61	**0.047**	0.16
Trunk muscle mass (kg)	42.76 ± 2.28	42.05 ± 1.90	41.05 ± 3.20	1.91	0.16	0.52	0.07	0.28
Arms muscle mass (kg)	10.35 ± 0.63	10.43 ± 0.74	9.94 ± 0.70	2.98	0.06	0.76	0.08	**0.04**

Table 2. Cont.

Variables	LEVEL OF SUCCESS			ANOVA		Post-hoc LSD Test (between Groups)		
	Higher (N = 13)	Medium (N = 13)	Lower (N = 31)			$p = *$		
	Mean ± SD	Mean ± SD	Mean ± SD	F	$p=$	1–2	1–3	2–3
Legs muscle mass (kg)	26.32 ± 1.06	26.11 ± 0.98	25.66 ± 1.54	1.32	0.28	0.68	0.14	0.31
Fat mass (kg)	13.47 ± 3.28	15.11 ± 2.52	13.06 ± 4.20	1.42	0.25	0.26	0.74	0.09
Trunk fat mass (kg)	7.28 ± 2.41	8.33 ± 1.90	7.08 ± 2.76	1.17	0.32	0.29	0.80	0.13
Arms fat mass (kg)	1.52 ± 0.43	1.58 ± 0.22	1.47 ± 0.44	0.36	0.70	0.66	0.75	0.40
Legs fat mass (kg)	4.72 ± 0.66	5.22 ± 0.68	4.63 ± 1.52	1.10	0.34	0.29	0.84	0.15
Biepicondilar humerus width (cm)	7.28 ± 0.29	7.12 ± 0.29	7.23 ± 0.47	0.52	0.60	0.33	0.73	0.42
Biepicondilar femur width (cm)	9.72 ± 0.43	10.00 ± 0.44	9.98 ± 0.66	1.11	0.34	0.22	0.17	0.93
Upper arm girth flexed and tensed (cm)	38.44 ± 1.65	38.96 ± 1.63	38.39 ± 2.49	0.33	0.72	0.54	0.94	0.42
Calf girth (cm)	40.93 ± 3.76	40.60 ± 4.14	41.31 ± 2.82	0.21	0.81	0.81	0.74	0.53
Sum of skinfolds (mm)	51.25 ± 21.45	63.13 ± 15.74	57.61 ± 19.23	1.27	0.29	0.12	0.32	0.38
Triceps skinfold (mm)	10.39 ± 3.02	13.30 ± 2.61	12.83 ± 4.47	2.34	0.11	0.058	0.059	0.71
Subscapular skinfold (mm)	14.79 ± 5.14	17.73 ± 4.80	16.85 ± 6.45	0.90	0.41	0.20	0.29	0.65
Supraspinale skinfold (mm)	14.16 ± 8.67	19.75 ± 9.82	15.26 ± 8.39	1.57	0.22	0.11	0.71	0.13
Medial calf skinfold (mm)	11.90 ± 8.22	12.35 ± 4.13	12.67 ± 5.25	0.08	0.92	0.85	0.70	0.87
Endomorphy rating	3.46 ± 1.22	4.40 ± 1.04	3.94 ± 1.19	2.09	0.13	**0.046**	0.22	0.24
Mesomorphy rating	5.28 ± 1.06	5.43 ± 1.38	5.62 ± 1.19	0.39	0.68	0.75	0.40	0.64
Ectomorphy rating	1.61 ± 0.69	1.42 ± 0.59	1.73 ± 0.82	0.83	0.44	0.50	0.64	0.21

Notes: SD—standard deviation; F—analysis of variance coefficient; $p =$ —level of statistical significance; $p = *$—level of statistical significance of Fisher LSD post hoc test between groups of Finn sailors according to their different levels of general success (1—higher; 2—medium; 3—lower).

By applying univariate analysis of differences, significant differences were found in the results of the arithmetic means for the variables *age* and *body mass* between the groups of elite sailors according to the general competitive success criterion.

Through post hoc analysis of differences, significant differences were found between groups of sailors at different levels of general competitive success for the variables *age* (higher vs. lower; medium vs. lower), *body mass* (higher vs. lower; medium vs. lower), *muscle mass* (higher vs. lower), *arms muscle mass* (medium vs. lower), and *endomorphy rating* (higher vs. medium).

The effect size [30] of these differences was high for the variable *age*, moderate for the variable *body mass*, and low for the other variables (*muscle mass*, *arms muscle mass*, and *endomorphy rating*).

Table 3 presents the classification of elite Finn sailors according to the somatotype category. The frequency and percentage of each somatotype category was calculated for the total sample.

Table 3. Frequency and ratio of somatotype categories of Finn sailors (N = 57).

Somatotype Categories	Frequency	Ratio (%)
Central	2	3.51
Balanced endomorph	1	1.75
Mesomorphic endomorph	2	3.51
Mesomorph–endomorph	6	10.53
Endomorphic mesomorph	39	68.42
Balanced mesomorph	5	8.77
Ectomorphic mesomorph	2	3.51

The analysis in Table 3 shows that out of the 13 possible somatotype categories, elite Finn sailors fit 7 categories. Just over 80% of the total sample of elite sailors fit the somatotype categories with the dominant *mesomorphic* component, 68.42% of which fit the *endomorphic mesomorph* category.

Figure 1 is graphic representation of the somatotype ratings of Finn class sailors divided into three groups according to their level of general competitive success: *higher level* (square), *medium level* (rhomb), and *lower level* (triangle).

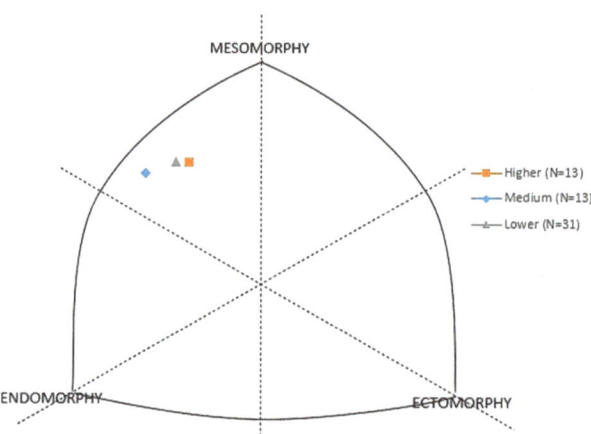

Figure 1. Somatochart.

4. Discussion

There are several major findings from this study: (a) anthropometric profiles of elite Finn class sailors have been determined; (b) somatotype profiles of elite Finn class sailors have been determined; and (c) significant differences between more-successful, medium, and less-successful sailors in some anthropometric parameters have been found. These findings require a more precise and detailed interpretation and will be further presented.

4.1. Finn Sailors Anthropometric Parameters Comparison to Previous Findings

The lack of scientific literature on a sample of elite Finn class sailors limits the possibility of quality comparison of the sample observed in this study to those of other authors. Furthermore, there are other problems: the research includes small subject samples, ranging from three to eight sailors [18,22,23,31,32], a small number of analyzed morphological characteristics [18,22–25,32], and a period in which the sailors were measured. Finn sailors in the available scientific literature were measured between 1995 and 2018, which would not be a problem if two new rules had not been adopted in this period that could affect sailors' morphological characteristics. The first rule was adopted in 1995 and it refers to prohibiting the use of the "weight jacket"; the second rule was adopted in 2000 and it refers to permitting pumping when sailing downwind.

Average body mass values in the observed sample of Finn sailors are ±1 kg compared to the body mass values recorded in other studies [22,24,32].

Finn sailors were from 8.6 kg to 7.4 kg lighter [18,23] before 1995, when the "weight jackets" were banned from sailing. By using the "weight jacket", a sailor could add weight to achieve better momentum in straightening the boat when sailing upwind, which ultimately allowed for greater speed in strong-wind conditions. On the other hand, in low-wind conditions, a sailor with lower body mass and without the "weight jacket" might be more agile and mobile when sailing and maneuvering. Furthermore, the positive impact of the reduced overall weight of the sailboat on the reduction in hydrodynamic resistance at lower speeds is also not negligible. Depending on the speed of the wind and the sailor's body mass, the "weight jacket" mass could range from 0.5 kg to 10 kg.

Pezelj et al. [15] also recorded lower body mass values. In their study, the body mass of U23 Finn sailors whose average age was 20.8 ± 1.27 years was 92.07 ± 5.66 kg. We may also interpret this difference in body mass by the fact that the subjects in the study conducted by Pezelj et al. [15] were, on average, 5 years younger than the observed sample and have not yet reached the "optimum" body mass for sailing in the Finn class.

Maiseti et al. [24] and Sanchez and Banos [31] recorded higher average body mass values of Finn sailors as compared to the observed sample. Finn sailors (n = 24) who participated in the 2000 Olympics had an average body mass of 97.5 ± 7.5 kg [24], whereas the members of the Spanish pre-Olympic team (n = 4) had an average body mass of 99.1 ± 7.3 kg [31].

We should take the comparison of body fat percentage between Finn sailors in the observed sample and those in studies conducted by other authors with reservations, considering that the methods of calculation in these studies are not identical. Cunningham [22] determined the body fat percentage of $18.6 \pm 3.0\%$ in Finn sailors (N = 8) by using the Durnin and Womersley method, whereas Sanchez and Banos [31] recorded $17.2 \pm 2.7\%$ (n = 4) by using the Carter method, and Pezelj et al. [15] used the bioelectric impedance method and recorded a body fat percentage of $13.01 \pm 4.02\%$.

The average stature values in the observed sample of Finn sailors are ± 1.5 cm as compared to the stature values determined in other studies [15,18,22–24,31,32].

Maiseti et al. [24] recorded 2.5 cm higher values of stature, whereas Bojsen et al. [18] recorded 3.4 cm lower average values of Finn sailors' stature as compared to the sample in our study.

4.2. Finn Sailor Anthropometric Parameters Comparison to Other Sailing Class Sailors Parameters

Comparing the anthropometric characteristics of Finn sailors to sailors in other Olympic classes, it is obvious why it is called the "heavy dinghy" class; in Finn sailors, almost all morphological characteristics have higher average values when compared to the sailors in other Olympic classes [11,17,20,21,23,24,26,32,33]. Average values of body height for Laser sailors recorded in the scientific literature range from 1.724 ± 0.64 m to 1.83 ± 0.3 m, whereas the values of body mass range from 75.6 ± 3.7 kg to 80.6 ± 2.8 kg [11,17,21,23,24,26,31–33]. In studies [11,26,31,33] on samples of Laser sailors, the authors have recorded a body fat percentage from $10.5 \pm 4.1\%$ to $23.2 \pm 12.1\%$. However, these results should be taken with reservations due to different methods of calculation.

The differences in morphological characteristics of Finn sailors are even more evident when compared to those of elite sailors in two-person Olympic classes: 470 and 49er. The average values of body height for sailors in these classes range from 1.75 m to 1.85 m, whereas their average body mass values range from 61.8 kg to 80.1 kg [31,32]. With their morphological characteristics, Olympic windsurfers in the RSX class can also fit into the stature and body mass range recorded in Laser, 470, and 49er sailors. In studies employing a sample of elite RSX sailors, the authors recorded average body height and body mass values of 1.78 ± 0.05 m and 75.4 ± 3.7 kg, respectively [20], and 1.79 ± 0.02 m and 72.9 ± 2.2 kg, respectively, with an average body fat percentage of $9.8 \pm 1\%$ [31].

4.3. Somatotype of Finn Sailors

Researchers have identified the *mesomorphic* somatotype component as the dominant component in all elite sailors sailing in Olympic and non-Olympic sailing classes [12,31,33]—even in young sailors in the Optimist class [14]. Elite Finn sailors are no exception. In this study, considering the average values of somatotype categories, it was determined that elite Finn sailors fit the *endomorphic mesomorph* somatotype category. Sailors in the men's one-person dinghy Olympic classes Laser and Finn [31,33] fit the same somatotype category, whereas sailors in the Olympic classes RSX and 470 fit the *ectomorphic mesomorph* category, with *balanced mesomorph* associated with the 49er class [31].

By analyzing the available literature, it can be noticed that the mesomorphic somatotype component is also the dominant somatotype component in elite athletes in many other Olympic disciplines, e.g., rowing [6], basketball [16], 100 m sprint [5], *off-road cycling* [8]; whereas Finn sailors share the *endomorphic mesomorph* somatotype category with kayakers [16] and rowers [7], and their average values of somatotype components are very similar to those recorded in water polo players of the Spanish national team [10].

4.4. Differences between Groups of Finn Sailors According to the General Sailing Achievement Level

For the best possible ranking in the World Sailing Rankings, which was used in this study to define general competitive success, a long-standing continuous participation in as many World Cup Regattas as possible is required. Young, non-established Finn sailors often lack the financial resources for participation in World Cup Regattas around the world; rather, they plan their regatta season more carefully by participating in lower-ranked regional competitions which may bring less points in the WSR rankings. Furthermore, it happens very often that elite sailor in the Laser class, amongst whom are Olympic champions as well, decide to change their sailing class and start competing in the Finn class. Considering that WSR rankings for the Laser and the Finn class are not connected, regardless of their number of points and ranking in the WSR rankings for the Laser class, sailors start their ranking in the Finn class competition with no points.

Through univariate analysis of difference and post hoc analysis, significant differences between more-successful, medium, and less-successful sailors in the variables *age, body mass, muscle mass, arm muscle mass*, and *endomorphy* rating were found.

These results indicate the possibility of selection processes and/or adaptation to sailing occurring in the Finn class. The homogeneity of Finn sailors in the parameters of longitudinal and transverse skeletal dimensions might reflect the selection process, whereas the determined impact and analyses of differences in the dimensions of soft tissue might reflect the adaptive process.

The development process of an elite sailor usually implies going through several sailing classes during his or her career. This transition from class to class follows the sailor's body growth and development to allow him or her to compete in the sailing class most suited to his or her morphological characteristics. In men's one-person dinghy, in most cases, this "journey" starts in the Optimist class, across the so-called transition classes, i.e., Laser 4.7 and Laser Radial, to the Olympic Laser Standard and Finn classes. When the height growth decelerates, i.e., stops around the age of 18, sailors start sailing in the Olympic classes. The class selection depends, among other things, upon morphological characteristics, and based on our results, we may conclude that even though they is not yet scientifically determined, the optimal values of body height and other longitudinal and transverse morphological characteristics required for successful sailing in the Finn class are defined quite clearly. Muscle mass and fat mass are morphological characteristics that can be changed by training operators. Thus, findings on the optimal values of soft tissue dimensions required for successful sailing in the Finn class, as well as their impact on competitive success, are extremely important to coaches and sailors. Sailors ranked among the first 40 competitors on the WSR rankings are approximately 5 years older, 3.5 kg heavier, and have greater muscle mass compared to the sailors with a lower ranking. Even though it is not possible to determine whether this is due to sailing in the Finn class or to some other training operators, it can be concluded that older and more-successful sailors have reached optimal values of body mass and muscle mass, whereas younger and less-successful sailors are yet to go through the period of body adaptation.

4.5. Limitations of the Study

In this study, only anthropometric parameters were measured. The analysis of morphological variables can only assume the influence of functional and motor abilities on competitive performance, but for a better and more complete analysis of competitive performance in sailing, in addition to morphological characteristics, it is necessary to carry out tests that assess the level of functional and motor abilities. It is unlikely that coaches and athletes would agree on such "stressful" tests prior the major competition, but scientist, coaches, athletes, and class leaders should look for such an option as the findings of such a study could have strong implications for the development of a specific sailing class and for the sailing sport in general.

The WSR is a measure of general sailing performance that expresses a summarized two-year general measure of performance in the Finn class. It is less dependent on, or influenced by, the situational conditions of sailing for this one regatta and the sailing conditions, like wind speed, water conditions, and other environmental factors, which were dominant in that racing week. But it would also be essential to establish differences in morphological parameters between different levels of situational competitive success. The study in question would be affected by all previously mentioned environmental factors, and the results could be interpreted considering wind speed and other sail racing parameters.

Even in this study, a couple of differences among international-level sailors were determined. Studies in which it could be possible to compare club-, national-, and international-level sailors would be beneficial for comparison with the "ideal" Finn class morphological profile. A wider performance range of sailors and possibly a larger number of participants could lead to more morphologically diverse groups; thus, the results might have different implications.

In this study, only univariate analysis was used, providing clear and understandable results and making it suitable for the wider sailing public. For future research, it would be advisable to use multivariate statistical analyses as discriminant analysis or multiple linear regression as it could provide more complex scientific information, especially at the level of latent anthropometric structures.

Future studies could use more demographic data like number of years of sailing in specific sailing class, first sailing class, age when started with sailing, previous sport, etc., and/or some non-sailing sport information pertaining to fitness training as all that information could be related to morphological status and anatomic adaptation to sailing in specific sailing class.

4.6. Possible Practical Applications

The values of anthropometric parameters determined for the sample of top Finn sailors may be of great help to coaches and young sailors when deciding on the selection of a senior Olympic class. If the sailors are already actively competing in the Finn class, they can compare their anthropometric characteristics to those of world-elite Finn sailors quite easily and possibly correct those parameters that can be changed under the influence of training, such as muscle mass and fat mass, i.e., body mass in total.

By comparing the anthropometric parameters of Finn sailors with those of sailors in other Olympic classes, it can be concluded that the elimination of the Finn class from the Olympic program could leave elite athletes with these anthropometric characteristics without the possibility of achieving top sports results in Olympic sailing. Thus, this article may serve as an argument in favor of making the decision to reinstate the Finn class in the Olympic program because the anthropologically "heavy-weight" sailors cannot compete successfully in any other current Olympic class.

To the best of our knowledge, this is the first study to determine the anthropometric and somatotype profile of elite Finn sailors or elite sailors in any other Olympic class. In the scientific literature, the impact of morphological characteristics on the general and situational competitive efficacy of elite athletes has been determined in different sports [5,7,8,11–16], and this study was conducted in an area of sport which has not yet been investigated—Finn sailing. The subject sample employed in this study does not only represent the sample in this particular population but also the majority of the population of world elite Finn sailors given that the study was conducted just before one of the biggest and most important competitions in the Finn class in a competitive season.

Sailing is sport that includes many sailing classes, of which four are part of the male Olympic sailing program. It would be essential for young sailors to establish and compare the anthropometric and somatotype profiles of elite sailors in each sailing class.

5. Conclusions

The anthropometric and somatotype profiles of elite Finn class sailors have been determined. This is the first time such a study has been conducted on sailors in any Olympic sailing class. Differences between groups of Finn sailors—grouped according to the level of general success—in some anthropometric parameters were determined. Anthropometric parameters, e.g., *body mass* and *muscle mass*, are clearly related to sailing performance and efficiency. Choosing a sailing class that is going to match the sailor's anthropometric profile is one of the most difficult issues for young sailors, so determining the relevant anthropometric parameters of each sailing class could be one of the most important scientific goals in the sailing field. Future research could focus on analyzing the differences among the sailors with respect to situational competitive success. Longitudinal studies could be beneficial to determine the process of anatomic adaptation in sailing at each sailing class.

Author Contributions: Conceptualization, L.P. and B.M.; methodology, L.P. and M.M.; field research, L.P. and M.M.; formal analysis, L.P., M.M. and B.M.; writing—original draft preparation, L.P., M.M. and B.M.; visualization, L.P. and B.M.; writing—review and editing, L.P. and B.M. All authors have read and agreed to the published version of the manuscript.

Funding: This research received no external funding.

Institutional Review Board Statement: This study was conducted in accordance with the general ethical principles of conducting research with human participants and approved by the Scientific Committee and by the Dean of the Faculty of Kinesiology, University of Split (21 April 2015). 2181-205-01-1-15-054.

Informed Consent Statement: Informed consent was obtained from all subjects involved in the study.

Data Availability Statement: The data presented in this study are available on request from the corresponding authors.

Acknowledgments: The authors gratefully acknowledge the support and help of the International Finn Association and the Yacht Club Labud, Split.

Conflicts of Interest: The authors declare no conflicts of interest.

References

1. Carter, J.E.L. *The Heath-Carter Anthropometric Somatotype—Instruction Manual*; San Diego State University, Department of Exercise and Nutritional Sciences: San Diego, CA, USA, 2002.
2. Wilmore, J.H. Validation of the first and second components of the Heath-Carter modified somatotype method. *Am. J. Phys. Anthropol.* **1970**, *32*, 369–372. [CrossRef] [PubMed]
3. Slaughter, M.H.; Lohman, T.G. Relationship of body composition to somatotype. *Am. J. Phys. Anthropol.* **1976**, *44*, 237–244. [CrossRef] [PubMed]
4. Olds, T. Body Composition and Sports Performance. In *Olympic Textbook of Science in Sport*; Maughan, R.J., Ed.; Wiley-Blackwell: London, UK, 2009; pp. 131–145.
5. Barbieri, D.; Zaccagni, L.; Babić, V.; Rakovac, M.; Mišigoj-Duraković, M.; Gualdi-Russo, E. Body composition and size in sprint athletes. *J. Sports Med. Phys. Fit.* **2017**, *57*, 1142–1146. [CrossRef] [PubMed]
6. Kaloupsis, S.; Bogdanis, G.C.; Dimakopoulou, E.; Maridaki, M. Anthropometric characteristics and somatotype of young Greek rowers. *Biol. Sport* **2008**, *25*, 57–69.
7. Mikulić, P.; Vučetić, V.; Matković, B.; Oreb, G. Morphological characteristics and somatotype of elite Croatian rowers. *Hrvat. Športskomed. Vjesn.* **2005**, *20*, 15–19.

8. Sanchez-Munoz, C.; Muros, J.J.; Zabala, M. World and Olympic mountain bike champions' anthropometry, body composition and somatotype. *J. Sports Med. Phys. Fit.* **2018**, *58*, 843–851. [CrossRef] [PubMed]
9. Shaw, G.; Mujika, I. Anthropometric Profiles of Elite Open-Water Swimmers. *Int. J. Sports Physiol. Perform.* **2018**, *13*, 115–118. [CrossRef] [PubMed]
10. Vila, H.; Ferragut, C.; Abraldes, J.A.; Rodríguez, N.; Argudo, F.M. Anthropometric characteristics of elite players in water polo. *Rev. Int. Med. Cienc. Act. Fís Deporte* **2010**, *10*, 652–663. Available online: http://cdeporte.rediris.es/revista/revista40/artcaracterizacion188.htm (accessed on 15 March 2024).
11. Caraballo, I.; Gonzalez-Montesinos, J.L.; Alias, A. Performance Factors in Dinghy Sailing: Laser Class. *Int. J. Environ. Res.* **2019**, *16*, 4920. [CrossRef]
12. Cortell-Tormo, J.M.; Perez-Turpin, J.A.; Cejuela-Anta, R.; Chinchilla-Mira, J.J.; Marfell-Jones, M.J. Anthropometric Profile of Male Amateur vs Professional Formula Windsurfs Competing at the 2007 European Championship. *J. Hum. Kinet.* **2010**, *23*, 97–101. [CrossRef]
13. Herbert-Losier, K.; Zinner, C.; Platt, S.; Stogl, T.; Holmberg, H.C. Factors that influence the performance of elite sprint cross-country skiers. *Sports Med.* **2017**, *47*, 319–342. [CrossRef]
14. Palomino-Martin, A.; Quintana-Santana, D.; Quiroga-Escudero, M.E.; Gonzales-Munoz, A. Incidence of anthropometric variables on the performance of top Optimist sailors. *J. Hum. Sport Exerc.* **2017**, *12*, 41–57. [CrossRef]
15. Pezelj, L.; Marinović, M.; Milavić, B. Morphological characteristics of elite U23 sailors—Finn European championship, Split 2015. *Sport Sci.* **2016**, *9*, 116–120.
16. Gutnik, B.; Zuoza, A.; Zuoziene, I.; Alekrinskis, A.; Nash, D.; Scherbina, S. Body physique and dominant somatotype in elite and low-profile athletes with different specializations. *Medicina* **2015**, *51*, 247–252. [CrossRef]
17. Blackburn, M. Physiological responses to 90 min of simulated dinghy sailing. *J. Sports Sci.* **1994**, *12*, 383–390. [CrossRef] [PubMed]
18. Bojsen, J.; Larsson, B.; Magnusson, S.P.; Aagaard, P. Strength and endurance profiles of elite Olympic class sailors. In *Human Performance in Sailing, Proceedings of the Incorporating the 4th European Conference on Sailing Sports Science and Sports Medicine and the 3rd Australian Sailing Science Conference, Auckland, New Zealand, 9–10 January 2003*; Massey University: Palmerston North, New Zealand, 2003; pp. 97–111.
19. Callewaert, M.; Geerts, S.; Lataire, E.; Boone, J.; Vantorre, M.; Bourgois, J. Development of an Upwind Sailing Ergometer. *Int. J. Sports Physiol. Perform.* **2013**, *8*, 663–670. [CrossRef]
20. Castagna, O.; Brisswalter, J.; Lacour, J.R.; Vogiatzis, I. Physiological demands of different sailing techniques of the new Olympic windsurfing class. *Eur. J. Appl. Physiol.* **2008**, *104*, 1061–1067. [CrossRef]
21. Cunningham, P.; Hale, T. Physiological responses of elite Laser sailors to 30 minutes of simulated upwind sailing. *J. Sports Sci.* **2007**, *25*, 1109–1116. [CrossRef]
22. Cunningham, P. The Physiological Demands of Elite Single-Handed Dinghy Sailing. Ph.D. Thesis, University of Chichester, Chichester, UK, 2004. Available online: http://eprints.chi.ac.uk/846/ (accessed on 15 March 2024).
23. Legg, S.J.; Miller, A.B.; Slyfield, D.; Smith, P.; Gilberd, C.; Wilcox, H.; Tate, C. Physical performance of New Zealand Olympic-class sailors. *J. Sports Med. Phys. Fit.* **1997**, *37*, 41–49.
24. Maisetti, O.; Guevel, A.; Iachkine, P.; Legros, P.; Briswalter, J. Sustained hiking position in dinghy sailing. Theoretical aspects and methodological considerations for muscle fatigue assessment. *Sci. Sports* **2002**, *17*, 234–246.
25. Pezelj, L.; Milavic, B.; Erceg, M. Respiratory Parameters in Elite Finn-Class Sailors. *Montenegrin J. Sports Sci. Med.* **2019**, *8*, 5–9. [CrossRef]
26. Vangelakoudi, A.; Vogiatzis, I.; Geladas, N. Anaerobic capacity, isometric endurance and Laser sailing performance. *J. Sports Sci.* **2007**, *25*, 1095–1100. [CrossRef] [PubMed]
27. Carter, J.E.L.; Heath, B. *Somatotyping—Development and Applications*; Cambridge University Press: Cambridge, UK, 1990.
28. Stewart, A.D.; Marfell-Jones, M.J.; Olds, T.; De Ridder, J.H. *International Standards for Anthropometric Assessment*; International Society for the Advancement of Kinanthropometry (ISAK): Lover Hut, New Zeland, 2011.
29. Kyle, U.G.; Boseaus, I.; De Lorenzo, A.D. Bioelectrical impedance analysis—Part II: Utilization in clinical practice. *Clin. Nutr.* **2004**, *23*, 1430–1453. [CrossRef] [PubMed]
30. Gamst, G.; Meyers, L.S.; Guarino, A.J. *Analysis of Variance Designs: A Conceptual and Computational Approach with SPSS and SAS*. Cambridge University Press: New York, NY, USA, 2008.
31. Sanchez, L.R.; Banos, V.M. Anthropometric profile and somatotype of sailors of the Spanish pre-olympic sailing team. *Sport TK* **2018**, *7*, 117–122.
32. Tanner, R.K.; Gore, C.J. (Eds.) *Physiological Tests for Elite Athletes*, 2nd ed.; Australian Institute of Sport: Lower Mitcham, Australia, 2013.
33. Marinović, M. Morphological characteristics of the sailmen in class laser and laser radial. *Hrvat. Športskomed. Vjesn.* **2001**, *16*, 16–20.

Disclaimer/Publisher's Note: The statements, opinions and data contained in all publications are solely those of the individual author(s) and contributor(s) and not of MDPI and/or the editor(s). MDPI and/or the editor(s) disclaim responsibility for any injury to people or property resulting from any ideas, methods, instructions or products referred to in the content.

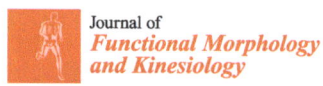
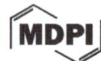

Article

Is Countermovement Jump an Indirect Marker of Neuromuscular Mechanism? Relationship with Isometric Knee Extension Test

Esteban Aedo-Muñoz [1], Jorge Pérez-Contreras [2,3], Alejandro Bustamante-Garrido [4], David Arriagada-Tarifeño [5], Jorge Cancino-Jiménez [5], Manuel Retamal-Espinoza [5], Rodrigo Argothy-Buchelli [6], Ciro Brito [1,7] and Pablo Merino-Muñoz [1,*]

[1] Escuela de Ciencias de la Actividad Física, El Deporte y la Salud, Facultad de Ciencias Médicas, Universidad de Santiago de Chile, Santiago 8370003, Chile; esteban.aedo@usach.cl (E.A.-M.); ciro.brito@usach.cl (C.B.)
[2] Escuela de Ciencias del Deporte y Actividad Física, Facultad de Salud, Universidad Santo Tomas, Santiago 8370003, Chile; jperez51@santotomas.cl
[3] Escuela de Doctorado de La Universidad de Las Palmas de Gran Canaria (EDULPGC), Las Palmas 35016, Spain
[4] Departamento de Educación Física, Deportes y Recreación, Facultad de Artes y Educación Física, Universidad Metropolitana de Ciencias de la Educación, Santiago 7760197, Chile; alejandrobustamanteg@gmail.com
[5] Escuela de Kinesiología, Facultad de Ciencias Médicas, Universidad de Santiago de Chile, Santiago 8370003, Chile; david.arriagada@usach.cl (D.A.-T.); jorge.cancino@usach.cl (J.C.-J.); manuel.retamal@usach.cl (M.R.-E.)
[6] Grupo de Investigación en Rendimiento Físico Militar (Renfimil), Escuela Militar de Cadetes "General José María Córdova", Bogotá 111211, Colombia; reargothyb@gmail.com
[7] Department of Physical Education, Federal University of Juiz de Fora, Governador Valadares 35010-180, Brazil
* Correspondence: pablo.merino@usach.cl; Tel.: +56955328751

Citation: Aedo-Muñoz, E.; Pérez-Contreras, J.; Bustamante-Garrido, A.; Arriagada-Tarifeño, D.; Cancino-Jiménez, J.; Retamal-Espinoza, M.; Argothy-Buchelli, R.; Brito, C.; Merino-Muñoz, P. Is Countermovement Jump an Indirect Marker of Neuromuscular Mechanism? Relationship with Isometric Knee Extension Test. *J. Funct. Morphol. Kinesiol.* **2024**, *9*, 242. https://doi.org/10.3390/jfmk9040242

Academic Editor: Pedro Miguel Forte

Received: 23 October 2024
Revised: 11 November 2024
Accepted: 13 November 2024
Published: 18 November 2024

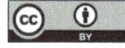

Copyright: © 2024 by the authors. Licensee MDPI, Basel, Switzerland. This article is an open access article distributed under the terms and conditions of the Creative Commons Attribution (CC BY) license (https://creativecommons.org/licenses/by/4.0/).

Abstract: Several studies have shown that force application is influenced by different neuromuscular mechanisms depending on the time of force application analysis in isometric knee extension test (IKE), and a countermovement jump (CMJ) has contributions from knee extension, so some CMJ variables could be indicators of such mechanisms. **Purpose:** The aim of this study was to determine the level of relationship of variables of IKE and bilateral CMJ tests. **Methods:** Male college soccer players (n = 25; corporal mass = 72 ± 8 kg; height = 171 ± 5 cm; age = 22 ± 2 years) performed the IKE at two angles (60° and 75°) on an isokinetic machine and the CMJ on two uniaxial force platforms. To determine the level of relationship, Pearson's correlation coefficient was analyzed between the test variables. **Results:** Trivial to moderate correlations (r = −0.45 to 0.62; $p < 0.05$) were found between CMJ variables and IKE in both knee angles (60° and 75°); **Conclusions:** The variables of IKE have a trivial to moderate correlation with the variables of CMJ, so the variables of CMJ could not be considered interchangeably with those of IKE and therefore considered indicators of neuromuscular mechanisms isolated from the knee extensor function. Longitudinal design (fatigue or training protocols) should be realized to corroborate these results.

Keywords: biomechanics; kinetic; kinematic; vertical jump; rate of force development

1. Introduction

The ability to generate force with the lower limbs is very important in sports actions, such as running, jumping, and changing direction; however, these actions that are performed in various sports or in daily living have a limited amount of time for application of force (50 to 400 ms depending on the technique and phases) [1]. This is why the assessment of force in the specific force-application times of sports or daily actions becomes crucial to evaluate sports performance [2]. To assess muscular strength, both dynamic or isometric and single-joint or multi-joints tests can be performed. Isometric single-joint tests have been used for more than five decades to measure muscle function due to their easy implementation and excellent reliability [3], and it has been evidenced that the application of force or torque over time, quantified as rate of force development (RFD) or rate torque development (RTD) and defined as the first derivative of force or torque over time, respectively, is influenced by different neuromuscular factors [3,4]. RTD and RFD in their early phase (<100 ms) are more influenced by neural mechanisms such as motor recruitment and motor unit discharge rate and in their late phase (>100 ms) by intrinsic muscle properties such as maximal force and muscle thickness [1,4,5]. This has been proven in several studies using isometric knee extension tests (IKE) [1,4–7]. This influence in different time intervals has been highlighted by several authors [6,7] due to the fact that changes and/or adaptations in different mechanisms could be analyzed without the need for the use of other equipment, such as, for example, the use of electromyography in order to analyze changes in muscle activation [4,8]. However, it cannot be assumed that the same mechanisms have similar influence during dynamic assessments of muscular strength [3,9].

In the dynamic assessments to evaluate the muscular strength of the lower limbs, vertical jumps are commonly used because they do not produce fatigue, are not invasive, and require little time to be applied [10], and countermovement jump (CMJ), which involves a stretch-shortening cycle (eccentric to concentric muscular contraction), is also widely used because it shows a strong relationship with other sport actions, such as acceleration, deceleration, and change of direction [11–13]. The jump height (JH), the most used variable from the CMJ and the easiest to calculate, has also been used to assess the neuromuscular state of athletes [14], but sometimes, it is too insensitive for detecting fatigue [15,16], mainly because athletes are able to maintain JH by altering their movement strategies [17]. An advantage offered by the assessment of CMJ using force platforms is that many kinetic variables can be derived from eccentric and concentric phases (sometimes called downward and propulsive phases) [18,19], and these, unlike JH, have been shown to be more sensitive for detecting acute and also chronic changes in the neuromuscular state of athletes, such as fatigue and detraining in specific phases of CMJ [15,20,21]. For this reason, and understanding that CMJ performance has contributions from the knee, some of its variables may have moderate to strong correlations with IKE [22]. Currently, in correlational studies between CMJ variables and IKE, the relationship between JH and the kinetic variables of isometric lower-body single-joint isometric tests on isokinetic machines has been mainly analyzed [22–24], and only one study analyzed the relationship between the RTD (i.e., IKE) and RFD (i.e., in CMJ), where it found trivial to small relationships with RTD in isometric single-joint test (hip, knee, and ankle), but it only analyzed the peak RTD and RFD in both tests [25], so the relationship between RTD in time intervals and other variables from CMJ is still unknown.

In the past, for coaches or sport scientists, access to technology such as isokinetic machines and laboratory force platforms has often been limited due to its size and cost; recently, much more economical and ecologically applicable field tools have emerged in sports, such as portable force platforms [26,27], which mainly, due to their low cost and easy transportation, are more accessible to technical teams and sports federations. So, the analysis of the relationship between CMJ variables and isometric tests could deliver information and values for some neuromuscular mechanisms (neural or muscular), delivering information from more applicable assessments within the area of sports biomechanics, physical activity sciences, and/or sports medicine that are more ecological, economical, and practical to perform in the field. From the background, the objective of the present study was to analyze the level of the relationship between different variables of different phases of CMJ and IKE.

2. Materials and Methods

2.1. Design

The present study was carried out through a quantitative approach with a non-experimental design of a cross-sectional type and correlational scope.

2.2. Procedures

The measurements were evaluated through two visits to the laboratory with one week of difference between visits. On the first visit of the laboratory, the informed consent was presented to the participants. Subsequently, familiarization of the experimental tests was carried out: bilateral countermovement jump (CMJ) and the isometric knee extension (IKE) tests, according to methodological recommendations involving RFD and RTD measures [3,28]. On the second visit, the subjects performed a standardized warm-up of 5 min of jogging on an electric treadmill at 8 km/h with no incline, followed by 20 squats and 10 front lunges per profile, followed by 2 min of dynamic lower-limb stretching, followed by a 3 min rest before jump evaluation [29] and later CMJ and IKE in this order. All subjects were informed of the risks, benefits, and objectives (first visit), and they completed an informed consent according to the Helsinki Agreement, which was approved by the local institutional ethics committee (code: 418/2023).

2.3. Sample

The sample comprised male college soccer players (n = 25; corporal mass = 72 ± 8 kg; height = 171 ± 5 cm; age = 22 ± 2 years). The players were in a competitive period where they underwent strength and conditioning training on Mondays and technical-tactical training on Tuesdays and Wednesdays and played an official match on Fridays. The inclusion criteria were (i) men with an age range of 18 to 30 years belonging to a university sports team, (ii) playing sports or physical exercise at least 3 times a week, and (iii) not having suffered a lower-limb injury during the last 6 months. The exclusion criterion was presenting any discomfort or pain during the study, either in the hours prior to the study, during warm-up, or during data recording.

2.4. Data Recording

2.4.1. Countermovement Jump Recording

Two portable PASPORT force plate platforms were used, namely model PS-2141 (PASCO® Scientific, Roseville, CA, USA), validated for vertical jumps [26,27], with a sample frequency of 1000 Hz with Pasco Capstone software version 2.3.1.1 (PASCO Scientific, Roseville, CA, USA). Their data were exported into a spreadsheet. Subjects were instructed to keep their hands on their hips (Figure 1) throughout the jump to focus only on the force generated by the lower extremities [30] and to jump as fast and as high as possible with their preferred depth [31], and they could choose the amplitude of the countermovement to avoid changes in the coordination pattern of the jump [32]. The subjects performed three attempts and rested for at least 15 s between attempts while data were stored.

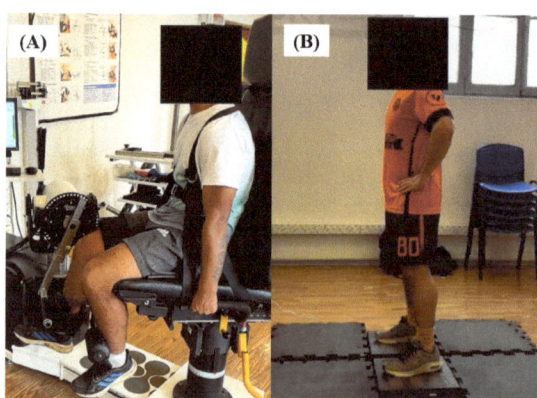

Figure 1. Start position in isometric knee extension (**A**) and countermovement jump (**B**).

2.4.2. Isometric Knee Extension Recording

The isokinetic equipment HUMAC NORM® testing and rehabilitation system (Model 502140, Stoughton, MA, USA) with a sample frequency of 1250 Hz was used for IKE. The positioning was performed according to the HUMAC NORM System User's Guide provided by the manufacturer. In each evaluation, each participant was positioned for alignment of the joint axis with the mechanical axis of the isokinetic equipment in relation to his anthropometric measurements, ensuring the participants' comfort and safety and the reliability of data collection. Each participant performed four attempts with a duration of 4 s with their dominant leg (preferred for kicking a soccer ball), with a 30 s pause between attempts and 3 min between angles with a knee angle of 60° and 75° because at these angles, the peak torque and RTD were higher compared to other angles [4]. The neutral approach indication was given to push as fast and hard as possible and place the hands on the equipment as shown (Figure 1).

2.5. Data Processing

2.5.1. Countermovement Jump Processing

The spreadsheets were processed through the MATLAB® software by a routine created by the authors (R2021a; The MathWorks, Inc., Natick, MA, USA). To detect the jump's onset, the method of three standard deviations and a time window of 2 s prior to the jump was used. For the identification of phases (unloading, yielding, braking, and concentric), the method proposed by Harry et al. [33] was used. For the analysis, the following variables were used: peak force, jump time, time for phases, mean force for phases, peak RFD for braking phase, and net impulse for phase (or defined integral). The jump height was calculated using impulse method [34]. For the analysis, the average of three attempts was used.

2.5.2. Isometric Knee Extension Processing

For the IKE, the signals were exported to a spreadsheet and finally processed through the MATLAB software by a routine created by the authors (R2021a; The MathWorks, Inc., Natick, MA, USA). The signal was resampled to 1000 Hz. The signal was filtered by a Butterworth low-pass filter of 4 orders with zero lag and a cut frequency of 20 Hz [35]. The first value at 1 newton was identified as the start of the test. For the analysis, the following variables were used: peak torque, RTD in windows of 50 ms up to 200 ms, and the instantaneous isometric peak RTD (PRTD). The attempt with the highest peak force was used for the analysis. The signal shape and variables are given visually in Figure 2.

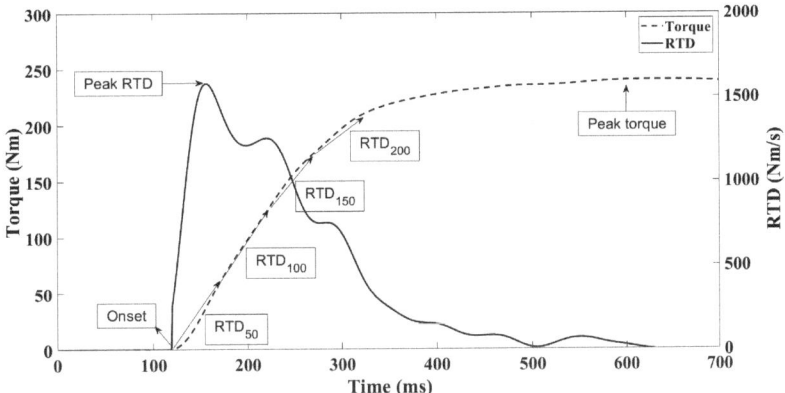

Figure 2. Signal shape and variables of isometric knee extension torque and isometric rate of torque development (RTD).

2.6. Statistical Analysis

The normality of the variables was analyzed using the Shapiro–Wilk test, where the assumption of normality was checked ($p > 0.05$). All descriptive statistics are presented as mean and standard deviation. The relationship between variables was analyzed through Pearson's correlation coefficient, where values were qualitatively categorized as trivial (0.00–0.09), weak (0.10–0.39), moderate (0.40–0.69), strong (0.70–0.89), and very strong (0.90–1.00) as well as negative values. The alpha was set at 0.05. All statistics were conducted in SPSS software version 25.

3. Results

In Table 1 are the descriptive statistics of both tests. In Table 2 are the correlation coefficients between kinematic-related variables of CMJ and IKE. Trivial to moderate correlations were found, and only moderate correlations showed statistical significance ($p < 0.05$).

Table 1. Descriptive statistics of CMJ and IKE test.

	Countermovement Jump (CMJ)				Isometric Knee Extension (IKE)		
	Variables	Mean	±SD		Variables	Mean	±SD
Kinematic	Jump height (m)	0.284	0.060	60 degrees	PT (N·m)	236	29
	Jump time (s)	0.688	0.076		PRTD (N·m/s)	5998	1546
	Time unloading (s)	0.167	0.039		RTD$_{50}$ (N·m/s)	1119	383
	Time yielding (s)	0.152	0.028		RTD$_{100}$ (N·m/s)	1077	260
	Time braking (s)	0.118	0.028		RTD$_{150}$ (N·m/s)	827	128
	Time concentric (s)	0.250	0.034		RTD$_{200}$ (N·m/s)	580	173
Kinetic	Peak force (N)	1649	228	75 degrees	PT (N·m)	216	33
	RFD unloading (N/s)	−53	13		PRTD (N·m/s)	5449	1682
	RFD yielding (N/s)	61	13		RTD$_{50}$ (N·m/s)	810	478
	RFD braking (N/s)	139	49		RTD$_{100}$ (N·m/s)	947	270
	PRFD (N/s)	8946	3741		RTD$_{150}$ (N·m/s)	811	224
	MF unloading (N)	342	56		RTD$_{200}$ (N·m/s)	571	167
	MF yielding (N)	412	66				
	MF braking (N)	705	132				
	MF concentric (N)	676	127				
	Impulse unloading (N·s)	56	12				
	Impulse yielding (N·s)	62	14				
	Impulse braking (N·s)	82	20				
	Impulse concentric (N·s)	166	21				

PT, peak torque; PRTD, peak rate of torque development; RTD50, rate of torque development 0–50 ms; RTD100, rate of torque development 50–100 ms; RTD150, rate of torque development 100–150 ms; RTD200, rate of torque development 150–200 ms; PRFD, peak rate of force development; RFD, rate of force development; MF, mean force.

Table 2. Correlation matrix between kinematic-related variables of CMJ and IKE at 60° and 75°.

		60° Knee Angle						75° Knee Angle					
Variables		PT	PRTD	RTD$_{50}$	RTD$_{100}$	RTD$_{150}$	RTD$_{200}$	PT	PRTD	RTD$_{50}$	RTD$_{100}$	RTD$_{150}$	RTD$_{200}$
Jump height	r	−0.15	−0.11	0.08	−0.28	−0.33	−0.07	−0.23	−0.13	0.25	−0.22	**−0.40**	−0.29
	p	0.47	0.59	0.71	0.17	0.11	0.76	0.28	0.53	0.23	0.30	**0.05**	0.17
Jump time	r	0.14	0.08	−0.12	0.00	**0.44**	**0.46**	0.05	0.03	−0.17	0.04	0.07	**0.46**
	p	0.50	0.70	0.57	0.99	**0.03**	**0.02**	0.81	0.91	0.42	0.86	0.74	**0.02**
Time unloading	r	−0.16	−0.07	−0.13	−0.11	0.26	0.00	0.06	−0.01	−0.17	0.05	0.23	0.25
	p	0.46	0.75	0.52	0.59	0.21	0.99	0.78	0.98	0.41	0.80	0.27	0.22
Time yielding	r	0.22	0.13	−0.03	0.06	0.33	**0.45**	0.14	0.13	0.07	0.09	−0.04	0.34
	p	0.29	0.54	0.87	0.78	0.10	**0.02**	0.50	0.53	0.75	0.69	0.86	0.10
Time braking	r	0.20	−0.01	−0.09	0.00	0.03	0.29	−0.09	−0.04	−0.07	−0.13	−0.14	0.04
	p	0.35	0.97	0.68	0.99	0.88	0.16	0.66	0.84	0.76	0.55	0.49	0.84
Time concentric	r	0.15	0.18	0.00	0.05	0.36	**0.41**	0.00	0.01	−0.16	0.02	0.02	**0.41**
	p	0.47	0.40	0.99	0.80	0.08	**0.04**	1.00	0.98	0.44	0.94	0.92	**0.04**

Bold values mean significant bilateral p-value <0.05; r, Pearson correlation coefficient; p-value; PT, peak torque; PRTD, peak isometric rate of torque development; RTD$_{50}$, rate of torque development 0–50 ms; RTD$_{100}$, rate of torque development 50–100 ms; RTD$_{150}$, rate of torque development 100–150 ms; RTD$_{200}$, rate of torque development 150–200 ms.

Table 3 shows the correlation coefficients between the related kinematic variables of CMJ and IKE. Trivial to moderate correlations were found, and only moderate correlations showed statistical significance ($p < 0.05$).

Table 3. Correlation matrix between force–time-related variables of CMJ and IKE at 60° and 75°.

Variables		60° Knee Angle						75° Knee Angle					
		PT	PRTD	RTD_{50}	RTD_{100}	RTD_{150}	RTD_{200}	PT	PRTD	RTD_{50}	RTD_{100}	RTD_{150}	RTD_{200}
Peak force	r	0.23	0.14	0.04	**0.41**	0.18	0.09	0.36	0.15	−0.17	0.27	**0.50**	0.15
	p	0.27	0.51	0.85	**0.04**	0.40	0.67	0.07	0.49	0.41	0.19	**0.01**	0.49
RFD unloading	r	−0.16	−0.20	−0.20	−0.19	0.22	0.08	0.10	−0.15	−0.33	0.14	0.23	0.40
	p	0.45	0.34	0.34	0.37	0.29	0.71	0.64	0.48	0.11	0.50	0.27	0.05
RFD yielding	r	−0.22	−0.07	0.03	0.14	−0.39	**−0.45**	0.03	0.08	0.20	0.04	0.06	−0.17
	p	0.29	0.73	0.89	0.50	0.06	**0.02**	0.88	0.71	0.35	0.87	0.77	0.43
RFD braking	r	−0.30	−0.09	0.00	0.15	−0.20	**−0.44**	0.01	−0.08	0.03	0.16	0.05	−0.02
	p	0.15	0.67	0.99	0.47	0.34	**0.03**	0.96	0.72	0.87	0.44	0.80	0.91
PRFD	r	0.01	0.13	0.18	0.40	−0.11	−0.33	0.26	0.09	−0.11	0.37	**0.39**	0.04
	p	0.97	0.55	0.40	0.05	0.60	0.11	0.20	0.68	0.61	0.07	**0.05**	0.84
MF unloading	r	0.37	0.37	0.32	**0.62**	0.07	0.02	**0.41**	0.19	0.00	**0.40**	0.35	0.17
	p	0.07	0.07	0.13	**<0.01**	0.74	0.91	**0.04**	0.35	0.99	**0.04**	0.08	0.41
MF yielding	r	0.32	0.39	0.35	**0.54**	0.15	−0.07	**0.41**	0.24	0.07	0.33	**0.44**	0.04
	p	0.12	0.06	0.09	**0.01**	0.47	0.73	**0.04**	0.24	0.73	0.11	**0.03**	0.85
MF braking	r	0.06	0.12	0.12	0.33	−0.01	−0.19	0.24	0.09	−0.18	0.24	**0.46**	0.04
	p	0.77	0.56	0.56	0.11	0.98	0.38	0.25	0.67	0.38	0.25	**0.02**	0.84
MF concentric	r	0.06	−0.03	0.07	0.06	−0.19	−0.09	0.13	0.10	0.22	0.02	0.02	−0.28
	p	0.78	0.88	0.75	0.76	0.37	0.68	0.54	0.65	0.29	0.91	0.94	0.17
Impulse unloading	r	0.07	0.16	0.06	0.30	0.32	0.04	0.36	0.14	−0.18	0.36	**0.51**	**0.40**
	p	0.75	0.44	0.79	0.15	0.12	0.86	0.08	0.50	0.39	0.07	**0.01**	**0.04**
Impulse yielding	r	**0.44**	**0.41**	0.27	**0.46**	0.38	0.29	**0.42**	0.27	0.12	0.28	0.29	0.29
	p	**0.02**	**0.04**	0.20	**0.02**	0.07	0.16	**0.03**	0.20	0.57	0.17	0.15	0.16
Impulse braking	r	0.24	0.08	0.01	0.23	0.04	0.16	0.04	−0.01	−0.19	0.00	0.17	0.03
	p	0.25	0.69	0.98	0.26	0.85	0.45	0.85	0.98	0.36	1.00	0.42	0.89
Impulse concentric	r	0.29	0.17	0.14	0.19	0.09	0.26	0.22	0.17	0.21	0.06	0.06	−0.05
	p	0.16	0.41	0.50	0.37	0.66	0.21	0.30	0.42	0.31	0.79	0.79	0.83

Bold values mean significant bilateral p-value <0.05; r, Pearson correlation coefficient; p value; PT, peak torque; PRTD, peak isometric rate of torque development; RTD_{50}, rate of torque development 0–50 ms; RTD_{100}, rate of torque development 50–100 ms; RTD_{150}, rate of torque development 100–150 ms; RTD_{200}, rate of torque development 150–200 ms; PRFD, peak rate of force development; RFD, rate of force development; MF, mean force.

4. Discussion

The present study aimed to determine the level of relationship between CMJ and IKE variables. The main findings showed trivial to moderate correlations between the variables of both tests.

Various studies have analyzed the relationship between CMJ and IKE, but most studies only analyze the JH [22–25], and to our knowledge, only one analyzed the correlation of other variables of CMJ with IKE [25]. Regarding the association between JH and IKE variables, some studies have found similar correlations [22,25] and other higher correlations [23,24]. The latter may have found this due to various methodological factors as well as data analysis. De Ruiter et al. (2006) found a moderate to strong correlation between JH and momentum at 40 ms normalized by time at peak torque, but the knee angle at the jump (90° and 120°) was controlled [24]. Laett et al. (2021) found trivial to moderate correlations ($p > 0.05$) between JH and the RTD accumulated in windows of 50 ms from onset to 250 ms. However, they found moderate correlations when the RTD was normalized by peak torque. On the other hand, they used an individualized angle to perform the isometric test (optimal angle through dynamic test) [23]. These methodological and data analysis differences could explain the differences compared to our results, where a controlled knee angle in the squat and adjusted knee angle in IKE could have increased the correlation between tests.

To our knowledge, only Van Hooren et al. (2022) analyzed the correlations between the kinetic variables of CMJ and IKE, finding trivial to weak correlations that agree with our findings. However, they only analyzed the relationship between PRFD and PRTD. They mentioned that their trivial to moderate correlations could be explained by motor control strategies, where subjects with poor inter-muscular coordination but with a great RTD may not be able to transfer their ability into movements that require greater coordination (dynamic multi-joint) [25]. For example, a recent review of the relationship between isometric and dynamic force showed moderate to very strong correlations between the kinetic variables (peak force and RFD) of isometric multi-joint tests, such as mid-thigh pull and isometric squat, with SJ jump height [36], showing an increase in correlation between tests due to biomechanical similarity (i.e., the same joints are involved in both tests). In the same line, the application of force in the vertical jump depends on three joints (hip, knee, and ankle) [37,38], so the dynamic RFD could have different contributions along with the added variability between subjects, where different joint contributions have been observed between good and bad jumpers (depending on jump height) [38]. In a recent study, the peak torque of hip was the variable with the strongest correlation with the JH during CMJ, corroborating this hypothesis [39].

Another factor that could explain the strength of the correlation is the type of contraction in the single-joint test, where studies have found weak to very strong correlations between dynamic knee extension tests (peak torque and power) and jump height [40,41], the same phenomenon that happens with the sprint, where IKE has a trivial correlation, and fast concentric has a moderate correlation [42]. Another study correlated knee isometric flexion PT and RTD with sprint performance at 30 m and found an explained variance of isometric in sprint between 0 and 28% [43]. That study analyzed the relationships between these variables and PRTD in knee extension and flexion and plantar flexion, finding trivial to weak correlations with JH, JT, TPF, and PRFD [25] and reaffirming that different physiological mechanisms modulate variables derived from dynamic and isometric actions [9], and therefore, monoarticular isometric testing would give poor information on RFD in sport movements [25,42–45].

One interesting aspect was that most moderate correlations were found between the eccentric variables of jump, and only concentric time had this correlation strength. One study found a similar neuromuscular response after eccentric and isometric exercise compared with concentric, explaining the torque–time integral between protocols [46]. This could explain our result, indicating more similarity between isometric and eccentric contractions than concentric. Also, the muscular strength of knee could be contributing more during eccentric phase and the ankle and hip during concentric phase [47].

One limitation of this research is the study design, and the results should be corroborated with an experimental and longitudinal design; for example, future research could simultaneously analyze both pre- and post-intervention tests (fatigue or training protocol). Other limitations correspond to methodological concerns about preferred depth countermovement in CMJ; because this affects the CMJ variables, it would be necessary to find a standardized methodology for assessment of CMJ. Also, unilateral CMJ should be tested since IKE was unilateral.

5. Conclusions

The variables of IKE have a trivial to moderate correlation with the variables of CMJ, so the variables of CMJ could not be considered interchangeably with those of IKE and therefore considered indicators of neuromuscular mechanisms isolated from the knee extensor function. A longitudinal design should be realized to corroborate these results.

Author Contributions: Conceptualization, P.M.-M., D.A.-T. and E.A.-M.; methodology, E.A.-M., J.P.-C., A.B.-G., P.M.-M., M.R.-E. and R.A.-B.; formal analysis, P.M.-M., A.B.-G., M.R.-E., C.B. and J.C.-J.; writing—original draft preparation, E.A.-M., P.M.-M., C.B. and J.P.-C.; writing—review and editing, E.A.-M., P.M.-M., D.A.-T., J.C.-J. and R.A.-B.; visualization, M.R.-E. and J.C.-J.; supervision, E.A.-M. and D.A.-T.; project administration, J.P.-C., M.R.-E. and R.A.-B.; funding acquisition, E.A.-M. All authors have read and agreed to the published version of the manuscript.

Funding: This research received no external funding.

Institutional Review Board Statement: The study was conducted in accordance with the Declaration of Helsinki and approved by the Institutional Ethics Committee of Universidad de Santiago de Chile (code: 418/2023).

Informed Consent Statement: Informed consent was obtained from all subjects involved in the study.

Data Availability Statement: Data will be made available under reasonable request.

Acknowledgments: Thanks to the USACH AYUDANTE_DICYT Project, Código 022304AM_Ayudante, Vicerrectoría de Investigación, Innovación y Creación.

Conflicts of Interest: The authors declare no conflicts of interest.

References

1. Andersen, L.L.; Aagaard, P. Influence of maximal muscle strength and intrinsic muscle contractile properties on contractile rate of force development. *Eur. J. Appl. Physiol.* **2006**, *96*, 46–52. [CrossRef] [PubMed]
2. Thomas, C.; Comfort, P.; Chiang, C.-Y.; Jones, P.A. Relationship between isometric mid-thigh pull variables and sprint and change of direction performance in collegiate athletes. *J. Trainology* **2015**, *4*, 6–10. [CrossRef] [PubMed]
3. Maffiuletti, N.A.N.; Aagaard, P.; Blazevich, A.; Folland, J.J.; Tillin, N.; Duchateau, J. Rate of force development: Physiological and methodological considerations. *Eur. J. Appl. Physiol.* **2016**, *116*, 1091–1116. [CrossRef] [PubMed]
4. Cossich, V.; Maffiuletti, N. Early vs. late rate of torque development: Relation with maximal strength and influencing factors. *J. Electromyogr. Kinesiol.* **2020**, *55*, 102486. [CrossRef]
5. D'Emanuele, S.; Tarperi, C.; Rainoldi, A.; Schena, F.; Boccia, G. Neural and contractile determinants of burst-like explosive isometric contractions of the knee extensors. *Scand. J. Med. Sci. Sports* **2022**, *33*, 127–135. [CrossRef]
6. Tillin, N.A.; Folland, J.P. Maximal and explosive strength training elicit distinct neuromuscular adaptations, specific to the training stimulus. *Eur. J. Appl. Physiol.* **2014**, *114*, 365–374. [CrossRef]
7. de Oliveira, F.B.D.; Rizatto, G.F.; Denadai, B.S. Are early and late rate of force development differently influenced by fast-velocity resistance training? *Clin. Physiol. Funct. Imaging* **2013**, *33*, 282–287. [CrossRef]
8. Place, N. Quantification of central fatigue: A central debate. *Eur. J. Appl. Physiol.* **2021**, *121*, 2375–2376. [CrossRef]
9. Krüger, R.L.; Aboodarda, S.J.; Jaimes, L.M.; MacIntosh, B.R.; Samozino, P.; Millet, G.Y. Fatigue and recovery measured with dynamic properties vs isometric force: Effects of exercise intensity. *J. Exp. Biol.* **2019**, *222*, jeb.197483. [CrossRef]
10. Lombard, W.; Starling, L.; Wewege, L.; Lambert, M. Changes in countermovement jump performance and subjective readiness-to-train scores following a simulated soccer match. *Eur. J. Sport Sci.* **2020**, *21*, 647–655. [CrossRef]
11. Merino-Muñoz, P.; Vidal-Maturana, F.; Aedo-Muñoz, E.; Villaseca-Vicuña, R. Relationship between vertical jump, linear sprint and change of direction in chilean female soccer players. *J. Phys. Educ. Sport* **2021**, *21*, 2737–2744.
12. Smajla, D.; Kozinc, Ž.; Šarabon, N. Associations between lower limb eccentric muscle capability and change of direction speed in basketball and tennis players. *PeerJ* **2022**, *10*, e13439. [CrossRef] [PubMed]
13. Villaseca-Vicuña, R.; Molina-Sotomayor, E.; Zabaloy, S.; Gonzalez-Jurado, J.A. Anthropometric profile and physical fitness performance comparison by game position in the Chile women's senior national football team. *Appl. Sci.* **2021**, *11*, 2004. [CrossRef]
14. Claudino, J.G.; Cronin, J.; Mezêncio, B.; McMaster, D.T.; McGuigan, M.; Tricoli, V.; Amadio, A.C.; Serrão, J.C. The countermovement jump to monitor neuromuscular status: A meta-analysis. *J. Sci. Med. Sport* **2017**, *20*, 397–402. [CrossRef]
15. Gathercole, R.; Sporer, B.; Stellingwerff, T.; Sleivert, G. Alternative Countermovement-Jump Analysis to Quantify Acute Neuromuscular Fatigue. *Int. J. Sports Physiol. Perform.* **2015**, *10*, 84–92. [CrossRef]
16. Silva, J.R.; Ascensão, A.; Marques, F.; Seabra, A. Neuromuscular function, hormonal and redox status and muscle damage of professional soccer players after a high-level competitive match. *Eur. J. Appl. Physiol.* **2013**, *113*, 2193–2201. [CrossRef]
17. Schmitz, R.J.; Cone, J.C.; Copple, T.J.; Henson, R.A.; Shultz, S.J. Lower-extremity biomechanics and maintenance of vertical-jump height during prolonged intermittent exercise. *J. Sport Rehabil.* **2014**, *23*, 319–329. [CrossRef]
18. Harry, J.R.; Barker, L.A.; Tinsley, G.M.; Krzyszkowski, J.; Chowning, L.D.; McMahon, J.J.; Lake, J. Relationships among countermovement vertical jump performance metrics, strategy variables, and inter-limb asymmetry in females. *Sport Biomech.* **2021**, 1–19. [CrossRef]
19. Merino-Muñoz, P.; Pérez-Contreras, J.; Aedo-Muñoz, E.; Bustamante-Garrido, A. Relationship between jump height and rate of braking force development in professional soccer players. *J. Phys. Educ. Sport* **2020**, *20*, 3614–3621. [CrossRef]

20. Cohen, D.D.; Restrepo, A.; Richter, C.; Harry, J.R.; Franchi, M.V.; Restrepo, C.; Poletto, R.; Taberner, M. Detraining of specific neuromuscular qualities in elite footballers during COVID-19 quarantine. *Sci. Med. Footb.* **2020**, *5*, 26–31. [CrossRef]
21. Merino-Muñoz, P.; Miarka, B.; Peréz-contreras, J.; Jofré, C.M. Relationship between external load and differences in countermovement jump in an official match of professional female soccer players. In Proceedings of the 40th International Society of Biomechanics in Sports Conference, Liverpool, UK, 19–23 July 2022; pp. 451–454.
22. Kozinc, Ž.; Šarabon, N. Measurements of Lower-limb Isometric Single-joint Maximal Voluntary Torque and Rate of Torque Development Capacity Offer Limited Insight into Vertical Jumping Performance Measurements of Lower-limb Isometric Single-joint Maximal Voluntary Torque. *Meas. Phys. Educ. Exerc. Sci.* **2021**, 1–12. [CrossRef]
23. Laett, C.T.; Cossich, V.; Goes, R.A.; Gavilão, U.; Rites, R.; de Oliveira, C.G. Relationship between vastus lateralis muscle ultrasound echography, knee extensors rate of torque development, and jump height in professional soccer athletes. *Sport Sci. Health* **2020**, *17*, 299–306. [CrossRef]
24. De Ruiter, C.J.; Van Leeuwen, D.; Heijblom, A.; Bobbert, M.F.; de Haan, A. Fast unilateral isometric knee extension torque development and bilateral jump height. *Med. Sci. Sports Exerc.* **2006**, *38*, 1843–1852. [CrossRef] [PubMed]
25. Van Hooren, B.; Kozinc, Ž.; Smajla, D.; Šarabon, N. Isometric single-joint rate of force development shows trivial to small associations with jumping rate of force development, jump height, and propulsive duration. *JSAMS Plus* **2022**, *1*, 100006. [CrossRef]
26. Lake, J.; Mundy, P.; Comfort, P.; McMahon, J.J.; Suchomel, T.J.; Carden, P. Concurrent Validity of a Portable Force Plate Using Vertical Jump Force–Time Characteristics. *J. Appl. Biomech.* **2018**, *34*, 410–413. [CrossRef]
27. Sands, W.A.; Bogdanis, G.C.; Penitente, G.; Donti, O.; McNeal, J.R.; Butterfield, C.C.; Poehling, R.A.; Barker, L.A. Reliability and validity of a low-cost portable force platform. *Isokinet. Exerc. Sci.* **2020**, *28*, 247–253. [CrossRef]
28. Rodríguez-Rosell, D.; Pareja-Blanco, F.; Aagaard, P.; González-Badillo, J.J. Physiological and methodological aspects of rate of force development assessment in human skeletal muscle. *Clin. Physiol. Funct. Imaging* **2018**, *38*, 743–762. [CrossRef]
29. Bishop, D. Warm up II: Performance changes following active warm up and how to structure the warm up. *Sport Med.* **2003**, *33*, 483–498. [CrossRef]
30. Lees, A.; Vanrenterghem, J.; De Clercq, D. Understanding how an arm swing enhances performance in the vertical jump. *J. Biomech.* **2004**, *37*, 1929–1940. [CrossRef]
31. Krzyszkowski, J.; Chowning, L.D.; Harry, J.R. Phase-Specific Verbal Cue Effects on Countermovement Jump Performance. *J. Strength Cond. Res.* **2021**, *36*, 3352–3358. [CrossRef]
32. Ugrinowitsch, C.; Tricoli, V.; Rodacki, A.L.; Batista, M.; Ricard, M.D. Influence of training background on jumping height. *J. Strength Cond. Res.* **2007**, *21*, 848–852. [CrossRef] [PubMed]
33. Harry, J.R.; Barker, L.A.; Paquette, M.R. A Joint Power Approach to Define Countermovement Jump Phases Using Force Platforms. *Med. Sci. Sports Exerc.* **2020**, *52*, 993–1000. [CrossRef] [PubMed]
34. Linthorne, N.P. Analysis of standing vertical jumps using a force platform. *Am. J. Phys.* **2001**, *69*, 1198–1204. [CrossRef]
35. Thompson, B.J. Influence of signal filtering and sample rate on isometric torque—Time parameters using a traditional isokinetic dynamometer. *J. Biomech.* **2019**, *83*, 235–242. [CrossRef] [PubMed]
36. Lum, D.; Haff, G.G.; Barbosa, T.M. The Relationship between Isometric Force-Time Characteristics and Dynamic Performance: A Systematic Review. *Sports* **2020**, *8*, 63. [CrossRef]
37. Bobbert, M.F.; Mackay, M.; Schinkelshoek, D.; Huijing, P.A.; Schenau, G.J.V.I. Biomechanical analysis of drop and countermovement jumps. *Eur. J. Appl. Physiol. Occup. Physiol.* **1986**, *54*, 566–573. [CrossRef]
38. Vanezis, A.; Lees, A. A biomechanical analysis of good and poor performers of the vertical jump. *Ergonomics* **2005**, *48*, 1594–1603. [CrossRef]
39. Shinchi, K.; Yamashita, D.; Yamagishi, T.; Aoki, K.; Miyamoto, N. Relationship between jump height and lower limb joint kinetics and kinematics during countermovement jump in elite male athletes. *Sports Biomech.* **2024**, 1–12. [CrossRef]
40. Iossifidou, A.; Baltzopoulos, V.; Giakas, G. Isokinetic knee extension and vertical jumping: Are they related? *J. Sports Sci.* **2005**, *23*, 1121–1127. [CrossRef]
41. Śliwowski, R.; Grygorowicz, M.; Wieczorek, A.; Jadczak, Ł. The relationship between jumping performance, isokinetic strength and dynamic postural control in elite youth soccer players. *J. Sports Med. Phys. Fitness* **2018**, *58*, 1226–1233. [CrossRef]
42. Hori, M.; Suga, T.; Terada, M.; Tanaka, M.; Kusagawa, Y.; Otsuka, M.; Nagano, A.; Isaka, T. Relationship of the knee extensor strength but not the quadriceps femoris muscularity with sprint performance in sprinters: A reexamination and extension. *BMC Sports Sci. Med. Rehabilitation* **2021**, *13*, 1–10. [CrossRef]
43. Ishøi, L.; Aagaard, P.; Nielsen, M.F.; Thornton, K.B.; Krommes, K.K.; Hölmich, P.; Thorborg, K. The Influence of Hamstring Muscle Peak Torque and Rate of Torque Development for Sprinting Performance in Football Players: A Cross-Sectional Study. *Int. J. Sports Physiol. Perform.* **2019**, *14*, 665–673. [CrossRef] [PubMed]
44. Diker, G.; Struzik, A.; Ön, S.; Zileli, R. The Relationship between the Hamstring-to-Quadriceps Ratio and Jumping and Sprinting Abilities of Young Male Soccer Players. *Int. J. Environ. Res. Public Heal.* **2022**, *19*, 7841. [CrossRef] [PubMed]
45. Morin, J.-B.; Samozino, P. Interpreting Power-Force-Velocity Profiles for Individualized and Specific Training. *Int. J. Sports Physiol. Perform.* **2016**, *11*, 267–272. [CrossRef]

46. Royer, N.; Nosaka, K.; Doguet, V.; Jubeau, M. Neuromuscular responses to isometric, concentric and eccentric contractions of the knee extensors at the same torque-time integral. *Eur. J. Appl. Physiol.* **2021**, *122*, 127–139. [CrossRef]
47. Kipp, K.; Kim, H. Relative contributions and capacities of lower extremity muscles to accelerate the body's center of mass during countermovement jumps. *Comput. Methods Biomech. Biomed. Eng.* **2020**, *23*, 914–921. [CrossRef]

Disclaimer/Publisher's Note: The statements, opinions and data contained in all publications are solely those of the individual author(s) and contributor(s) and not of MDPI and/or the editor(s). MDPI and/or the editor(s) disclaim responsibility for any injury to people or property resulting from any ideas, methods, instructions or products referred to in the content.

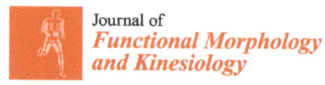

Article

Similarity Index Values in Fuzzy Logic and the Support Vector Machine Method Applied to the Identification of Changes in Movement Patterns During Biceps-Curl Weight-Lifting Exercise

André B. Peres [1,2], Tiago A. F. Almeida [2,3], Danilo A. Massini [2,3], Anderson G. Macedo [2,3,4], Mário C. Espada [5,6,7,8,9,10], Ricardo A. M. Robalo [5,7,9], Rafael Oliveira [9,10], João P. Brito [9,10] and Dalton M. Pessôa Filho [2,3,*]

1. Instituto Federal de Educação, Ciência e Tecnologia de São Paulo (IFSP), Piracicaba 13414-155, SP, Brazil; andreperes@ifsp.edu.br
2. Graduate Programme in Human Development and Technologies, São Paulo State University (UNESP), Rio Claro 13506-900, SP, Brazil; tiagofalmeida.w@gmail.com (T.A.F.A.); dmassini@hotmail.com (D.A.M.); andersongmacedo@yahoo.com.br (A.G.M.)
3. Department of Physical Education, School of Sciences (FC), São Paulo State University (UNESP), Bauru 17033-360, SP, Brazil
4. Post-Graduation Program in Rehabilitation Sciences, Institute of Motricity Sciences, Federal University of Alfenas (UNIFAL), Alfenas 37133-840, MG, Brazil
5. Instituto Politécnico de Setúbal, Escola Superior de Educação (CIEQV—Setúbal), 2914-504 Setúbal, Portugal; mario.espada@ese.ips.pt (M.C.E.); ricardo.robalo@ese.ips.pt (R.A.M.R.)
6. Sport Physical Activity and Health Research & INnovation CenTer (SPRINT), 2040-413 Rio Maior, Portugal
7. Centre for the Study of Human Performance (CIPER), Faculdade de Motricidade Humana, Universidade de Lisboa, 1499-002 Cruz Quebrada, Portugal
8. Comprehensive Health Research Centre (CHRC), Universidade de Évora, 7004-516 Évora, Portugal
9. School of Sport, Santarém Polytechnic University, Av. Dr. Mário Soares, 2040-413 Rio Maior, Portugal; rafaeloliveira@esdrm.ipsantarem.pt (R.O.); jbrito@esdrm.ipsantarem.pt (J.P.B.)
10. Research Centre in Sport Sciences, Health Sciences and Human Development (CIDESD), Santarém Polytechnic University, 2040-413 Rio Maior, Portugal
* Correspondence: dalton.pessoa-filho@unesp.br

Abstract: Background/Objectives: Correct supervision during the performance of resistance exercises is imperative to the correct execution of these exercises. This study presents a proposal for the use of Morisita–Horn similarity indices in modelling with machine learning methods to identify changes in positional sequence patterns during the biceps-curl weight-lifting exercise with a barbell. The models used are based on the fuzzy logic (FL) and support vector machine (SVM) methods. **Methods**: Ten male volunteers (age: 26 ± 4.9 years, height: 177 ± 8.0 cm, body weight: 86 ± 16 kg) performed a standing barbell bicep curl with additional weights. A smartphone was used to record their movements in the sagittal plane, providing information about joint positions and changes in the sequential position of the bar during each lifting attempt. Maximum absolute deviations of movement amplitudes were calculated for each execution. **Results:** A variance analysis revealed significant deviations ($p < 0.002$) in vertical displacement between the standard execution and execution with a load of 50% of the subject's body weight. Experts with over thirty years of experience in resistance-exercise evaluation evaluated the exercises, and their results showed an agreement of over 70% with the results of the ANOVA. The similarity indices, absolute deviations, and expert evaluations were used for modelling in both the FL system and the SVM. The root mean square error and R-squared results for the FL system ($R^2 = 0.92$, r = 0.96) were superior to those of the SVM ($R^2 = 0.81$, r = 0.79). **Conclusions:** The use of FL in modelling emerges as a promising approach with which to support the assessment of movement patterns. Its applications range from automated detection of errors in exercise execution to enhancing motor performance in athletes.

Keywords: pattern recognition; motor activity; theoretical models; resistance training

1. Introduction

Monitoring the movement of the barbell is common in weightlifting exercises to assess the performance of the practitioner [1]. In the bicep-curl exercise, supervision of the barbell movement by a professional tends to prevent injuries resulting from improper loads, postures, and executions [2].

The supervision of resistance exercises by a personal trainer plays an important role in preventing injury and in promoting the physical development of practitioners. The involvement of an experienced professional ensures that exercises are performed with proper technique, with postures and loads adjusted as necessary. This personalized attention not only minimizes the risk of injuries that can occur due to improper execution but also maximizes the benefits of training [3].

One of the main obstacles to adhering to supervised physical exercise is the high cost of personal training services. Studies show that hiring a professional for individualized support can be financially unfeasible for a large portion of the population, leading many to abandon regular exercise programs [4].

With the advancement of technology, fitness apps have become increasingly popular as alternatives to personal training services. These apps offer a variety of features, including personalized workout plans and progress tracking, at a lower cost [5].

However, the accuracy of these apps has been questioned. Several studies indicate that the accuracy of data collected by digital devices can vary significantly, raising uncertainties about their reliability compared to professional supervision. Research suggests that many users may not achieve the expected results due to errors in algorithms or in the interpretation of the collected information [5].

In summary, while digital apps provide an accessible solution for monitoring physical exercise, the costs associated with professional supervision and uncertainties regarding the accuracy of emerging technologies continue to be significant barriers to effective adherence. The combination of these factors suggests an urgent need to develop solutions that integrate the best of both worlds: professional support and digital technologies.

Increasing the load on the bar during bicep-curl exercises can change movement patterns. Werner et al. [6] investigated how different loads (60%, 85%, and 95% of an athlete's one-repetition maximum—1 RM) influence movement patterns. The results indicated that relative load has a significant effect on movement patterns. This suggests that as the load increases, athletes may adopt different movement patterns, which is relevant for training, especially for younger athletes who are perfecting their technique. Furthermore, the study highlighted that while lighter loads may allow for more repetitions, this could lead to the risk of developing movement patterns that are not ideal for maximum loads.

The trajectories of joint movements during exercise execution can serve as a basis for the analysis of movement patterns. These analyses help in identifying aberrant movement behaviours and evaluating sports technique. The goal is to provide quantitative and reliable feedback on movement quality, assisting coaches in making more accurate decisions regarding athlete performance and safety. Additionally, they can be used to investigate the relationships between movement patterns and injury risk [7].

Generally, motion data describe movement trajectories, each consisting of a temporal sequence of recorded locations for an object. In this work, we utilize the trajectory of a marker on the bar to analyse its movement trajectory [8]. Analysing human movement trajectories as time series is not uncommon and is part of current research [9].

Despite technological advancements, form analysis during practice of resistance exercises remains a rare feature of monitoring apps. There are some available apps that perform video motion analysis, such as OpenCap, Mirror AR, Runmatic, Spark Motion, Onform, and PhysioMaster. However, this functionality, coupled with immediate feedback at the end of each execution, could bring enormous benefits for training safety and effectiveness. Automatic analysis of exercise form, for example, would greatly reduce the risk of injuries and could enable feedback to be provided after each repetition of a resistance exercise [10].

To implement this feature, it is necessary to employ mathematical methods for movement analysis. The trajectory of a movement, as previously mentioned, can be analysed as a time series that can be compared to a good movement reference and analysed for needed alterations. To this end, a similarity test can be employed to identify pattern changes between different executions of an exercise and a standard model established according to the guidelines and protocols of the National Strength and Conditioning Association (NSCA) [11].

The Morisita–Horn (MH) dispersion or overlap index [12] is a measure of similarity or difference between two data sets. The index ranges from 0 (no similarity) to 1 (complete similarity). It is a measure used in ecology to quantify the overlap between two communities or species samples. It is particularly useful for assessing the similarity in species composition between different habitats or populations, allowing for an understanding of how species share resources or occupy similar niches [12]. In the present study, this index was adapted for the analysis of two bar-movement trajectories during the execution of the biceps-curl weight-lifting exercise.

The values obtained for the MH index for correct executions, within an acceptable range of variation, can be taken as a reference for comparison with executions involving additional load; these data can then be subjected to an analysis of possible changes. However, to identify changes in exercise execution patterns (changes in spatial trajectory), a mathematical model based on fuzzy logic (FL) has shown good results [13]. In this case, the values obtained with the MH index were used to establish degrees of membership and rule sets for the FL system.

FL has demonstrated good performance in modelling human thought processes and is capable of handling uncertainty [14]. It can be designed to simulate how humans think and make decisions, especially in situations where information is imprecise or incomplete [15]. This is particularly relevant in healthcare and also in physical training, where assessments often rely on subjective interpretations by the professional making the diagnosis [16]. As the values of the MH index vary on a scale from 0 to 1, a regression model based on machine learning called the Support Vector Machine (SVM) model was also applied to quantify the accuracy of movement, and its performance was compared with that of the model obtained using FL.

SVM is a machine learning algorithm used for classification and regression that seeks to find the optimal hyperplane that separates different classes of data. It can be applied to classify and recognize movement patterns, such as physical activities or gestures [17], aiding in areas such as rehabilitation [18], sports [19], and human–computer interaction [20]. Additionally, it has a significant advantage in movement analysis: its ability to handle high-dimensional data and robustness against overfitting (high accuracy on training data but poor prediction on unseen data) makes it effective for analysing complex movement data [21,22].

In this study, we aimed to analyse the suitability of the MH index for training a machine learning procedure to identify movement-pattern alterations during a weight-lifting exercise. To design the model, a common single-joint exercise (biceps curl with a barbell) was modelled based on the hypothesis that deviations from the Cartesian coordinates of the bar position in the sagittal plane (e.g., horizontal and vertical displacements) that may reflect significant pattern alterations due to load increase can be automatically detected using FL analysis associated with the MH scale. Moreover, the deviations in displacement measured through traditional means (such as absolute deviations) can be related to similarity changes detected by the MH index to quantify the degree of similarity between executions using SVM algorithms. In addition, variance analyses between groups (ANOVA) and human evaluators might increase the confidence associated with using similarity indices in modelling with FL and SVM regression, resulting in a viable approach to employing mathematical models in automated movement analysis.

2. Materials and Methods

2.1. Participants

Twelve male volunteers, all with more than six months of experience in resistance training, participated in the study. At the beginning of the tests, the volunteers self-reported their training sessions, with 8 to 10 maximum repetitions, 3 to 4 sets per exercise, and 6 to 9 exercises per session, 3 to 5 times per week. Two volunteers were excluded because they were unable to complete all the repetitions. The remaining ten (age: 26 ± 4.9 years, height: 177 ± 8.0 cm, body weight: 86 ± 16 kg) completed all the proposed repetitions. The study was approved by the ethics committee of the local university (protocol: 17486119.0.0000.5398).

2.2. Procedures

Data collection was conducted in the Laboratory of Human Sports Performance Optimization (LABOREH). Participants used a green semi-spherical marker measuring 25 mm in diameter that was fixed to the barbell.

The volunteers performed a sequence of three complete repetitions of a biceps-curl weight-lifting exercise using only the barbell (9 kg/considered no load). After a ten minute rest, they performed three more repetitions of the exercise with a load (using the barbell with weights) of 25% of their body weight. This was followed by another break and three additional repetitions of the biceps-curl weight-lifting exercise with a load of 50% of their body weight [8]. Volunteers were instructed to perform each set with a similar cadence and were told this cadence should be close to that used in their daily routine to avoid unusual performance conditions. Additional guidelines for the performance of the biceps curl were as follows: (i) the inter-hand distance was measured during the first set and maintained throughout the attempts; (ii) the exercise was performed with a full range of movement (with ascending and descending phases), using an external focus; (iii) the participants were instructed to avoid sagittal oscillations of the trunk and barbell, any movement or impulse of lower limbs, and exaggerated elevation of the scapulae; and (iv) the technique was controlled by the researchers via feedback for the participant when a correct technique was observed [23]:

For the collection of temporal positional data during resistance exercises, a digital video camera attached to a Galaxy S9 smartphone (Samsung®, Suwon-si, Gyeonggi-do, Korea) with 12 megapixels and UHD 4K resolution was used. The camera was stationary, with its optical axis perpendicular to the participant's sagittal plane, as shown in Figure 1 [8].

The procedure for calibrating the measurements was based on distances between markers in the background (forming a right triangle) and in a plane coincident with the participant's sagittal plane. Additionally, actual measurements of some body segments of the volunteers (upper arm, forearm) and their actual heights were used to verify the measurements. This approach made it possible to determine displacement measurements from the two-dimensional coordinates of the participant in the plane they occupied [8,9].

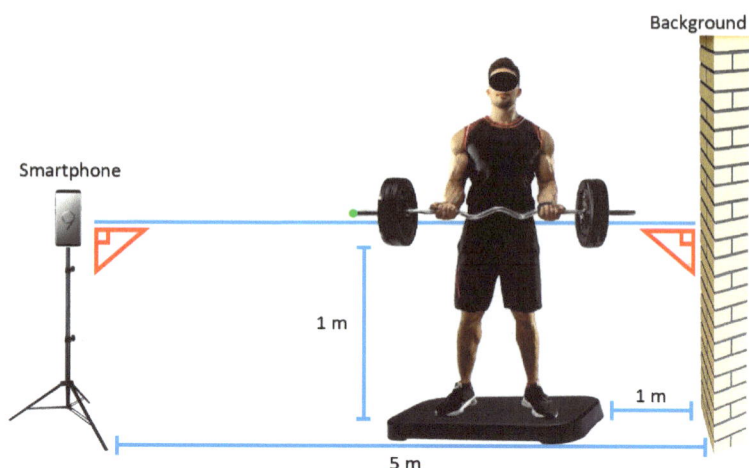

Figure 1. Scheme for capturing videos. Image partly generated by AI in: https://firefly.adobe.com/generate/images (accessed on 14 September 2024).

Video capture in MPEG-4 format was conducted for three complete executions of the proposed exercises for each of the three load variations. The recordings were made at a frequency of 30 frames per second [24,25], and the video acquisition time corresponded to three executions of the respective exercise for each load [8].

Digital processing of the videos was performed using Wondershare Filmora version 9 (Wondershare Filmora, Hong Kong, China) [26] to apply a Chroma Key effect [27] on the colour of the markers and to apply an Alpha channel [28] to better contrast the markers with the rest of the environment in the scene. Kinovea 0.8.27 software (Kinovea, Bordeaux, France) [29] was used for semi-automatic tracking of the markers, and their coordinates were exported to Extensible Markup Language files. The origin of the Cartesian coordinate system was assigned to the centre of the marker located on the bar at the beginning of the upward movement [8].

2.3. Obtaining Displacement Measurements

Displacement measurements were taken from the marker located on the bar and calculated from its movement in relation to the x-axis, as follows:

$$\Delta x = x_f - x_i \tag{1}$$

where Δx is the displacement, x_f is the x-value of the coordinate at the end point, and x_i is the x-value of the coordinate at the origin.

Displacement in relation to the y-axis was calculated as follows:

$$\Delta y = y_f - y_i \tag{2}$$

where Δy is the displacement, y_f is the y-value of the coordinate at the endpoint, and y_i is the y-value of the coordinate at the origin.

2.4. Human Evaluators

To obtain a qualitative analysis for comparisons that reflects what is common in physical assessments, two specialists with over 30 years of experience (experts in evaluation) visually analysed the performances of the exercises executed with different load variations. They observed the exercises performed by the volunteers through videos, and their data were used as an observational reference for statistical/mathematical models. They used as a reference the execution performed with only the bar, without added load. When they observed the executions performed with two different loads, they attempted to identify any changes in horizontal and vertical displacements versus the reference exercise execution (i.e., the silhouette of motion for the repetitions with no load added) [9]. For this observational analysis, the observer recorded the part of the silhouette that differed from the reference motion The results of the observer analysis were further tested by ANOVA (see section below) to determine whether the standard deviation from the reference motion coordinate was significant and therefore corroborated the results of the observer's analysis by the observer; these results were then used to determine whether the alteration in movement patterns should be incorporated into the movement modelling using FL.

2.5. Statistical Analysis

The descriptive statistics, normality tests, and analysis of variance of the data were obtained using SPSS® version 22.0.0 (SPSS, Corp, Armonk, NY, USA) [30]. A one-way ANOVA was conducted to verify the existence of significant differences in the maximum displacement (vertical and horizontal) during the lifting phase of the exercise as the average of three full-range joint repetitions with each load. Tukey's post-hoc test was applied with a significance level of $p < 0.05$. Using the maximum values of absolute deviations of the displacements, a one-way ANOVA was conducted with Tukey's post-hoc test at a significance level of $p < 0.05$ to verify the existence of significant differences in displacement among the three different loads.

Morisita–Horn Index

The MH index was calculated using Equation (3), which was presented by Horn [12], as follows:

$$I_{MH} = \frac{2\sum_{i=1}^{S} x_i y_i}{\left(\frac{\sum_{i=1}^{S} x_i^2}{X^2} + \frac{\sum_{i=1}^{S} y_i^2}{Y^2}\right) XY} \quad (3)$$

where x_i is the abundance of species i in sample x; y_i is the abundance of species i in sample y; and X and Y are the number of species for the samples. The equation was implemented using the average of the maximum displacement values from the three no-load executions (with only the bar) as a reference and compared to the maximum values obtained in the other executions. The no-load executions (training for correct execution) Ex1, Ex2, and Ex3 generated the average value of maximum displacements, MMD0. This average value was compared to the other executions, here designated as follows: Ex1_25, Ex2_25, Ex3_25 for the load of 25% of the subject's body weight and Ex1_50, Ex2_50, and Ex3_50 for the load of 50% of the subject's body weight. The absolute and relative deviation values in relation to the mean were also obtained.

The results obtained from ANOVA, which showed significant differences in displacement, along with the analysis by the specialists, provided the criteria for modelling marker positioning data using FL based on the MH indices and absolute deviations found. The chosen model for identification was Sugeno with 18 inference rules, considering the maximum absolute deviation obtained via computer vision and the load used (0%, 25%, or 50%). The FL system, which was implemented using the Fuzzy Logic Designer app, employed the weighted average defuzzification method.

Since the values of the MH index present a similarity scale, regression was also performed using SVM. The results obtained from ANOVA, which showed significant differences in displacement, were also utilized. The entire regression process conducted by SVM was developed using the Regression Learner app, comparing the following models: linear SVM, quadratic SVM, cubic SVM, fine Gaussian SVM, medium Gaussian SVM, and coarse Gaussian SVM. In all cases, cross-validation for five groups was used to protect against overfitting. Pearson correlation calculations, polynomial fit, Morisita–Horn indices, fuzzy modelling, and SVM modelling were all performed using Matlab® 24.1.0 software (Matlab, Portola Valley, CA, USA) [31].

3. Results

The averages of the maximum displacement values of the bar during the upward phase of the exercise for all participants were calculated in centimetres. For a load of 0%, using only the bar, the average horizontal displacement was 23.7 ± 5.9 cm. For a load of 25%, it was 23.6 ± 5.0 cm, and for a load of 50%, it was 24.9 ± 4.3 cm. The average vertical displacement was 56.8 ± 7.7 cm for a load of 0%, 59.6 ± 8.5 cm for a load of 25%, and 64.0 ± 9.0 cm for a load of 50%.

The maximum values of absolute deviations (in cm) obtained in each execution with loads of 25% (Ex1_25, Ex2_25, and Ex3_25) and 50% (Ex1_50, Ex2_50, and Ex3_50), using the average of the maximums from the first three executions (MMD0) as a reference, are displayed in Tables 1 and 2.

Table 1. Maximum values of absolute horizontal deviations for each volunteer/load.

	Absolute Horizontal Deviation Values (cm)									
Exec.	V01	V02	V03	V04	V05	V06	V07	V08	V09	V10
Ex1_25	4.20	10.41	0.88	4.56	3.90	6.71	9.23	4.33	0.55	4.44
Ex2_25	4.07	4.69	5.03	3.82	0.97	2.48	2.62	0.13	4.27	3.78
Ex3_25	5.25	0.98	4.10	5.32	1.35	1.82	0.5	2.73	7.79	4.18
Ex1_50	6.12	4.58	2.47	4.57	5.61	0.15	4.38	1.24	1.45	2.99
Ex2_50	5.42	3.58	0.89	4.98	4.03	10.15	1.39	3.03	0.44	5.63
Ex3_50	7.55	2.30	0.69	7.63	6.86	4.35	3.63	0.93	1.94	4.05

Ex1_25, execution one at 25% of the subject's body weight; Ex2_25, execution two at 25% of the subject's body weight; Ex3_25, execution three at 25% of the subject's body weight; Ex1_50, execution one at 50% of the subject's body weight; Ex2_50, execution two at 50% of the subject's body weight; Ex3_50, execution three at 50% of the subject's body weight.

Table 2. Maximum values of absolute vertical deviations for each volunteer/load.

	Values of Absolute Vertical Deviations (cm)									
Exec.	V01	V02	V03	V04	V05	V06	V07	V08	V09	V10
Ex1_25	1.29	5.61	2.11	0.87	4.25	10.88	18.32	6.03	5.31	10.00
Ex2_25	0.64	5.02	6.27	4.03	3.11	4.43	7.59	1.49	12.01	7.63
Ex3_25	0.68	9.27	5.82	6.31	2.58	3.95	3.01	3.21	9.44	5.03
Ex1_50	7.14	2.82	6.53	15.45	6.51	24.43	15.19	7.94	17.35	15.23
Ex2_50	5.62	6.36	1.48	16.03	4.60	13.69	12.27	3.92	11.87	18.06
Ex3_50	11.8	9.08	0.53	13.78	14.48	18.63	13.82	3.80	11.23	18.54

Ex1_25, execution one at 25% of the subject's body weight; Ex2_25, execution two at 25% of the subject's body weight; Ex3_25, execution three at 25% of the subject's body weight; Ex1_50, execution one at 50% of the subject's body weight; Ex2_50, execution two at 50% of the subject's body weight; Ex3_50, execution three at 50% of the subject's body weight.

In a comparison of the average maximum horizontal displacement values from the first three executions (using only the bar) with the executions at 25% and 50% of the subject's body weight, no significant difference was found within the group. The same comparisons for vertical displacement showed a significant difference within the group only when the displacement values with the no-load exercises were compared to displacement values with the repetitions at 50% of the subject's body weight, yielding a p-value of $p = 0.002$.

Thus, MH indices were calculated for the maximum vertical displacements for each volunteer for each execution/load. Table 3 displays these index values with comparisons between MMD0 and the maximum values from executions performed at 50% load.

Table 3. Morisita–Horn/Volunteer Indices (vertical).

	Morisita–Horn/Volunteer Indices (Vertical)									
Exec.	V01	V02	V03	V04	V05	V06	V07	V08	V09	V10
Ex1_50	0.99807	0.99948	0.99709	0.98621	0.99712	0.97582	0.98924	0.99626	0.98587	0.98458
Ex2_50	0.99877	0.99744	0.99983	0.98526	0.99853	0.99155	0.99277	0.99904	0.99299	0.97906
Ex3_50	0.99507	0.99495	0.99998	0.98882	0.98705	0.98510	0.99097	0.99910	0.99369	0.97806

The human evaluators conducted a qualitative analysis of the exercises recorded on video with respect to the load variations. Using as a reference the exercise performed without added load (with only the bar), they were able to perceive variations only when the no-load executions were compared with those performed at 50% of the subject's body weight. When the assessments by Ev.01 and Ev.02 of the difference between individual attempts were compared to the ANOVA results, the following results were obtained: ANOVA and Ev.01 showed 70% agreement, and ANOVA and Ev.02 showed 80% agreement.

As a result, only the values of deviations and MH indices in the comparison between MMD0 and 50% load were used to create the mathematical models. Figure 2 displays the graph of MH values and absolute deviations with a trendline given by the quadratic equation, as follows:

$$y = -3.1026 \times 10^{-5} x^2 - 4.1535 \times 10^{-4} x + 1.0013 \tag{4}$$

with an R-squared value of 0.92 and a Pearson correlation coefficient of 0.96.

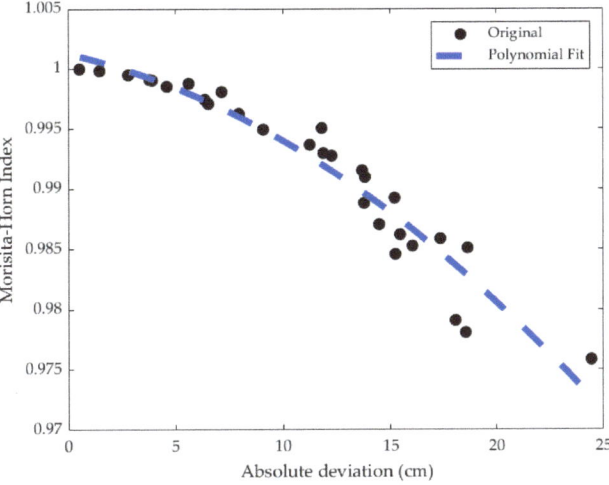

Figure 2. Scatterplot of MH index values vs. absolute deviation values.

Based on the evaluations of the specialists, a range of absolute deviation values was established for the identification of statistically significant changes in movement patterns as a result of increased load. These deviation values, along with the MH index values, served as the basis for modelling the FL system. A deviation range was established within the closed interval of [0, 25], with zero representing no error and 25 representing the maximum deviation value relative to the mean of the initial position. Figure 3 displays how the system was created: two inputs, the maximum deviation value from the execution and the load value (the system was assigned load variation even though no significant difference was observed by ANOVA), were used. The variation in deviation was subdivided into six parts using Gaussian functions (Figure 4).

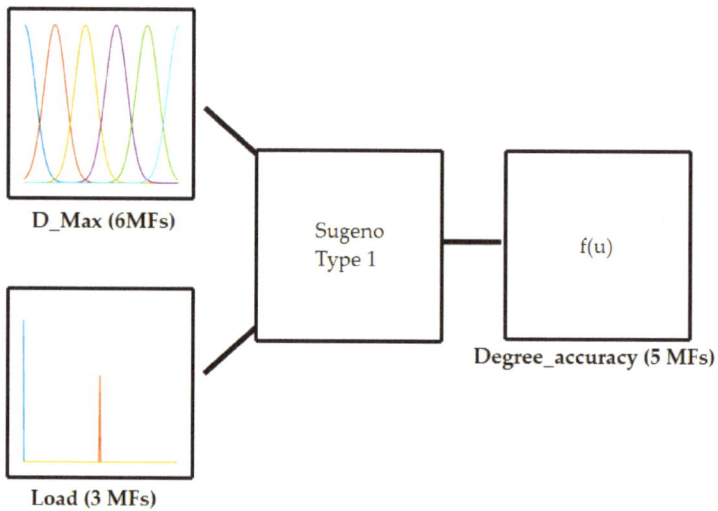

Figure 3. Fuzzy Inference System model.

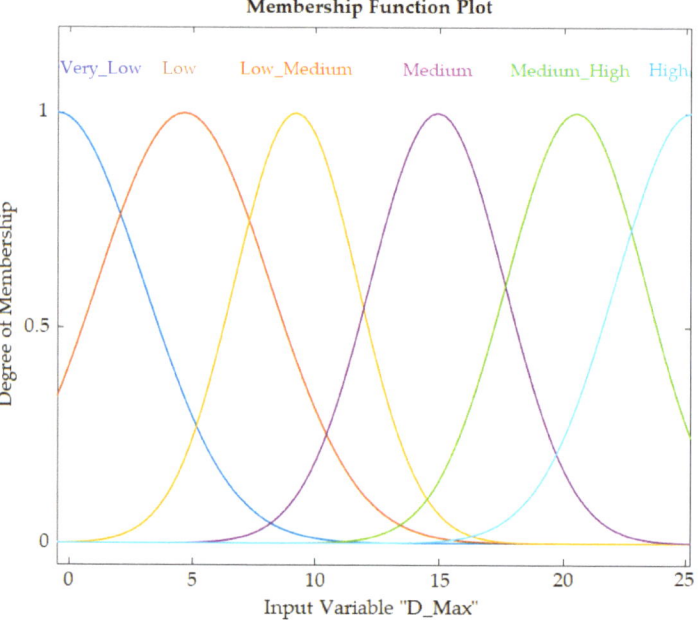

Figure 4. Variation in the values of the absolute deviations at the system input.

The output values were modelled with the MH variation within a range of 97 to 100% (0.97, 1.0) similarity between the comparisons. The values obtained from the FL system and the original values are displayed in Figure 5. The Pearson correlation coefficient for the two sets of values was 0.96, and R-squared = 0.92.

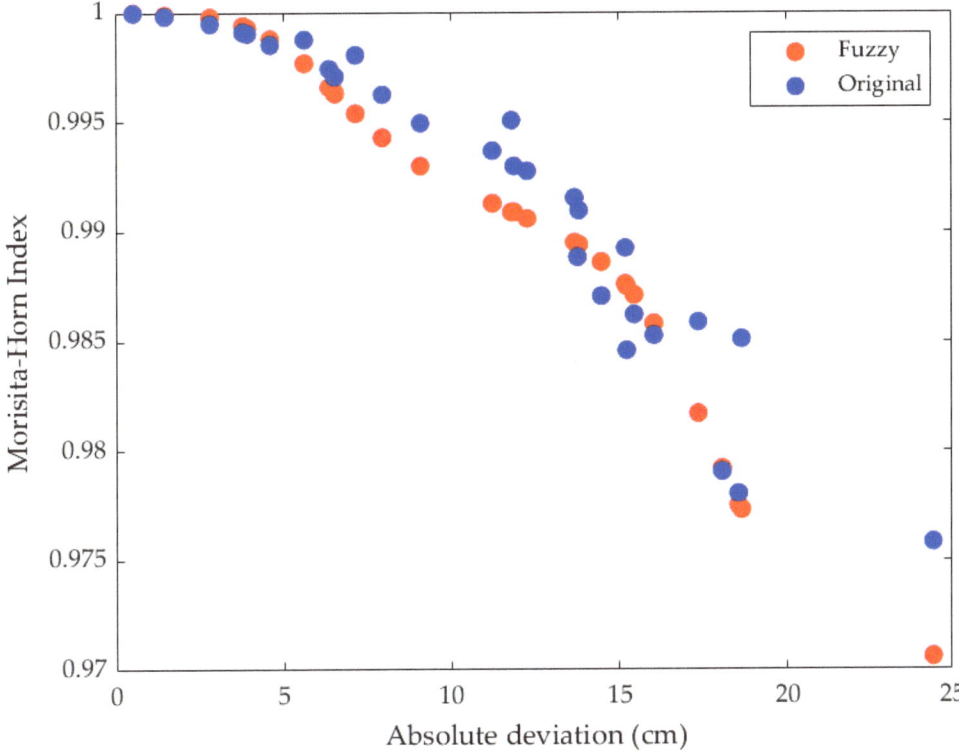

Figure 5. Comparison between original Morisita–Horn data and data obtained from the fuzzy logic model.

To compare the methods, a regression model using SVM was also employed. The model was trained with the absolute deviation values and MH indices for the comparisons of MMD0 with the executions at 50% load. The following models were trained: linear SVM, quadratic SVM, cubic SVM, fine Gaussian SVM, medium Gaussian SVM, and coarse Gaussian SVM. The root mean square error (RMSE) and R-squared values are displayed in Table 4.

Table 4. RMSE and R-squared values for the different SVM models.

	Linear	Quadratic	Cubic	Fine Gaussian	Medium Gaussian	Coarse Gaussian
RMSE	0.0038507	0.0071847	0.0053830	0.0041965	0.0040772	0.0031715
R-squared	0.72	0.02	0.45	0.66	0.68	0.81

RMSE, root mean square error.

As shown in Table 4, the best SVM model was the coarse Gaussian. With this model, we obtained the comparison between the original values and those obtained from the model (Figure 6). The Pearson correlation coefficient for the two sets of values was 0.79.

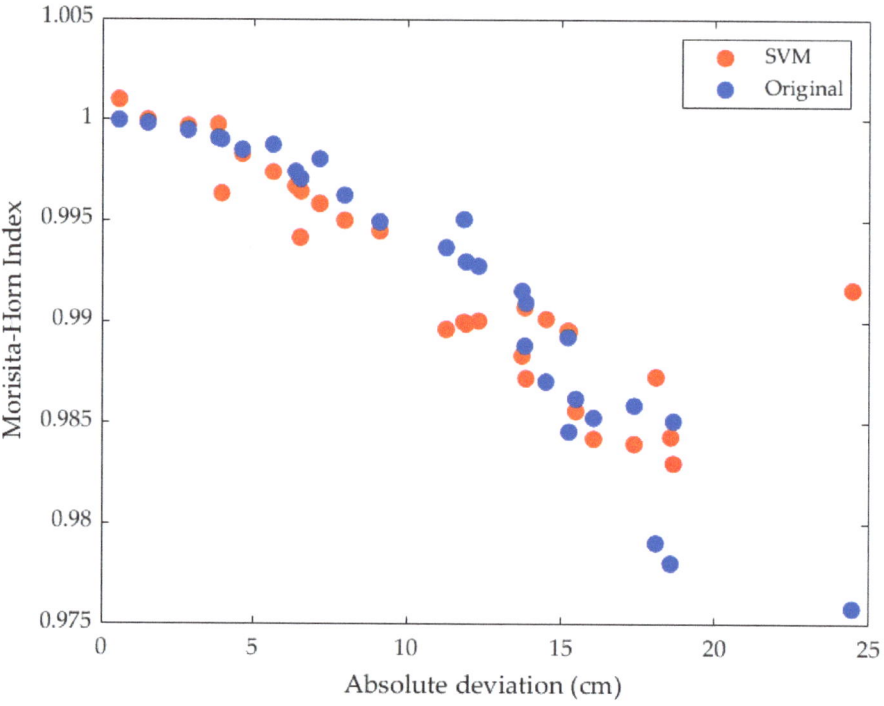

Figure 6. Comparison between original Morisita–Horn data and data obtained by the coarse Gaussian SVM model.

4. Discussion

This study identified disturbances in movement due to increased load during the execution of a barbell bicep-curl exercise using a similarity index. The use of maximum absolute deviation for the analyses is justified by the need to identify significant changes in movement patterns, with the no-load execution serving as the reference. The maximum absolute deviation values were used to verify the existence of significant differences in range of motion with the different loads utilized, an approach similar to that used in the work by Peres et al. [8]. This allows for an assessment of an individual's ability to lift a certain load while utilizing muscular contraction to overcome resistance and control sources of joint instability and thereby ensuring safety and effectiveness in training.

In the biceps-curl weight-lifting exercise, the primary movement is elbow flexion, which primarily involves the biceps brachii muscle. When weight is added, the force required to perform the movement increases, resulting in a change in vertical displacement during the exercise; vertical displacement is thus more sensitive than horizontal displacement to load variations [32]. In contrast, horizontal movement involves rotational movements that are not the primary focus of the bicep curl. During this exercise, the involved joints, especially the elbow, do not perform significant movements [8]. The bicep curl is predominantly a uniaxial movement focused on elbow flexion and extension and does not involve the lateral or rotational displacements that would be necessary to generate significant differences in horizontal displacement [23].

Only the comparisons that showed significant differences in displacement were subjected to similarity analysis. The use of the similarity index allowed for the comparison of two executions of the bar movement as time series. In this study, the MH index was used to compare the movement performed with only the bar to the movements executed with added load. The index ranges in value from 0 to 1, where 0 indicates no similarity and 1 indicates complete similarity [12]. A high index value suggests that the maximum deviations of the movements are very similar among the analysed individuals, indicating consistent technical execution. Lower values may indicate significant variations in technique or movement execution, which could be relevant for adjustments in training or for developing personalized rehabilitation or performance programs. The analysis using the MH index provided a quantitative approach to identifying changes in movement patterns due to load variations, contributing to a better understanding of the variables that influence practitioner performance [33]. Table 3 displays the similarity values of the MH index. The variation of the index ranged from 0.97582 to 0.99998, encompassing absolute deviation variations within the range of 0.53 to 24.43 cm. This result reflects that the execution movements are similar, but the load variations identified as significantly altering the movement fall within this range.

The human evaluators, when analysing movement with reference to the execution performed without added load, were able to observe variations only for executions with a load of 50% of the subject's body weight, a result corroborated by the ANOVA results. The percentage agreement between ANOVA and evaluators for responses identifying or not identifying significant displacements relative to the established reference (no load) and other executions (with load) varied between 70% and 80%, while agreement among evaluators was equal to 90%. In the comparison of the results obtained from ANOVA and human evaluators, there was good agreement both between the evaluators and the model and among evaluators in some cases. Good agreement among evaluators indicates consistency in error perception in human assessment [9,34]. However, evaluating exercise quality via human judgment is subjective and time-consuming [35].

The results obtained from the MH indices, along with the values of maximum absolute deviations, are displayed in Figure 2 in a scatterplot with a trendline described by a quadratic function generated by Matlab® version 24.1.0 [31], which showed an R-squared value of 0.92, within acceptable limits for model fitting. This fit would already serve to relate observed values of absolute motion deviations with significance index values of MH; however, as this work aimed to incorporate characteristics of human experts into movement assessment, FL was used for modelling and relating load, vertical absolute deviation, and similarity index, which was taken to indicate movement disturbance.

With the MH variation values ranging from 0.97582 to 0.99998 and absolute deviation variations within the range of 0.53 to 24.43 cm, a comparison of results from ANOVA and human evaluators established a similarity-index variation of 97 to 100% (0.97, 1.0) for identifying changes in movement patterns, with maximum absolute deviation values between 0 and 25 cm, where zero indicates no error and 25 represents the maximum deviation relative to the mean of the initial position.

The FL system was created using the Sugeno inference method, relating the maximum absolute deviation values from each execution for different loads (0%, 25%, or 50%), even though significant differences (as measured with similarity index values) were observed only when the 50% load variation was compared with the 0% load variation. These similarity index values indicate, within the presented scale, the accuracy of the movement compared to the no-load reference. This variation can be associated with the degree of accuracy in performing the movement described in Figure 4, which includes six execution levels (very low, low, low medium, medium, medium high, and high), represented in the system by Gaussian functions. In this case, these levels allow for feedback at the end of the upward execution of the exercise, where the feedback is based on classifying the executed movement.

Siow, Chin, and Kubota [35] similarly proposed an FL system to evaluate simple exercises based on human skeleton poses. Their goal was to provide a more objective and efficient way to assess exercise quality for older adults. The researchers' approach consisted of four steps: (1) converting video into a sequence of human skeleton poses; (2) extracting essential poses from the sequence; (3) generating FL membership functions based on pose similarity and exercise completeness; and (4) performing rule inference and defuzzification to obtain an exercise score. The method was evaluated across four types of execution: (1) correct exercise, (2) incorrect pose, (3) incomplete sequence, and (4) different exercise. In our work, we opted to classify performance into five categories: (1) Total Error, (2) Medium Error, (3) Average Execution, (4) Medium Accuracy, and (5) Total Accuracy. The authors concluded that their method could distinguish between different types of exercise executions and provide a reasonable exercise score. They concluded that this method presents a promising technique for evaluating simple exercises using human skeleton poses.

Work by Huang et al. [36] also proposed evaluating rehabilitation exercises through joint tracking in an intelligent system based on FL that was capable of tracking and quantifying joint-movement effectiveness in patients. The evaluation system was developed to address inaccuracies and uncertainties in joint movements. The inputs from joint movements were transformed into degrees of membership by projecting numerical input values into a set of membership functions using FL set inference.

After results were obtained with the FL system and compared with polynomial fitting performed earlier, an additional test was conducted to compare different machine learning methods: one based on evaluations from experts in resistance-exercise assessment (fuzzy) and one based solely on similarity related to maximum absolute deviation (using the same values for fitting presented in Figure 2). Thus, a regression model using SVM was employed. The RMSE and R-squared results displayed in Table 4 show that the linear and coarse Gaussian models yielded the best results. The coarse Gaussian model yielded an R-squared value of 0.81, which was superior to that of the linear model (0.72). The Pearson correlation coefficient was also calculated for the data obtained from the coarse Gaussian model and the observed data from original MH indices, yielding a value of 0.79.

A comparison of the initial quadratic fit with the FL model and the SVM models reveals that in terms of R-squared and Pearson correlation coefficients, both quadratic fit and FL models outperform SVM models. Both quadratic fit and FL models yielded R-squared values equal to 0.92 and correlation coefficients equal to 0.96, while the best SVM yielded an R-squared of 0.81 and a correlation coefficient of 0.79.

FL is particularly effective in dealing with uncertainties and variabilities in data. Unlike polynomial fitting, which assumes a precise and deterministic relationship between variables, as noted by Fouzia, Khenfer, and Boukezzoula [37], FL modelling allows for working with imprecise or vaguely defined information, better reflecting the complexity of human joint movements, which can be influenced by multiple nonlinear factors and complex interactions.

FL modelling offers a more flexible framework for capturing nonlinear relationships. These models can be adjusted for different conditions or contexts without the need to rewrite the underlying mathematical function. This is especially useful in biomedical applications, where data characteristics can vary significantly among individuals or situations [38].

The FL model, particularly the Takagi–Sugeno model, is considered a universal approximator and has proven to be very accurate in modelling nonlinear systems, often outperforming polynomial models in terms of accuracy and interpretability. Furthermore, the flexibility of FL models allows for better adaptation to uncertainties and nonlinearities compared to traditional polynomial models. Therefore, in many cases, the FL model may be more advantageous [39].

Regarding FL modelling and SVM, although it has already been shown that there are differences in RMSE and R-squared values that favour the FL model in this case, there are still additional advantages to the FL model over SVM for modelling human movement data. According to Apostolopoulos and colleagues [40], many practical applications related to the control and modelling of dynamic systems, such as human movements, often see FL-based systems outperform SVM. This is due to the ability of FL models to handle uncertainties and model complex relationships between variables, which is crucial in dynamic and nonlinear contexts like those associated with human movements, as corroborated by the work of Andújar and Zaitseva [38,39].

FL-based systems are particularly effective at capturing interactions and dependencies among different factors that influence human behaviour, allowing for more intuitive and interpretable modelling. Additionally, they can be easily adapted to include new information or variables, which is an advantage in dynamic environments where conditions can change rapidly. In contrast, while SVMs are powerful in classification and regression tasks, they may not be as effective at modelling complex dynamic relationships without significant pre-processing and careful feature selection [40]. Therefore, in contexts where modelling dynamic systems and interpreting relationships between variables are essential, FL models may be a superior choice compared to SVMs.

Besides this, the current study did not aim to design a universal reference movement for a biceps curl from which the model could recognize imperfections in performance by anyone (e.g., skilled or non-skilled subjects, subjects with disabilities) or dysfunctional executions. The findings apply only to the alteration of position from the beginning to the end of an exercise with a load increment. For example, the ascendent (lift) phase was considered essential in functional terms, since it is based on the ability of the contractile mechanisms of muscle to produce concentric torque; the muscles must be able to overcome resistance and perform the exercise with control of the degrees of instability (i.e., keeping load and body parts within the trajectory expected for the movement), therefore ensuring optimal performance and safety [41]. In addition, since the analysis of human movement by human observation is based on large-scale features, with a low level of detail (i.e., spatial accuracy and temporal resolution), the size of an alteration of movement that could be detected by visual examination is dependent on a priori knowledge of the type of movement or the viewpoint from which the movement is observed [42]. Moreover, advanced motor performance might show functional variability and that an experienced observer might judge these functional particularities to be qualitatively different [43]. Therefore, the support of an automated analysis applying a machine learning algorithm can improve correspondence among judges, assisting them in judging a movement when no body model is available. To that end, a direct relationship between execution and the reference motion must be established [44,45].

One limitation of the present method lies in the fact that it evaluates movement displacement in a two-dimensional (2D) manner. In contrast, three-dimensional (3D) analyses provide a more comprehensive view of movement across different planes, allowing for the assessment of changes in joint position that may occur to maintain proper posture under increased load. Moreover, a 3D model including the sagittal plane would provide more accurate data by avoiding parallax and perspective errors often associated with 2D analyses [8]. It is important to note, however, that the barbell bicep curl predominantly occurs in the sagittal plane rather than in the transverse and frontal planes. While the 3D approach presents advantages over 2D analysis, two-dimensional analyses like those conducted in this study still allow for movement evaluation using data obtained from any type of video recording. Other limitations are the small sample size, small number of evaluators, and low temporal recording resolution (30 Hz). Regarding the temporal resolution, it is important to note that the movement cadence was not high, so the 30 Hz video recording was probably sufficient to avoid loss of temporal positional data during the biceps curl. In addition, it is important to consider that the influence of frame resolution on automatized image analysis remains to be addressed. Finally, the expert visual analysis of variations in the trajectory of the movement may be a source of systematized error, since the level of correspondence between the different trajectories is associated with the accuracy of the cognitive representation of the movement pattern to be analysed [46]. Therefore, additional information on the movement to be analysed, such as might be collected via a third evaluator, detailed kinematics, and inertial information could contribute further insights on the features to be observed, hence improving confidence in the human analysis [42,44,47].

Future research should consider analysing individuals' movements across different planes beyond the sagittal plane using three-dimensional coordinates (3D). This approach will enable a more detailed investigation into the positional sequence of joints and objects while allowing for an expansion of the FL system beyond the results obtained through two-dimensional analysis. Furthermore, future studies using human expertise for visual examination of movement should try to minimize the sources of errors by assisting the observation process with the following: (i) more one independent evaluator, since alignment between three evaluators trends to increase confidence in the analysis; (ii) detailed kinematics information (e.g., relative and absolute angle-to-angle curves) regarding limb position and joint coordinate during the movement; and (iii) the inertial information (e.g., 3-D vectors of limb or barbell temporal and spatial parameters, as measured using accelerometer, gyroscope, and magnetometer signals) to quantitatively interpret the causes of movement alterations. Thus, modelling using FL presents itself as a promising tool to assist in diagnosing motor patterns, with applications ranging from identifying errors in movement execution during exercise to optimizing motor performance in athletes.

5. Conclusions

The results of the present study indicate that the MH similarity index can be utilized to identify changes in movement patterns due to increased load during the execution of the biceps-curl weight-lifting exercise. Furthermore, the indices provide sufficient information for modelling in automated exercise evaluation systems. It was observed that variations due to increased load in the horizontal axis are not significant for the biceps-curl weight-lifting exercise. The comparison between two machine learning models, FL and SVM, demonstrated the superiority of FL modelling in applications involving human movement. The analysis conducted here showed that an FL system can provide more accurate information about movement patterns than human visual observation. Since the work was carried out using standard video recordings on a smartphone, this highlights that the use of the FL model can be easily implemented on mobile devices, emphasizing the practicality of automated supervision for monitoring movement using smartphone cameras.

Author Contributions: Conceptualization, A.B.P. and D.M.P.F.; methodology, A.B.P. and D.M.P.F.; formal analysis, A.B.P., M.C.E. and D.M.P.F.; investigation, A.B.P., M.C.E. and D.M.P.F.; supervision, A.B.P. and D.M.P.F.; data curation, A.B.P., M.C.E., A.G.M., D.A.M. and D.M.P.F.; writing—original draft preparation, A.B.P., M.C.E., A.G.M., T.A.F.A., D.A.M., R.A.M.R., R.O., J.P.B. and D.M.P.F.; writing—review and editing, A.B.P., M.C.E., T.A.F.A., D.A.M., R.A.M.R., R.O., J.P.B., R.O. and D.M.P.F.; visualization, A.B.P., M.C.E., T.A.F.A., D.A.M., R.A.M.R., R.O., J.P.B., R.O. and D.M.P.F.; funding acquisition, M.C.E. and D.M.P.F. All authors have read and agreed to the published version of the manuscript.

Funding: This work was supported by the São Paulo Research Foundation (FAPESP), under Grant (number 2017/23717-9). This research was also funded by the Foundation for Science and Technology, I.P., Grant/Award Number UIDB/04748/2020 and by the Instituto Politécnico de Setúbal. R.O. and J.P.B. are research members of the Research Center in Sports Sciences, Health and Human Development (CIDESD) which was funded by National Funds by FCT-Foundation for Science and Technology under the following project UI/04045. The funders had no role in the design of the study; in the collection, analyses, or interpretation of data; in the writing of the manuscript, or in the decision to publish the results.

Institutional Review Board Statement: This study was conducted in accordance with the Declaration of Helsinki and was approved by the UNESP ethics committee under number 17486119.0.0000.5398.

Informed Consent Statement: All subjects signed an informed consent form prior to participation in the research.

Data Availability Statement: The data that support the findings of this study are available from the last author (dalton.pessoa-filho@unesp.br) upon reasonable request.

Acknowledgments: The author A.G.M. would like to thank the scholarship from the Brazilian Federal Agency for Support and Evaluation of Graduate Education (CAPES—Finance Code 001). The scholarship of the author T.A.F.A. was granted by the Brazilian Federal Agency for Support and Evaluation of Graduate Education (CAPES), in the scope of the Program CAPES-PrInt, process number 88887.310463/2018-00, Mobility number 88887.580265/2020-00. All the authors would like to thank the São Paulo Research Foundation (FAPESP—process 2017/23717-9) for the financial support, as well as the National Council for Scientific and Technological Development—CNPq (process: 150328/2024-9).

Conflicts of Interest: The authors declare no conflicts of interest.

References

1. Chavda, S.; Sandau, I.; Bishop, C.; Xu, J.; Turner, A.N.; Lake, J.P. Validity and Reliability of a Commercially Available Inertial Sensor for Measuring Barbell Mechanics During Weightlifting. *Appl. Sci.* **2024**, *14*, 7397. [CrossRef]
2. Gray, S.E.; Finch, C.F. The Causes of Injuries Sustained at Fitness Facilities Presenting to Victorian Emergency Departments—Identifying the Main Culprits. *Inj. Epidemiol.* **2015**, *2*, 6. [CrossRef] [PubMed]
3. Lu, Y.; Leng, X.; Yuan, H.; Jin, C.; Wang, Q.; Song, Z. Comparing the impact of personal trainer guidance to exercising with others: Determining the optimal approach. *Heliyon* **2024**, *10*, e24625. [CrossRef] [PubMed]
4. Collado-Mateo, D.; Lavín-Pérez, A.M.; Peñacoba, C.; Del Coso, J.; Leyton-Román, M.; Luque-Casado, A.; Gasque, P.; Fernández-Del-Olmo, M.Á.; Amado-Alonso, D. Key Factors Associated With Adherence to Physical Exercise in Patients with Chronic Diseases and Older Adults: An Umbrella Review. *Int. J. Environ. Res. Public Health* **2021**, *18*, 2023. [CrossRef] [PubMed]
5. Angosto, S.A.; García-Fernández, J.; Grimaldi-Puyana, M. A Systematic Review of Intention to Use Fitness Apps (2020–2023). *Humanit. Soc. Sci. Commun.* **2023**, *10*, 512. [CrossRef]
6. Werner, I.; Szelenczy, N.; Wachholz, F.; Federolf, P. How do movement patterns in weightlifting (clean) change when using lighter or heavier barbell loads? A Comparison of Two Principal Component Analysis-Based Approaches to Studying Technique. *Front Psychol.* **2021**, *11*, 606070. [CrossRef] [PubMed]
7. Zhao, X.; Ross, G.; Dowling, B.; Graham, R.B. Three-Dimensional Motion Capture Data of a Movement Screen from 183 Athletes. *Sci. Data* **2023**, *10*, 235. [CrossRef]
8. Peres, A.B.; Espada, M.C.; Santos, F.J.; Robalo, R.A.M.; Dias, A.A.P.; Muñoz-Jiménez, J.; Sancassani, A.; Massini, D.A.; Pessôa Filho, D.M. Accuracy of Hidden Markov Models in Identifying Alterations in Movement Patterns during Biceps-Curl Weight-Lifting Exercise. *Appl. Sci.* **2023**, *13*, 573. [CrossRef]
9. Peres, A.B.; Sancassani, A.; Castro, E.A.; Almeida, T.A.F.; Massini, D.A.; Macedo, A.G.; Espada, M.C.; Hernández-Beltrán, V.; Gamonales, J.M.; Pessôa Filho, D.M. Comparing Video Analysis to Computerized Detection of Limb Position for the Diagnosis of Movement Control during Back Squat Exercise with Overload. *Sensors* **2024**, *24*, 1910. [CrossRef]
10. Coates, W.; Wahlström, J. LEAN: Real-Time Analysis of Resistance Training Using Wearable Computing. *Sensors* **2023**, *23*, 4602. [CrossRef]
11. National Strength and Conditioning Association (NSCA). *Exercise Technique Manual for Resistance Training*; Human Kinetics: Champaign, IL, USA, 2022.
12. Horn, H.S. Measurement of "Overlap" in Comparative Ecological Studies. *Am. Nat.* **1966**, *100*, 419–424. [CrossRef]

13. Lim, C.H.; Vats, E.; Chan, C.S. Fuzzy human motion analysis: A review. *Pattern Recognit.* **2015**, *48*, 1773–1796. [CrossRef]
14. Zadeh, L.A. Fuzzy Sets. *Inf. Control* **1965**, *8*, 338–353. [CrossRef]
15. Wu, H.; Xu, Z. Fuzzy Logic in Decision Support: Methods, Applications and Future Trends. *Int. J. Comput. Commun. Control* **2020**, *16*, 4044. [CrossRef]
16. Ahmadi, H.; Gholamzadeh, M.; Shahmoradi, L.; Nilashi, M.; Rashvand, P. Diseases Diagnosis Using Fuzzy Logic Methods: A Systematic and Meta-Analysis Review. *Comput. Methods Programs Biomed.* **2018**, *161*, 145–172. [CrossRef]
17. Nguyen, P.; Ngoc, T. Hand Gesture Recognition Algorithm Using SVM and HOG Model for Control of Robotic System. *J. Robot.* **2021**, *2021*, 3986297. [CrossRef]
18. Bouteraa, Y.; Abdallah, I.B.; Boukthir, K. A New Wrist–Forearm Rehabilitation Protocol Integrating Human Biomechanics and SVM-Based Machine Learning for Muscle Fatigue Estimation. *Bioengineering* **2023**, *10*, 219. [CrossRef]
19. Surasak, T.; Praking, P.; Kitchat, K. Leveraging Support Vector Machine for Sports Injury Classification. In Proceedings of the 15th International Conference on Information Technology and Electrical Engineering (ICITEE), Chiang Mai, Thailand, 26–27 October 2023; pp. 234–238. [CrossRef]
20. Wang, Y. Research on the Construction of Human-Computer Interaction System Based on a Machine Learning Algorithm. *J. Sens.* **2022**, *2022*, 3817226. [CrossRef]
21. Guido, R.; Ferrisi, S.; Lofaro, D.; Conforti, D. An Overview on the Advancements of Support Vector Machine Models in Healthcare Applications: A Review. *Information* **2024**, *15*, 235. [CrossRef]
22. Carter, J.A.; Rivadulla, A.R.; Preatoni, E. A Support Vector Machine Algorithm Can Successfully Classify Running Ability When Trained with Wearable Sensor Data from Anatomical Locations Typical of Consumer Technology. *Sports Biomech.* **2022**, *23*, 2372–2389. [CrossRef]
23. Coratella, G.; Tornatore, G.; Longo, S.; Toninelli, N.; Padovan, R.; Esposito, F.; Cè, E. Biceps Brachii and Brachioradialis Excitation in Biceps Curl Exercise: Different Handgrips, Different Synergy. *Sports* **2023**, *11*, 64. [CrossRef] [PubMed]
24. Yang, T.H.; Wu, C.H.; Huang, K.Y. Coupled HMM-based Multimodal Fusion for Mood Disorder Detection Through Elicited Audio-visual Signals. *J. Ambient. Intell. Hum. Comput.* **2017**, *8*, 895–906. [CrossRef]
25. Zimmermann, M.; Ghazi, M.M.; Ekenel, H.K.; Thiran, J.P. Visual Speech Recognition Using PCA Networks and LSTMs in a Tandem GMM-HMM System. *Lect. Notes Comput. Sci.* **2017**, *10117*, 264–276. [CrossRef]
26. Wondershare Filmora. Available online: https://filmora.wondershare.com/pt-br/ (accessed on 15 March 2022).
27. Van Den Bergh, F.; Lalioti, V. Software Chroma Keying in an Immersive Virtual Environment: Research Article. *S. Afr. Comput. J.* **1999**, *24*, 155–162.
28. Matlani, P.; Shrivastava, M. Hybrid Deep VGG-net Convolutional Classifier for Video Smoke Detection. *Comput. Model. Eng. Sci.* **2019**, *119*, 427–458. [CrossRef]
29. Kinovea. Available online: https://www.kinovea.org/ (accessed on 20 May 2022).
30. IBM Brasil. Análise de Dados com Software SPSS—IBM Brasil. Available online: https://www.ibm.com/br-pt/analytics/spss-statistics-software (accessed on 6 August 2024).
31. MathWorks Inc. *MATLAB*, version R2024a; The MathWorks Inc.: Natick, MA, USA, 2024.
32. Coratella, G.; Tornatore, G.; Longo, S.; Esposito, F.; Cè, E. Bilateral Biceps Curl Shows Distinct Biceps Brachii and Anterior Deltoid Excitation Comparing Straight vs. EZ Barbell Coupled with Arms Flexion/No-Flexion. *J. Funct. Morphol. Kinesiol.* **2023**, *8*, 13. [CrossRef]
33. Petre, I.M.; Boscoianu, M.; Oancea, B.; Chicomban, M.; Turcu, I.; Simion, G. Analysis of the Physiognomy of Unique Sets in the Maximum Number of Repetitions Strategy—The Case of One-Arm Scott Machine Seated Bicep Curls. *Appl. Sci.* **2022**, *12*, 8308. [CrossRef]
34. Porz, N.; Knecht, U.; Sick, B.; Murina, E.; Barros, N.; Schucht, P.; Herrmann, E.; Gralla, J.; Wiest, R.; El-Koussy, M.; et al. Computer-Aided Radiological Diagnostics Improves the Preoperative Diagnoses of Medulloblastoma Pilocytic Astrocytoma and Ependymoma: A Reproducibility Study. *Clin. Transl. Neurosci.* **2018**, *2*, 2514183X18786602. [CrossRef]
35. Siow, C.Z.; Chin, W.H.; Kubota, N. Evaluating Simple Exercises with a Fuzzy System Based on Human Skeleton Poses. In Proceedings of the 2023 IEEE International Conference on Fuzzy Systems (FUZZ), Incheon, Republic of Korea, 13–17 August 2023; pp. 1–6. [CrossRef]
36. Huang, Y.P.; Kuo, W.L.; Basanta, H.; Lee, S.-H. Evaluating Power Rehabilitation Actions Using a Fuzzy Inference Method. *Int. J. Fuzzy Syst.* **2021**, *23*, 1919–1933. [CrossRef]
37. Fouzia, M.; Khenfer, N.; Boukezzoula, N.E. Robust Adaptive Tracking Control of Manipulator Arms with Fuzzy Neural Networks. *Eng. Technol. Appl. Sci. Res.* **2020**, *10*, 6131–6141. [CrossRef]
38. Zaitseva, E.; Levashenko, V.; Rabcan, J.; Kvassay, M. A New Fuzzy-Based Classification Method for Use in Smart/Precision Medicine. *Bioengineering* **2023**, *10*, 838. [CrossRef]
39. Andújar, J.M.; Barragán, A.J.; Vivas, F.J.; Enrique, J.M.; Segura, F. Iterative Nonlinear Fuzzy Modeling of Lithium-Ion Batteries. *Batteries* **2023**, *9*, 100. [CrossRef]

40. Apostolopoulos, I.D.; Papandrianos, N.I.; Papathanasiou, N.D.; Papageorgiou, E.I. Fuzzy Cognitive Map Applications in Medicine over the Last Two Decades: A Review Study. *Bioengineering* **2024**, *11*, 139. [CrossRef] [PubMed]
41. Reiser, R.F., II; Mackey, D.T.; Overman, J.W. Between the Beginning and End of a Repetition: How Intrinsic and Extrinsic Factors Influence the Intensity of a Biceps Curl. *Strength Cond. J.* **2007**, *29*, 64–76. [CrossRef]
42. Gavrila, D.M. The Visual Analysis of Human Movement: A Survey. *Comput. Vis. Image Underst.* **1999**, *73*, 82–98. [CrossRef]
43. Giblin, G.; Farrow, D.; Reid, M.; Ball, K.; Abernethy, B. Perceiving Movement Patterns: Implications for Skill Evaluation, Correction and Development [Percepción de los patrones de movimiento]. *Rev. Int. Cienc. Deporte* **2014**, *11*, 5–17. [CrossRef]
44. Poppe, R. Vision-Based Human Motion Analysis: An Overview. *Comput. Vis. Image Underst.* **2007**, *108*, 4–18. [CrossRef]
45. Aggarwal, J.K.; Cai, Q. Human Motion Analysis: A Review. *Comput. Vis. Image Underst.* **1999**, *73*, 428–440. [CrossRef]
46. Carroll, W.R.; Bandura, A. Role of timing of visual monitoring and motor rehearsal in observational learning of action patterns. *J. Mot. Behav.* **2013**, *17*, 269–281. [CrossRef] [PubMed]
47. O'Reilly, M.A.; Whelan, D.F.; Ward, T.E.; Delahunt, E.; Caulfield, B.M. Classification of deadlift biomechanics with wearable inertial measurement units. *J. Biomech.* **2017**, *58*, 155–161. [CrossRef]

Disclaimer/Publisher's Note: The statements, opinions and data contained in all publications are solely those of the individual author(s) and contributor(s) and not of MDPI and/or the editor(s). MDPI and/or the editor(s) disclaim responsibility for any injury to people or property resulting from any ideas, methods, instructions or products referred to in the content.

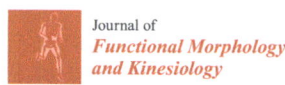 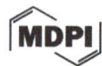

Brief Report

A Comparison of Paddle Forces between Whitewater and Flatwater Training in C1 Canoe Slalom

James M. Wakeling [1,*], Stanislava Smiešková [1], Matej Vajda [2] and Jan Busta [3]

[1] Department of Biomedical Physiology and Kinesiology, Simon Fraser University, Burnaby, BC V5A 1S6, Canada
[2] Hamar Institute for Human Performance, Faculty of Physical Education and Sports, Comenius University, 814 99 Bratislava, Slovakia; matej.vajda@gmail.com
[3] Faculty of Physical Education and Sport, Charles University, 110 00 Prague, Czech Republic; buster@centrum.cz
* Correspondence: wakeling@sfu.ca

Abstract: Background/Objectives: Becoming an elite canoe slalom athlete requires thousands of hours of training, spread over many years. It is difficult to assess the correct balance between flatwater and whitewater training because differences in the paddle forces on these terrains are not known. The aim of this study was to describe paddle forces during canoe slalom training on flatwater and whitewater courses for the C1 canoe category. Methods: Paddle forces for twenty C1 canoe slalom athletes were quantified during all-out figure-of-eight tests on a flatwater course and during race simulations on a whitewater course. Paddle forces were measured using strain gauges embedded in the paddle shaft and quantified by their force, impulse, and stroke durations. Results: The mean force during the pull phase of the paddle strokes was not significantly different between the flatwater and whitewater courses; however, the longer pull phase durations led to a greater pull phase impulse when paddling on the whitewater course. Conclusions: This study indicates that training for all-out runs on a whitewater course is more demanding for canoe slalom athletes than performing all-out trials on a flatwater figure-of-eight course. This evidence may help to develop effective training plans that are essential to reach the highest levels of the sport.

Keywords: canoe slalom; force; paddle; stroke; training

Citation: Wakeling, J.M.; Smiešková, S.; Vajda, M.; Busta, J. A Comparison of Paddle Forces between Whitewater and Flatwater Training in C1 Canoe Slalom. *J. Funct. Morphol. Kinesiol.* **2024**, *9*, 167. https://doi.org/10.3390/jfmk9030167

Academic Editor: Pedro Miguel Forte

Received: 7 August 2024
Revised: 3 September 2024
Accepted: 10 September 2024
Published: 17 September 2024

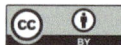

Copyright: © 2024 by the authors. Licensee MDPI, Basel, Switzerland. This article is an open access article distributed under the terms and conditions of the Creative Commons Attribution (CC BY) license (https://creativecommons.org/licenses/by/4.0/).

1. Introduction

Canoe slalom is an Olympic discipline in which athletes race down a whitewater course in the fastest time possible while having to negotiate a series of gates that are hung over the course. Some gates must be negotiated in a downstream direction and some in an upstream direction, and penalties are accrued for touching or missing the gates. Success in canoe slalom requires the ability to paddle a boat fast and to manoeuvre effectively and precisely through the turbulent water features in order to navigate a route through the gates.

Becoming an elite canoe slalom athlete requires an individual to undertake thousands of hours of training, spread over many years in the sport. The most important factor in performance is technique, especially the paddling technique. Performance tests performed on flatwater are highly correlated with race performance on whitewater [1,2]. However, in canoe slalom, the characteristics of straight paddling in terms of basic biomechanical parameters have still not been described sufficiently. Studies were always conducted on flatwater, focused on the kayaking category only [3,4] or aimed at studying asymmetries [5].

The description of both kinematic (paddling strokes: stroke rate, stroke length; boat acceleration; boat velocity: peak velocity, mean velocity) and kinetic (paddle forces: peak force, mean force, impulse) parameters influencing canoe slalom performance is still lacking, especially on whitewater and in the C1 category (canoe category where athletes kneel in the boat and use single-bladed paddle).

In canoe sprint (flatwater speed canoeing), the biomechanical parameters of paddling have been repeatedly investigated and described (e.g., [6–8]), but due to the completely different boats (slalom boats are shorter, slower, turn easier, and have greater hydrodynamic drag), significantly different values can be expected in canoe slalom on the flatwater and even more on the whitewater. Because we do not know the comparison of the forces acting on flatwater and whitewater, we often cannot objectively assess the correct balance between flatwater and whitewater training. Knowing these biomechanical indicators can help to develop an effective training plan which is essential to reach the highest levels of the sport, and this requires an understanding of the correct balance and effectiveness of training on flatwater and on whitewater terrains. We would hypothesise that even when athletes paddle all-out during flatwater or whitewater training, the additional complexity of paddling in whitewater will cause greater biomechanical demands during paddling.

Therefore, the aim of this study was to describe the biomechanical parameters of flatwater and whitewater paddling in men and women in the scientifically less-monitored C1 category.

2. Materials and Methods

This study is part of a larger project, with the flatwater methods and initial findings published elsewhere [6]. For this study, twenty C1 canoe slalom athletes were tested (13 males: age 22.0 ± 6.9 years, height 180.0 ± 5.2 m, weight 73.8 ± 8.3 kg; and 7 females: age 18.0 ± 3.4 years, height 168.4 ± 5.9 m, weight 60.4 ± 7.2 kg (mean $\pm$ standard deviation)). The athletes were mostly from the Czech junior and senior national teams, with several younger athletes from the local club also participating. Athletes were only considered if they were 15 years or older. All athletes trained regularly and competed internationally in the testing season. The younger athletes were in the Developmental to National level [9] and the older athletes were Elite to World-class [9], including 7 who had won medals at canoe slalom European Championships, World Championships, or Olympic Games. The athletes all provided oral consent to take part in the study, in accordance with requirements from the University Office of Research Ethics. Athlete testing occurred on flatwater and whitewater sections of the canoe slalom training facility at Roudnice na Labem in Czechia.

Athletes initially did their regular warm-up that included dry land stretching and at least 10 min of paddling (technical strokes, short bouts of speed and acceleration, and getting accustomed to the testing equipment). Athletes then paddled two sets of figure-of-eight time trials around two slalom poles that were part of two slalom gates that were hanging above the water; athletes had a 10 min rest between trials. Athlete times were started when their torso passed the first pole, they paddled nine lengths (from one pole to the other), turning to the left around the second pole, and then to the right around the first pole. The time was stopped when their torso passed the second pole at the end of the ninth length. Athletes then paddled 1 or 2 timed runs on the whitewater course (14 downstream and 6 upstream gates), with at least a 15 min rest before each run. The arrangement of gates on a slalom course is changed for every competition and is influenced by the water features at each specific site. For this study, a typical competition course was set by experienced canoe slalom coaches, with the goal of having the fastest time of about 90 s. The performance goal for each of these runs was to achieve the fastest time possible (including 2 s time penalties for touching the gates).

Details of the equipment calibration, data collection, and processing have been described elsewhere [5]. In brief, each athlete paddled their own boat and wore a high-speed satellite positioning system (10 Hz GPS and GLONAS systems, Glo 2, Garmin, Switzerland) strapped to their helmet to measure position and speed, and an inertial measurement unit (recording rate 25 Hz; MetamotionRL, Mbientlab, CA, USA) taped inside their boat to measure boat orientation and acceleration. Paddle forces were measured using strain gauges that were embedded in a spigot that was secured in the paddle shafts between the positions of the top and bottom hands (recording rate 100 Hz; Canoe Power Meter 2nd Gen., One Giant Leap, Nelson, New Zealand), and they were filmed using a 60 Hz video.

GPS data were recorded directly onto an Android phone placed in the cockpit, and the IMU and paddle data were stored on these respective devices and downloaded onto a computer after each test. The paddle was equipped with medium-sized blades (Revolution, G'Power, Opatowek, Poland). The strain gauges on the paddle were calibrated at the beginning of the study by hanging weights from the shaft [5] so that the force acting at the centre of the area of the paddle blade could be related to the strain in the paddle shaft and the hand position of the athlete ($r^2 > 0.99$).

All data processing was conducted in custom software (Wolfram Research, Inc., Mathematica version 13, Champaign, IL, USA). The baseline strain measurements for the paddles were taken as the mode of the recorded strains, and this is the typical strain during the out-of-water transition phase when the paddle is unloaded. Post-processing divided the data into individual paddle strokes. All types of paddle strokes (on-side or off-side and left or right) were pooled together. Paddle forces were quantified when their absolute force exceeded 60 N. Athletes sometimes used back sweep strokes for the upstream gates, which resulted in negative paddle forces; these strokes accounted for less than 1% of the paddle strokes and were excluded from further analysis. Paddle strokes were quantified by their mean paddle force [N] and impulse [N s] during the pull phase, the mean force [N] during the whole stroke cycle, the pull duration [s] (the time spent pulling on the paddle in the water during the paddle stroke), and the transition duration [s] (the time between the pull phases, most often with the paddle out of the water).

The paddle stroke parameters were visualized by their distributions (subdivided by athletes and flat/white water). For this visualization, the athletes were ranked by the median paddle force that they achieved on the flatwater course. The paddle stroke parameters were statistically evaluated by analysis of variance (ANOVA) using the SPSS version 27 statistical package. Flat/white water was included as a factor, and athlete was included as a random factor. Effects were deemed to be statistically significant at the $p < 0.05$ level. The paddle stroke parameters are described by their estimated marginal means (with standard error of the mean) that emerged from these ANOVAs.

3. Results

The mean time to complete the flatwater course was 97.45 ± 7.18 s (mean ± s.d.) and for the whitewater course was 103.41 ± 11.23 s (raw time, not including penalties); the times were not significantly different between the flatwater and whitewater courses. A total of 2106 paddle strokes were measured for the flatwater tests, and 1927 strokes for the whitewater tests (Figures 1 and 2).

The mean force during the pull phase of the paddle strokes was not significantly different between the flatwater and whitewater courses: 138.0 ± 0.57 N and 137.7 ± 0.59 N, respectively. However, there was a significant difference in the duration of the pull phase: 0.48 ± 0.007 s for the flatwater and 0.61 ± 0.007 s for the whitewater course. This led to a significantly lower impulse for the pull phase of 68.8 ± 1.05 N s for the flatwater than 87.2 ± 1.09 for the whitewater course.

The transition duration (between the pull phases) was not significantly different between the flatwater and whitewater courses: 0.45 ± 0.005 s and 0.44 ± 0.005 s, respectively. Thus, the pull phase was a smaller proportion of the whole stroke cycle for the flatwater course, resulting in a lower mean force for the whole stroke cycle of 73.2 ± 0.64 N for the flatwater compared to 81.8 ± 0.66 N for the whitewater course. The paddle stroke frequency (calculated from the combined pull and transition durations) was 1.08 Hz for the flatwater course and 0.95 Hz for the whitewater course.

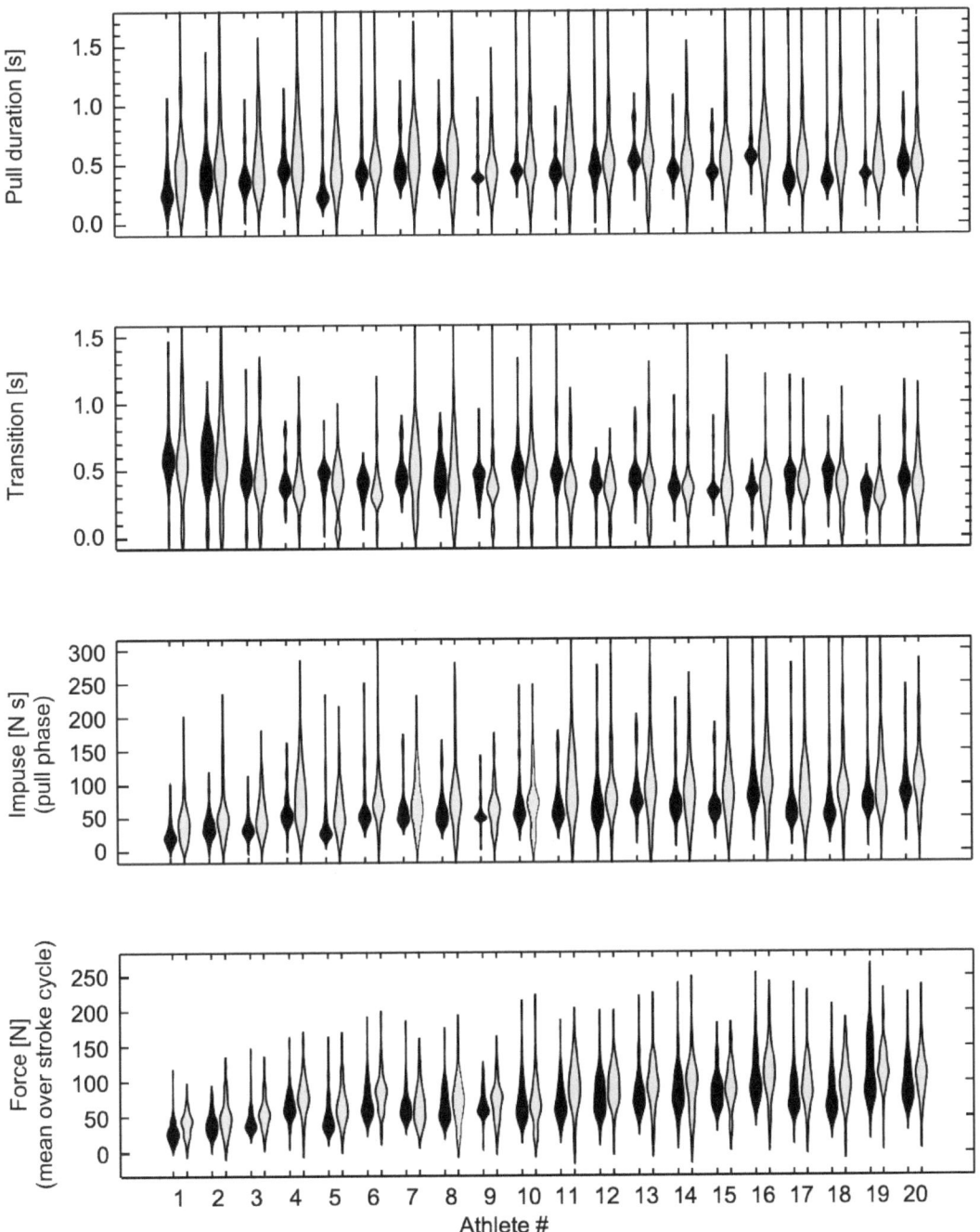

Figure 1. Distribution of pull duration, transition time, impulse, and paddle force for the twenty athletes. Strokes for flatwater training are shown in black, and those for whitewater training are in grey.

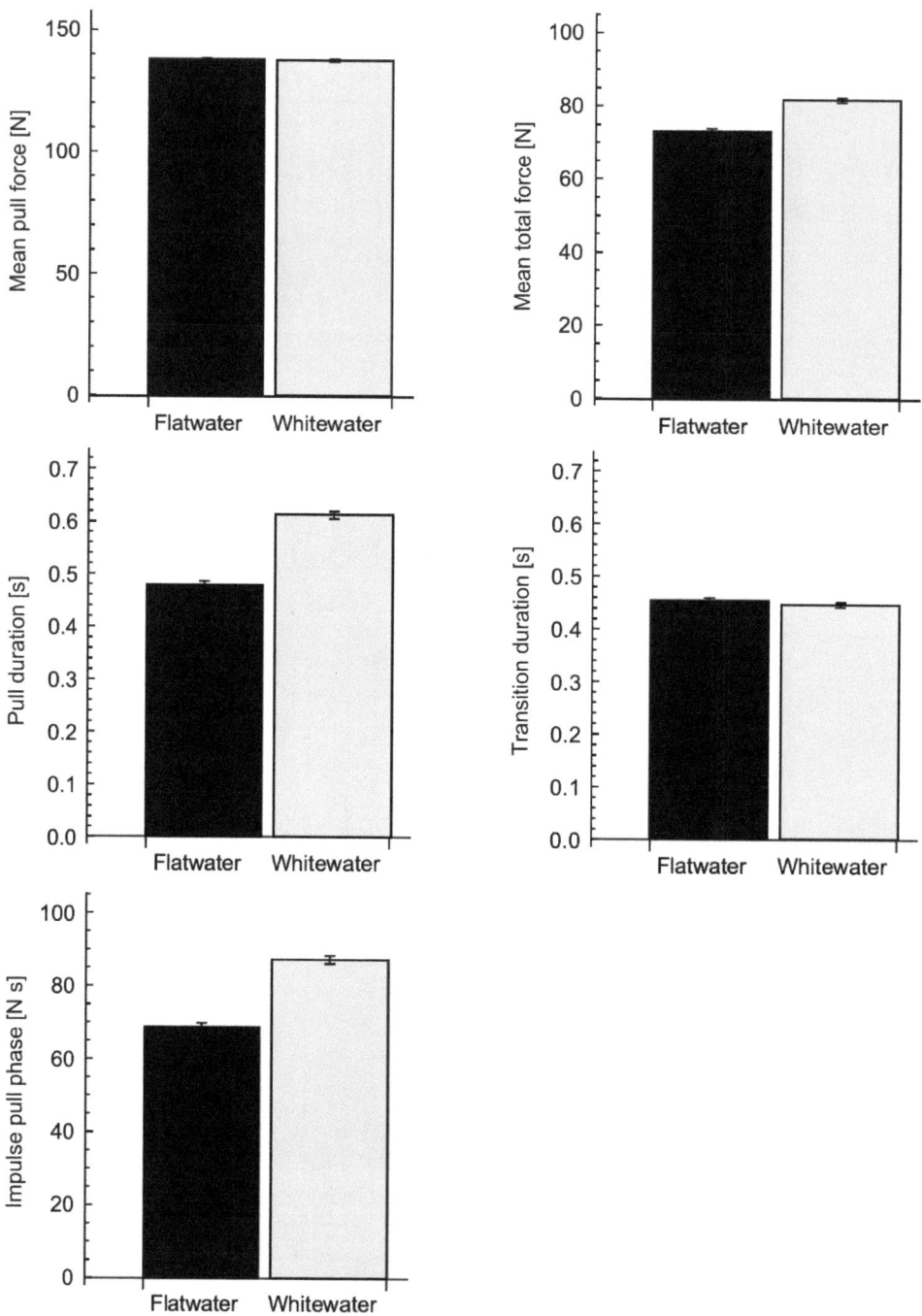

Figure 2. Mean stroke parameters (with standard error of mean). Strokes for flatwater training are shown in black, and those for whitewater training are in grey.

4. Discussion

Comparison of athletes' metabolic energy sources between straight flatwater and slalom whitewater paddling showed that the energy sources (aerobic versus anaerobic) were remarkably similar, but the absolute metabolic energy costs are difficult to compare due to energy requirement being neither maximal nor constant during whitewater slalom paddling [10]. The mechanical power output during flatwater slalom tests has been determined by using sensors to measure the force, angular velocity, and acceleration in the paddle shaft [3]; however, the mechanical power on whitewater additionally depends on the water velocity, which varies continuously throughout a whitewater slalom course, and so comparisons of mechanical power between flatwater and whitewater courses cannot be made using only such equipment. In this study, we report the mean paddle force and pull phase impulse that are measured from instrumented paddle shafts. These parameters have previously been reported for slalom paddling [3–5,11] and can be directly compared between flatwater and whitewater situations.

The female athletes completed run times that were on average 9% slower than the male times. We previously reported [5] that the (flatwater) paddle forces from this study were lower for female athletes and increased with athlete age (that is partly a proxy of experience). Nonetheless, the median paddle forces for each athlete in this report showed a coefficient of determination $r^2 = 0.94$ between the flatwater and whitewater scenarios. Thus, athletes with strong paddle forces on flatwater likely also produce strong paddle forces on whitewater, regardless of their sex, age, or experience (Figure 1).

Even though the flatwater course involved both straight sections and turning around gates, the whitewater course was technically more complex due to the addition of the moving water. The athletes would have to continuously negotiate through whitewater features (waves, stoppers, and current differentials) and this requires a more complex set of paddle strokes. Despite this complexity, we found that the mean paddle forces during the pull phase of each stroke were similar for the flatwater and whitewater courses (Figures 1 and 2). The duration of the pull phase was significantly longer for the whitewater course (Figures 1 and 2). In order to accomplish the myriad of different moves on a whitewater course, canoe slalom athletes mostly use a range of turning and blended strokes, which have longer durations than forward strokes [12]. The longer pull phase durations combined with the similar paddle forces resulted in a greater impulse being applied during each pull phase. The transition durations between the pull phases of each stroke were not significantly different between the flatwater and whitewater courses, and thus the longer pull durations occupied a larger proportion of the whole stroke duration for whitewater; this can be termed the duty cycle. Thus, the mean paddle force was greater when expressed over the whole stroke cycle for the whitewater course (Figure 2).

In this study, whitewater testing was always conducted after flatwater testing, leading to a potential bias for fatigue-based reductions in performance on the whitewater courses. Despite this, the mean paddle forces in the drive phase were not reduced, and indeed the overall mean force was higher on the whitewater courses due to the greater duty cycles. Additionally, athletes must endure the additional stress and challenge of the varying water features and currents when on a whitewater course. Successfully negotiating whitewater courses requires additional technical and psychological skills to manage the challenging water conditions; indeed, flatwater performance becomes less of a predictor of whitewater performance as the water difficulty increases [2] and these additional demands become more prominent.

A limitation of this study is that it used one instrumented paddle for all athletes. The length of the paddle was adjusted to be the same as the athlete's regular paddle; however, the paddle may have had a different blade size, mass, and profile than the athlete's own paddle (for instance, the instrumentation added 33 g to the mass of the paddle). Thus, the paddle may have been more similar to some athletes' paddles than to others. This aspect of the paddle performance would contribute to variance in the subject factor used in the ANOVA. However, the main effects of the type of water are independent of this factor and would be largely insensitive to the influence of the paddle. Additionally, all the other parts of the athlete's equipment were their own, and the testing sessions were kept as realistic as possible.

5. Conclusions

During canoe slalom training on all-out trials in a C1 canoe, a greater impulse is used for paddle strokes on whitewater compared to flatwater. This finding suggests that training for all-out runs on a whitewater course is more demanding for canoe slalom athletes than performing all-out trials on a flatwater figure-of-eight course. This provides more support for the suggestion that athletes and coaches should consider the importance of training and preparation races, in advance of important competitions, on whitewater terrain, particularly on water difficulty that resembles where the competitions will be held [2].

Author Contributions: Conceptualization, J.M.W. and S.S.; methodology, J.M.W. and S.S.; software, J.M.W.; validation, J.M.W.; formal analysis, J.M.W.; investigation, J.M.W.; resources, J.M.W., S.S., M.V. and J.B.; data curation, J.M.W.; writing—original draft preparation, J.M.W. and J.B.; writing—review and editing, J.M.W., S.S., M.V. and J.B.; visualization, J.M.W.; supervision, J.M.W.; project administration, J.M.W. and S.S.; funding acquisition, J.M.W. and M.V. All authors have read and agreed to the published version of the manuscript.

Funding: This research was funded by an NSERC of Canada Discovery Grant to JW (RGPIN/7015-2020), and VEGA of Slovakia for financial support to MV (#1/0573/22).

Institutional Review Board Statement: This study was conducted in accordance with the Declaration of Helsinki, and approved by the Ethics Committee of Simon Fraser University (protocol code (#30000761, approved: 21 December 2021).

Informed Consent Statement: Informed consent was obtained from all subjects involved in the study.

Data Availability Statement: The original contributions presented in the study are included in the article, further inquiries can be directed to the corresponding author.

Acknowledgments: We thank the custodians of the slalom course at Roudnice-nad-Labem for the use of their facilities. We thank Felix Krupa, Jaylene Pratt, and Hannah Wood for technical assistance with the data collection.

Conflicts of Interest: The authors declare no conflicts of interest. The funders had no role in the design of the study; in the collection, analyses, or interpretation of data; in the writing of the manuscript; or in the decision to publish the results.

References

1. Baláš, J.; Busta, J.; Bílý, M.; Martin, A. Technical skills testing of elite slalom canoeists as a predictor of competition performance. *Int. J. Perform. Anal. Sport* **2020**, *20*, 870–878. [CrossRef]
2. Vajda, M.; Piatrikova, E. Relationship between flat-water tests and canoe slalom performance on 4 different grades of water terrain difficulty. *Int. J. Sports Physiol. Perform.* **2022**, *17*, 185–194. [CrossRef] [PubMed]
3. Macdermid, P.W.; Fink, P.W. The Validation of a Paddle Power Meter for Slalom Kayaking. *Sports Med. Int. Open* **2017**, *1*, E50–E57. [CrossRef] [PubMed] [PubMed Central]
4. Macdermid, P.W.; Olazabal, T. The relationship between stroke metrics, work rate and performance in slalom kayakers. *Biomechanics* **2022**, *2*, 31–43. [CrossRef]
5. Wakeling, J.M.; Smiešková, S.; Pratt, J.S.; Vajda, M.; Busta, J. Asymmetries in paddle force influence choice of stroke type for canoe slalom athletes. *Front. Physiol.* **2023**, *14*, 1227871. [CrossRef]
6. Gomes, B.B.; Ramos, N.V.; Conceição, F.A.V.; Sanders, R.H.; Vaz, M.A.; Vilas-Boas, J.P. Paddling Force Profiles at Different Stroke Rates in Elite Sprint Kayaking. *J. Appl. Biomech.* **2015**, *31*, 258–263. [CrossRef] [PubMed]
7. Nilsson, J.E.; Rosdahl, H.G. Contribution of Leg-Muscle Forces to Paddle Force and Kayak Speed During Maximal-Effort Flat-Water Paddling. *Int. J. Sports Physiol. Perform.* **2016**, *11*, 22–27. [CrossRef] [PubMed]
8. Gomes, B.B.; Ramos, N.V.; Conceição, F.A.V.; Sanders, R.H.; Vaz, M.A.; Vilas-Boas, J.P. Paddling time parameters and paddling efficiency with the increase in stroke rate in kayaking. *Sports Biomech.* **2022**, *21*, 1303–1311. [CrossRef] [PubMed]
9. McKay, A.K.; Stellingwerff, T.; Smith, E.S.; Martin, D.T.; Mujika, I.; Goosey-Tolfrey, V.L.; Sheppard, J.; Burke, L.M. Defining Training and Performance Caliber: A Participant Classification Framework. *Int. J. Sports Physiol. Perform.* **2022**, *17*, 317–331. [CrossRef] [PubMed]

10. Zamparo, P.; Tomadini, S.; Didonè, F.; Grazzina, F.; Rejc, E.; Capelli, C. Bioenergetics of a slalom kayak (k1) competition. *Int. J. Sports Med.* **2006**, *27*, 546–552. [CrossRef] [PubMed]
11. Macdermid, P.W.; Gilbert, C.; Jayes, J. Using a kayak paddle power-meter in the sport of whitewater slalom. *J. Hum. Sport Exerc.* **2020**, *15*, 105–118. [CrossRef]
12. Hunter, A.; Cochrane, J.; Sachlikidis, A. Canoe slalom competition analysis. *Sports Biomech.* **2008**, *7*, 24–37. [CrossRef] [PubMed]

Disclaimer/Publisher's Note: The statements, opinions and data contained in all publications are solely those of the individual author(s) and contributor(s) and not of MDPI and/or the editor(s). MDPI and/or the editor(s) disclaim responsibility for any injury to people or property resulting from any ideas, methods, instructions or products referred to in the content.

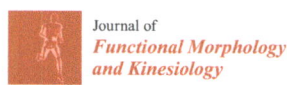

Article

Upper-Limb Muscle Fatigability in Para-Athletes Quantified as the Rate of Force Development in Rapid Contractions of Submaximal Amplitude

Gennaro Boccia [1,2], Paolo Riccardo Brustio [1,2,*], Luca Beratto [2,3], Ilaria Peluso [4], Roberto Ferrara [5], Diego Munzi [6], Elisabetta Toti [4], Anna Raguzzini [4], Tommaso Sciarra [5,6] and Alberto Rainoldi [3,4]

[1] Department of Clinical and Biological Sciences, University of Turin, 10043 Turin, Italy; gennaro.boccia@unito.it
[2] Neuromuscular Function Research Group, School of Exercise and Sport Science, University of Turin, 10126 Turin, Italy; luca.beratto@unito.it
[3] Department of Medical Sciences, University of Turin, 10126 Turin, Italy; alberto.rainoldi@unito.it
[4] Research Centre for Food and Nutrition (CREA-AN), 00178 Rome, Italy; ilaria.peluso@crea.gov.it (I.P.); elisabetta.toti@crea.gov.it (E.T.); anna.raguzzini@crea.gov.it (A.R.)
[5] Rehabilitation Medicine Department, Italian Army Medical Hospital, 00143 Rome, Italy; robertoferrara85@gmail.com (R.F.); sciarratommaso@hotmail.com (T.S.)
[6] Joint Veteran Defence Center, 00184 Rome, Italy; diego.munzi@gmail.com
* Correspondence: paoloriccardo.brustio@unito.it

Citation: Boccia, G.; Brustio, P.R.; Beratto, L.; Peluso, I.; Ferrara, R.; Munzi, D.; Toti, E.; Raguzzini, A.; Sciarra, T.; Rainoldi, A. Upper-Limb Muscle Fatigability in Para-Athletes Quantified as the Rate of Force Development in Rapid Contractions of Submaximal Amplitude. *J. Funct. Morphol. Kinesiol.* **2024**, *9*, 108. https://doi.org/10.3390/jfmk9020108

Academic Editor: Pedro Miguel Forte

Received: 29 April 2024
Revised: 13 June 2024
Accepted: 14 June 2024
Published: 20 June 2024

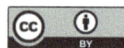

Copyright: © 2024 by the authors. Licensee MDPI, Basel, Switzerland. This article is an open access article distributed under the terms and conditions of the Creative Commons Attribution (CC BY) license (https://creativecommons.org/licenses/by/4.0/).

Abstract: This study aimed to compare neuromuscular fatigability of the elbow flexors and extensors between athletes with amputation (AMP) and athletes with spinal cord injury (SCI) for maximum voluntary force (MVF) and rate of force development (RFD). We recruited 20 para-athletes among those participating at two training camps (2022) for Italian Paralympic veterans. Ten athletes with SCI (two with tetraplegia and eight with paraplegia) were compared to 10 athletes with amputation (above the knee, N = 3; below the knee, N = 6; forearm, N = 1). We quantified MVF, RFD at 50, 100, and 150 ms, and maximal RFD (RFDpeak) of elbow flexors and extensors before and after an incremental arm cranking to voluntary fatigue. We also measured the RFD scaling factor (RFD-SF), which is the linear relationship between peak force and peak RFD quantified in a series of ballistic contractions of submaximal amplitude. SCI showed lower levels of MVF and RFD in both muscle groups (all p values ≤ 0.045). Despite this, the decrease in MVF (Cohen's d = 0.425, $p < 0.001$) and RFDpeak (d = 0.424, $p = 0.003$) after the incremental test did not show any difference between pathological conditions. Overall, RFD at 50 ms showed the greatest decrease (d = 0.741, $p < 0.001$), RFD at 100 ms showed a small decrease (d = 0.382, $p = 0.020$), and RFD at 150 ms did not decrease ($p = 0.272$). The RFD-SF decreased more in SCI than AMP ($p < 0.0001$). Muscle fatigability impacted not only maximal force expressions but also the quickness of ballistic contractions of submaximal amplitude, particularly in SCI. This may affect various sports and daily living activities of wheelchair users. Early RFD (i.e., ≤ 50 ms) was notably affected by muscle fatigability.

Keywords: explosive strength; fatigability; sport; disability

1. Introduction

Manual wheelchair use involves many physical challenges for the upper limbs, mainly because of rapid force requirements and prolonged usage resulting in neuromuscular fatigue [1]. Additionally, the inefficiency of manual wheelchair propulsion as a mode of ambulation has been highlighted; indeed, in comparison to the legs, arm work is less efficient and more strenuous, resulting in a diminished physical capacity [2]. Neuromuscular fatigue due to extended wheelchair use may result in muscle coordination changes with a shift in joint power from the shoulder joint to the elbow [3]. This may result in excessive strain on elbow flexors and extensor muscles.

Neuromuscular fatigue is commonly evaluated as the exercise-induced decline in a muscle's maximal force-generating capacity. The most widely used indicator is the isometric maximal voluntary contraction force (MVF) [4]. MVF is calculated over 3 to 5 s maximal isometric contractions. However, in sports and the daily living of para-athletes, such prolonged contractions are likely never adopted. This lack of task specificity could lead to an inaccurate estimation of the magnitude of neuromuscular fatigue.

In addition to MVF, the rate of force development (RFD) has recently gained popularity as a measure of explosive strength in various contexts. RFD is calculated from the ascending part of the force–time curve during an explosive contraction, either as a mean time-locked value or a maximal slope of force signal (RFDpeak). This measure has been studied extensively [5,6], and it is more functionally relevant than pure maximal strength [7,8]. RFD has been shown to be more sensitive than MVF in detecting chronic changes caused by factors such as disuse [9], strength training [10], and rehabilitation [11], as well as acute adjustments associated with exercise [12], muscle damage [13], and pain [14]. RFD, especially early RFD ($\leq$50 ms), has been suggested to be largely influenced by neural mechanisms, mainly in relation to motor unit behaviour [15]. This physiological feature of RFD may explain why this variable is often more sensitive to changes than MVF [16], especially when the fatiguing task comprises rapid force production [17]. The analysis of muscle excitation in the first 50 ms of contraction employing high-density electromyography (HD-EMG) might provide even more insights into the causes of possible decrement of early RFD [17–19].

In this context, the protocol normally used to calculate RFD in submaximal amplitude contractions is the so-called RFD scaling factor (RFD-SF) [20–23]. The protocol consists of a series of fast, i.e., burst-like, contractions performed at different sub-maximal intensities (i.e., from 20 to 80% MVF) [24–26]. This means the participants aim to reach a submaximal force level as rapidly as possible. Such motor tasks mimic, in isometric conditions, the brief muscle excitation profiles typically observed in locomotion [27,28]. The adoption of RFD-SF has emerged as an informative measure to quantify the neuromuscular quickness of submaximal contractions [20,29–31]. For these reasons, we consider it more appropriate to detect muscle fatigability in real-life conditions [32].

This study aimed to compare neuromuscular fatigability of the elbow flexors and extensors between athletes with amputation (AMP, being above the knee, below the knee, or at the level of the forearm) and athletes with spinal cord injury (SCI, either paraplegia or tetraplegia) for maximum isometric muscle strength and RFD, and between time intervals for RFD and electromyographic signal amplitude. Comparing SCI and AMP para-athletes will help foster a more comprehensive understanding of disability sport performance, leading to better support, training, equipment, and inclusivity for athletes of all abilities.

2. Materials and Methods

2.1. Recruitment and Characteristics of Athletes

The study was conducted in accordance with the Declaration of Helsinki, and the protocol was approved by the Ethics Committee of the Italian Army Medical Hospital. All participants read and signed the informed consent form and knew they could withdraw at any time. A convenience sample of 20 athletes (10 with AMP and 10 with SCI) participating in two training camps (May and September 2022, Jesolo) for Italian Paralympic veterans was recruited for this study. The presence of SCI or AMP was applied as inclusion criteria. Data characterising the volunteers was collected through questionnaires [33]. The Joint Veteran Defence Center, Scientific Department, Army Medical Center, Rome, Italy, provided the health condition of each athlete. The main characteristics of athletes are depicted in Table 1. Wheelchair users typically adopted manual wheelchairs with propulsion assist devices in their leisure time.

Table 1. Characteristics of athletes.

	AMP	SCI
Age, years	43.3 ± 2.8	44.6 ± 3.4
Lesion level (incomplete for SCI, prosthesis for AMP)	Above knee, n = 3 Below knee, n = 6 Forearm, n = 1 Wheelchair users (2/10)	Tetraplegia (C6-C7), n = 3 Paraplegia (T7-T12), n = 7 Wheelchair users (10/10)
Sport practiced	Athletics, Basketball, Cycling, Sitting volleyball, Swimming, Tennis	Athletics, Archery, Hand-bike, Sitting Volleyball, Swimming, Power Soccer
Training/h week	5.3 ± 0.9	5.2 ± 1.0
Television/h week	12.0 ± 3.6	11.8 ± 2.6
Screening/h week	27.9 ± 7.7	22.4 ± 4.1
Sleeping/h day	7.1 ± 0.3	7.6 ± 0.2
Neurogenic bowel, %	-	40%
Neurogenic bladder, %	-	40%

AMP: athletes with amputation, SCI: athletes with a spinal cord injury.

2.2. Anthropometric Measurements

Body mass was measured on an electronic scale with an accuracy of 0.01 kg (Wunder RW 02, Trezzo sull'Adda, Italy) and calculated by subtracting the weight of the wheelchair/prosthesis and clothes (weighted separately) from total mass.

2.3. Neuromuscular Function Evaluation

2.3.1. Setup

The participants utilised an identical setup to that previously employed by the authors [34]. In summary, the athletes with AMP were seated on a chair while athletes with SCI were seated on their wheelchair. All participants had their right arm flexed at a 90° angle from full extension and slightly abducted from the trunk (approximately 15°). The wrist was immobilised using non-elastic straps and a custom-built telescopic support. A strain gauge load cell (Model TF 022, CCt transducers, Turin, Italy) was connected to record compression and extension forces. The hand and forearm were positioned neutrally, and real-time visual feedback was displayed on a 48 cm × 27 cm computer screen. The force and EMG signals were sampled at a rate of 2048 Hz and converted to digital data using a 16-bit A/D converter (Sessantaquattro, OT Bioelettronica, Turin, Italy).

2.3.2. High-Density Surface Electromyography

Two bidimensional HD-sEMG matrices of 32 electrodes each (4 rows × 8 columns, 8 mm inter-electrode distance, gold-coated; model: GR08MM0805, OT Bioelettronica, Turin, Italy) were placed over the right upper limb. The first was placed over the long head of the biceps brachii, and the second over the later head of the triceps brachii [35]. The reference electrode (24 mm, model: CDE-S. OT Bioelettronica, Turin, Italy) was placed on the acromion of the same limb; a strap ground electrode, dampened with water, was placed around the wrist. Before the array application, the skin was prepared to remove body hair, slightly abraded with an abrasive paste, and finally cleaned with water [36].

To ensure proper electrode–skin contact, the electrode cavities of the matrices were filled with 20–30 lL of conductive paste (Spes-Medica, Battipaglia, Italy). The electrode arrays were fixed with an extensible dressing. The EMG signals were amplified (gain 150), sampled at 2048 Hz, bandpass filtered (20–450 Hz, Butterworth 4th order) and converted to digital data with a 16-bit A/D converter (Sessantaquattro; OT Bioelettronica, Turin, Italy). Signals, in single-differential configuration, were visualised during acquisition and then stored on a personal computer using OT BioLab+ software version 1.5.5.0 (OT Bioelettronica, Turin, Italy) for further analysis.

2.3.3. Procedures

The experimenters paid particular attention to avoiding movement in the torso and shoulders during the execution of contractions. Additionally, participants were instructed to avoid activating their trapezius muscles during elbow flexion and leaning their body forward during elbow extension. All test sessions were conducted by the same investigators, and participants were given standardised verbal encouragement during the execution of maximal voluntary and rapid contractions.

The protocol started with a warm-up comprising 10 submaximal isometric contractions ranging from 20% to 80% of the perceived maximum force and the familiarisation with ballistic contractions (details to follow). Then, participants performed two maximal voluntary isometric contractions and the RFD-SF protocol before (PRE) and immediately after (POST) a graded arm cranking test, until task failure. The POST session started on average 3 ± 1 min after the end of the graded test.

To measure MVF at PRE, two 5 s maximal voluntary contractions were performed if the difference in MVF between the two trials was greater than 5%.

The RFD-SF protocol (Figure 1, left panel) began two minutes after the last maximal voluntary contractions. The original RFD-SF protocol requires the performance of 125 ballistic (burst-like, see Figure 1, right panel) isometric contractions across a full range of submaximal amplitudes [29]. The study utilised a shortened version of the original protocol, which consisted of at least 36 contractions and demonstrated reliable results [37]. Participants were instructed to perform 12 ballistic isometric contractions, interspersed by 5 s, at 20%, 40%, 60%, and 80% of their MVF, totalling 48 contractions. The levels of force required were randomised between participants and kept withing participants between PRE and POST. They were required to produce rapid contractions with peak forces reaching approximately $\pm 10\%$ of the target force. Each pulse was controlled by standardised acoustic cues. If a ballistic isometric contraction was not performed correctly, it was repeated. No changes in content were made. The computer screen displayed the range force as a horizontal band with a width of 20% MVF. Participants were instructed to perform each isometric torque pulse as quickly as possible and then relax immediately. The focus was on the speed of the contraction rather than the precision.

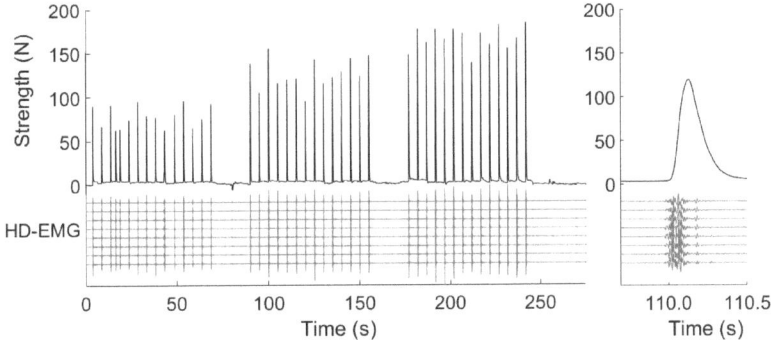

Figure 1. In the left panel, the upper part of the graph shows a representative example of the force signal recorded during the evaluation of the elbow extensor muscles of an amputee subject. The lower part of the graph shows the electromyographic (HD-EMG) signals from one of the four columns of electrodes that are part of the array placed on the triceps brachii (lateral head). In the right panel, the magnification of one repetition is plotted. As can be seen, the active phase of the muscle contraction lasts about 200 ms.

2.4. Incremental Arm-Cranking Graded Test

Athletes used an incremental graded arm-cranking ergometer to voluntary fatigue [23,24]. The purpose of the graded test was only to induce muscle fatigability; however, cardiorespiratory measurements were obtained using the wearable metabolic system K5 metabolimeter

(COSMED, Rome, Italy) and under continuous heart rate monitoring (data not presented herein).

2.5. Signal Processing

2.5.1. Onset Determination and Time Windows

The signal processing was performed using custom-written software in MATLAB (ver. 2023a, he MathWorks Inc., Natick, MA, USA). Force onsets were automatically detected through a hand-customised MATLAB code [7,38]. In the case that contractions presented countermovement or pretension, they were removed from the analysis. On average, no more than 3 contractions were removed from voluntary contraction at each time point (i.e., PRE and POST) for each subject. The EMG time windows were calculated from EMG onset, whilst force time windows were calculated from force onset. Therefore, EMG and force time windows (i.e., the windows of 50, 100, and 150 ms) were shifted by the time difference between EMG and force onsets (i.e., electromechanical delay), which we arbitrarily set to 15 ms based on previous studies on voluntary contractions [17].

2.5.2. Force Signal

The force signals were low-pass filtered at 100 Hz using a fourth-order zero-lag Butterworth. MVF was measured from the 5 s maximum voluntary contractions, and it was defined as the highest force over the two trials performed at PRE and the single trial performed at POST. All RFD parameters were calculated from the burst-like contractions of the RFD-SF protocol. RFD (Δforce/Δtime) was estimated at 50, 100, and 150 ms (defined as RFD50, RFD100, RFD150). Maximum RFD (RFDpeak) was calculated as the maximum first derivative of the force signal from the onset of contraction using a 20 ms moving average window [39].

To calculate the RFD-SF, the force signal was pre-processed using an overlapping moving window of 0.1 s [20,32,40]. The use of a moving window was preferred over a 5 Hz low-pass filter to avoid introducing aberrations in the signals, which are typically evident as a force signal below zero just before the onset of contraction. Next, the RFD signal was obtained by computing the first derivative of the force signal. The peak force and RFDpeak (the local maximum of the RFD signal) were determined for each ballistic contraction. The RFD-SF was calculated by determining the linear regression slope between peak force and peak RFD for each contraction. RFD-SF measures how RFD scales with force in a range of submaximal contractions, providing a quantification of quickness across a span of intensities. Outliers were identified and removed using the Cook distance methodology to improve the fit of the linear regression [41].

2.5.3. High-Density Surface Electromyography

EMG channels with excessive noise or artefacts were removed after visual analysis. Then, we identified the innervation zone for each matrix of electrodes and selected the channels with propagating action potentials. Single-differential EMG signals were calculated for each column and visually inspected. Four to eight single-differential EMG channels with clear motor unit action potential propagation without shape change from the nearest innervation zone to the distal tendon were chosen for the analysis.

The amplitude of voluntary HD-sEMG signals was assessed as the root mean square (RMS) across all available channels. RMS calculated at 50, 100, and 150 ms from EMG onset (defined as RMS50, RMS100, RMS150) was then averaged across channels to obtain a single value for each muscle. This procedure produces more reliable results in voluntary and evoked contractions [42].

2.6. Statistical Analysis

Statistical analysis was performed in R (ver. 3.5.2, R Development Core Team, 2009) and JASP (JASP team, version 0.18.3). First, we adopted a series of repeated-measure ANOVAs to compare the trend of each mechanical and EMG variable in time (PRE vs. POST), between conditions (SCI vs. AMP), and between time intervals (50, 100, and 150 ms).

Then, to answer the main experimental question, we analysed the peakRFD with multilevel mixed linear regression analysis through the package lme4 Version 1.1.19. Linear mixed-effects models are particularly suitable in this experimental design, as participants performed dozens of contractions with each muscle group, and the model accounts for such a hierarchical data structure. We adopted the peak force reached in each contraction, time (PRE vs. POST), muscle group (elbow flexors vs. extensors), and condition (SCI vs. AMP) as fixed factors, and we considered the random intercept over participants and the random slope of muscle group (as each muscle group, within each participant, may have different levels of strength):

$$\text{peakRFD} \sim \text{peak force} \times \text{time} \times \text{muscle} \times \text{condition} + (\text{muscle} \mid \text{subjects})$$

Paired, two-tailed Student's t-tests were used to compare the other parameters between PRE vs. POST. The Kolmogorov–Smirnov normality test was used to assess distribution normality. Post hoc analysis was adjusted with Bonferroni corrections. The level of statistical significance was set to $p < 0.05$. In graphs, data are reported as mean and 95% confidence intervals (C.I.). The effect size in ANOVA analysis was reported as partial eta squared η^2. The magnitude of the difference between PRE vs. POST was calculated as Cohen's d effect size. Threshold values for effect size statistics were <0.2, trivial; ≥0.2, small; ≥0.5, moderate; ≥0.8, large; and ≥1.4, very large.

3. Results

3.1. Incremental Arm-Cranking Graded Test

AMP reached greater peak power output than SCI (AMP: 128.0 ± 6.1 W, SCI 88.0 ± 9.0 W, $p < 0.001$). AMP also reached greater peak HR (AMP: 171.5 ± 5.4 beats/min, SCI 131.7 ± 14.5 beats/min, $p < 0.05$) and VO_{2peak} (AMP: 34.4 ± 2.8 mL/kg/min, SCI 23.1 ± 1.2 mL/kg/min, $p < 0.001$).

3.2. Neuromuscular Function Differences between AMP and SCI

As shown in Figure 2, SCI showed lower levels of maximum strength and explosive force capacity compared to AMP. In particular, SCI showed lower MVF in both elbow flexor muscles (d = 0.460, $p = 0.045$) and extensor muscles (d = 0.700, $p = 0.003$). Similarly, RFD in SCI was lower in both elbow flexor muscles (d = 0.400, $p = 0.045$) and extensor muscles (d = 0.500, $p = 0.032$).

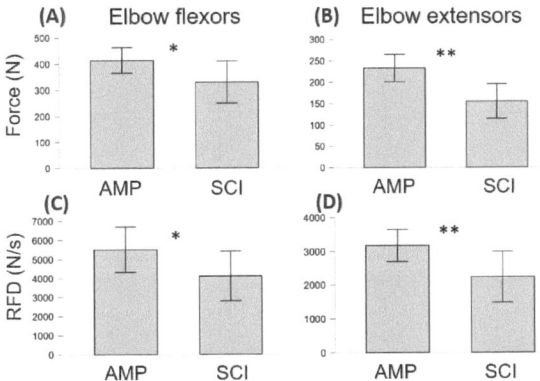

Figure 2. The level of maximum voluntary force (MVF) and rate of force development (RFD) of the elbow flexor and extensor muscles in athletes with amputation (AMP) and athletes with a spinal cord injury (SCI) for elbow flexors (**A**,**C**) and elbow extensors (**B**,**D**). * $p < 0.05$, ** $p < 0.01$.

3.3. Fatigability Effect on Neuromuscular Function

As can be seen in Figure 3A,B, there was a significant effect of the fatiguing task on MVF (F = 19.4, η_p^2 = 0.520, p < 0.001) both in SCI and AMP. There was no statistically significant interaction between the groups in fatigue susceptibility (group × time interaction: F = 1.3, η_p^2 = 0.067, p = 0.269). However, as can be seen in Figure 2D, SCI appeared to have no signs of fatigue on the elbow extensor muscles, as force levels remained constant (PRE 155 ± 56 N; POST: 155 ± 69 N). As can be seen in Figure 4C,D, there was a moderate effect of the fatiguing task on RFD (F = 12.0, η_p^2 = 0.401, p = 0.003). In fact, RFD force decreased in both groups (p < 0.01 for all muscle groups, see Figure 4C,D). There was no statistically significant interaction between groups in fatigue susceptibility (group × time interaction: F = 1.3, η_p^2 = 0.007, p = 0.719).

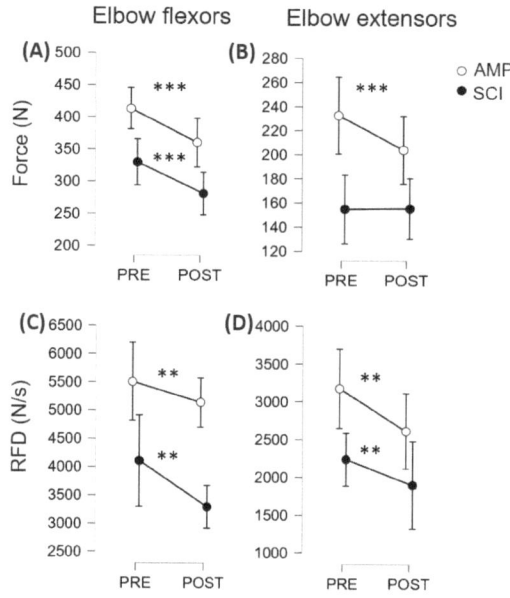

Figure 3. Maximum voluntary force (MVF) and rate of force development (RFDpeak) of the elbow flexor and extensor muscles in athletes with amputation (AMP) and athletes with a spinal cord injury (SCI) are reported for PRE and POST for elbow flexors (**A,C**) and elbow extensors (**B,D**). ** p < 0.01, *** p < 0.001.

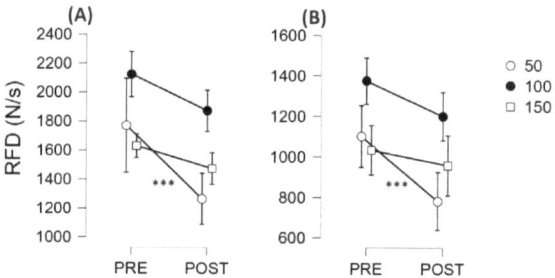

Figure 4. Rate of force development (RFD) values (mean and 95% CI) before (PRE) and after (POST) a maximal arm ergometer test (fatiguing task) are reported. Values are shown for the elbow flexor (**A**) and elbow extensor (**B**) muscles and are reported separately for 50, 100, and 150 ms time intervals. As the condition did not emerge as a significant factor, the two groups (AMP and SCI) were merged. *** p < 0.001.

The time-locked analysis of RFD showed that there was no interaction with the condition (SCI vs. AMP, all p values greater than 0.185); therefore, the results are presented by merging the two groups together (Figure 4). There was not an interval × muscle × time interaction ($p = 0.576$), but there was an interval × time interaction (F = 11.2, $\eta_p^2 = 0.385$, $p < 0.001$) suggesting that the two muscle groups behaved similarly, but some time intervals were more susceptible to fatigue than others. Post hoc analysis showed that RFD50 showed the greatest decrease (d = 0.741, $p < 0.001$), RFD100 showed a small decrease (d = 0.382, $p = 0.020$), and RFD150 did not decrease ($p = 0.272$). The post hoc results within each muscle group are reported in Figure 4.

The time-locked analysis of RMS showed that there was not any interaction with the condition (SCI vs. AMP, all p values greater than 0.122); therefore, the results are presented by merging the two groups together (Figure 5). There was no interval × muscle × time interaction ($p = 0.922$), but there was an interval × time interaction (F = 7.0, $\eta_p^2 = 0.293$, $p = 0.003$), suggesting that the two muscle groups behaved similarly, but some time intervals were more susceptible to fatigue than others. However, post hoc analysis did not detect any significant differences, even though the RMS50 tended to decrease with time and RMS100 and RMS150 tended to increase with time (see Figure 5).

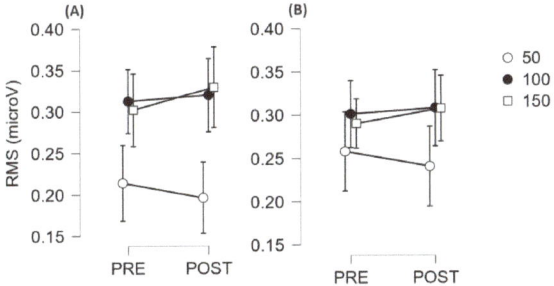

Figure 5. Electromyographic signal amplitude (RMS) values (mean and 95% CI) before (PRE) and after (POST) a maximal arm ergometer test (fatiguing task) are reported. Values are shown for the elbow flexor (**A**) and elbow extensor (**B**) muscles and are reported separately for 50, 100, and 150 ms time intervals. As the condition did not emerge as a significant factor, the two groups (AMP and SCI) were merged.

At POST, participants reached lower levels of force (−12%, d = 0.257, $p = 0.002$) during the rapid burst-like contractions compared to PRE (see Figure 6, F = 12.6, $\eta_p^2 = 0.414$). There was no interaction with the muscle group or condition ($p = 0.837$).

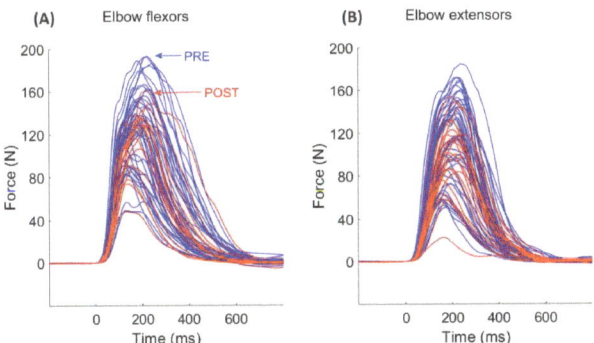

Figure 6. Representative example of the force recorded during all explosive muscle contractions performed before (blue) and after (red) the fatiguing task in an amputee subject in elbow flexors (**A**) and extensors (**B**).

The linear hierarchical model analysing RFD in the RFD-SF protocol showed that there was a peak force × time interaction (F = 72.3, $p < 0.0001$), meaning that the linear relationship between the peak force and RFD reached in each contraction changed between PRE and POST (Figure 7). Indeed, the estimate of RFD-SF merging all participants, i.e., the slope of the linear regression between peak force and peak RFD of all contractions and participants, decreased after the fatiguing task (Figure 7). There was also a significant peak force × time × condition (F = 20.8, $p < 0.0001$), showing that SCI had a larger decrease in RFD-SF than AMP. In particular, RFD-SF decreased from 15.0 to 14.1 in elbow extensors of AMP (Figure 7A), from 18.4 to 16.8 in elbow flexors of AMP (Figure 7B), from 17.0 to 14.3 in elbow extensors of SCI (Figure 7C), and from 16.6 to 13.6 in elbow flexors of SCI (Figure 7D).

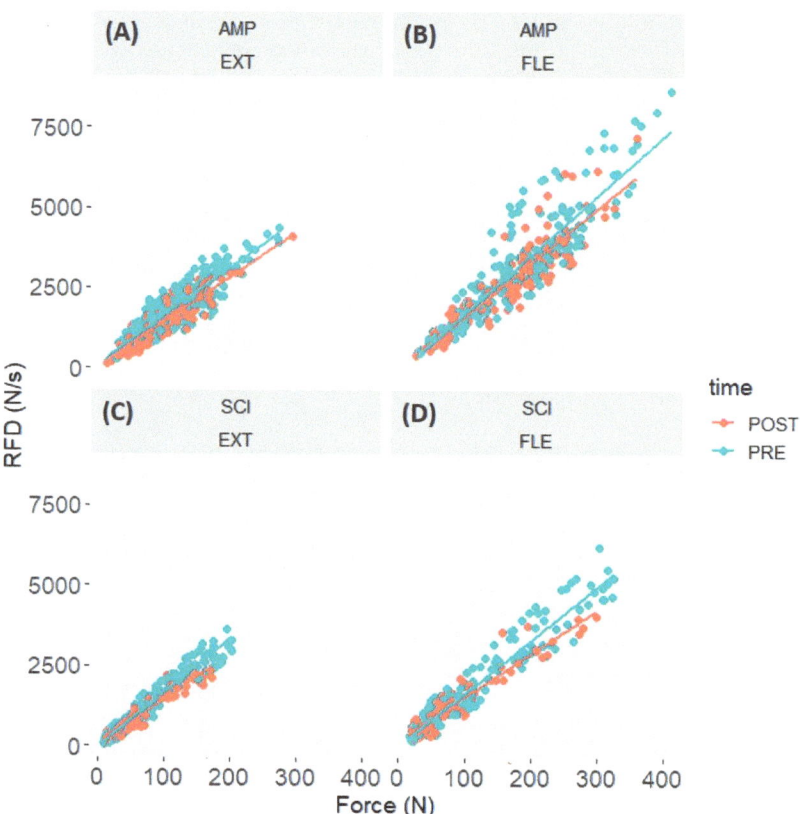

Figure 7. Peak rate of force development (RFD) is plotted against the peak force reached in each contraction of the RFD-SF protocol before (PRE) and after (POST) the fatiguing task. Values are shown for the elbow extensor (EXT, (**A,C**)) and elbow flexor muscles (FLE, (**B,D**)) separately for subjects with amputation (AMP, (**A,B**)) and with spinal cord injury (SCI, (**C,D**)).

4. Discussion

This study aimed to assess neuromuscular fatigue by comparing rapid force production between athletes with amputation (AMP) and spinal cord injury (SCI) in their elbow flexors and extensors. The present experimental setup involved a series of rapid isometric contractions at various submaximal intensities, mimicking brief muscle excitation profiles observed in various daily life activities. This approach aimed to provide a more functionally relevant measure of muscle fatigue. The participants, comprising AMP and SCI athletes, underwent neuromuscular function evaluations before and after a graded arm cranking test to voluntary fatigue. We found that (1) at PRE, SCI had lower MVF and RFDpeak values than AMP (all d values were ≈ 0.4–0.5); (2) after the fatiguing task, SCI and AMP showed a similar decrease of both MVF and RFDpeak (all d values were ≈0.4); (3) in the time-locked analysis of RFD, both groups showed a larger reduction in RFD50 (d = 0.7) compared to RFD100 (d = 0.4) and RFD 150 (not affected); (4) overall, the amplitude of HD-EMG did not change in all time intervals (Figure 5); (5) at POST, the RFD-SF decreased, more in SCI than in AMP, meaning that the quickness of ballistic contractions of submaximal amplitude decreased after the fatiguing task (Figures 6 and 7).

4.1. Differences and Similarities between SCI and AMP

The SCI athletes exhibited lower MVF and RFD levels than AMP athletes in both elbow flexors and extensors (Figure 2). These findings underscore the differential impact of spinal cord injury versus limb amputation on the neuromuscular function of the upper limb. Additionally, both groups demonstrated decreased RFD and MVF following the fatiguing task (Figure 3), suggesting similar susceptibility to fatigue across populations, albeit by varying degrees. Interestingly, while both groups exhibited fatigue, SCI athletes showed no signs of fatigue in the elbow extensor muscles, as force levels remained constant. This observation could suggest differential fatigue patterns between muscle groups or adaptations specific to the SCI population. More likely, many SCI athletes in our sample could barely activate their elbow extensor (as can be seen from the force produced, see Figure 2). Therefore, that muscle group probably did not perform sufficient muscle work during the fatigue test to generate signs of muscle fatigue. In other words, elbow extensors did not fatigue through exercise because they were not activated enough to disturb the metabolic condition. Further investigations are warranted to elucidate these findings.

4.2. Fatigability Expressed as Reduction of MVF or RFDpeak

The study highlighted the importance of task specificity in evaluating neuromuscular fatigue, particularly in para-athletes whose daily activities may not involve prolonged maximal contractions. While MVF is a standard measure, it may not accurately reflect the fatigue experienced during more functional tasks. RFD, especially early RFD ($\leq$50 ms from the contraction onset), has been suggested to be more sensitive to changes in neuromuscular function due to fatigue [16,43,44], potentially because of its reliance on neural mechanisms related to motor unit behaviour [45]. The time-locked analysis of RFD revealed a significant decrease across time intervals, with the greatest decrease observed at RFD50, followed by a smaller decrease at RFD100, and no change at RFD150. This pattern suggests that the early phase of force production is particularly susceptible to fatigue, which aligns with previous research highlighting the importance of early rapid force generation in the fatigued condition [17]. Of note, those reductions were similar in SCI and AMP, suggesting the two groups of para-athletes had similar susceptibility to fatigue induced by an incremental test at the arm ergometer.

4.3. Contraction Quickness in Ballistic Contractions of Submaximal Amplitude

The adoption of RFD-SF to quantify neuromuscular quickness [46] has been applied to detect asymmetries [34,47,48], ageing [29,49], and neuromuscular disorders [50]. Nevertheless, using the RFD-SF, two previous studies failed to detect neuromuscular [30] or mental fatigue [49]. In the present study, we demonstrated for the first time that RFD-SF is susceptible to neuromuscular fatigability induced by an incremental arm-cranking test. Beyond the fact that the previous study was conducted on the lower limbs [30], the shorter recovery in the present study (≈3 min) compared to the previous one (5–8 min) may have limited the recovery of fatigue, thus allowing its detection through RFD-SF protocol.

Here, we found that the capacity to perform ballistic contractions of submaximal amplitude is altered in the presence of fatigue (Figure 7). While the present study cannot identify the physiological cause for this impairment (as the HD-EMG amplitude did not change over time, Figure 5), it is possible to speculate on the consequences of this finding. Neuromuscular fatigability has always been detected using maximal contractions because it was operationally defined as a decrease in muscle strength/power [4]. However, the fact that the maximal strength decreases does not necessarily mean that the strength available in rapid contractions of submaximal force levels decreases. Therefore, it would be relevant to directly measure the reduction in capacities of performing short rapid contractions, much shorter than those required to measure MVF, like the ones typically used in the stroke to push a wheelchair. With the RFD-SF protocol, we demonstrated a quickness reduction in muscle contraction modality that is more relevant for both athletic performance and daily activities, particularly among para-athletes. Furthermore, we demonstrated that people with spinal cord injury might be more susceptible to fatigability in this specific task (Figure 7). The present findings contribute to our understanding of neuromuscular fatigue in para-athletes and underscore the importance of task-specific assessments. Future research should explore the physiological roots of this behaviour, considering the unique challenges posed by different impairments.

4.4. Electromyographic Parameters

The muscle activation, measured as the RMS of the HD-EMG signal, was calculated in 50 ms time intervals from the onset of muscle contractions. The fact that the amplitude of the EMG signal did not decrease (Figure 5) can be explained in two ways: (1) there was no decrease in the neural command under fatigue conditions; (2) there was a decrease in the neural command, but the amplitude estimation was affected by confounding factors intrinsic to the electromyographic evaluation (such as the phenomenon of amplitude cancellation) that overestimate the amplitude of the signal under fatigue conditions. In any case, the fact that the amplitude of the EMG signal did not decrease suggests that there was no appreciable decrease in neural activation during the explosive contractions and, therefore, central fatigue was limited. Consequently, the decrease in rapid force production that herein reported is probably due to factors of peripheral origin (e.g., decreased muscle contractility).

4.5. Limitations

The sample size of the present study is small in absolute terms. However, considering the small number of people in the reference population, i.e., Italian paralympic veterans, which comprises a few dozen people, the number of participants recruited in the present study was considerable. Furthermore, the presence of two wheelchair users in the group with amputation might have slightly confused the results. It would have been useful to test the fatigability of the shoulder muscles as well. However, we had to reduce the number of muscles tested in order to reduce the testing time, especially at POST. This is because increasing the number of muscles tested would have increased the recovery time, i.e., the time between the end of the exercise and the test, thus invalidating the measures of fatigue. Furthermore, measuring the actual torque instead of force would have improved the reliability of our results.

5. Conclusions

We firstly demonstrated that muscle fatigability impacts not only maximal force expression, i.e., maximal strength (i.e., MVF) and maximal quickness (RFDpeak), but also the quickness of ballistic contractions of submaximal amplitudes, especially in para-athletes with spinal cord injury. Consequently, the effects of muscle fatigability can be seen also during many sports and daily living activities of wheelchair users. We also found that early RFD, i.e., the quickness of the first 50 ms of muscle contraction, were particularly affected by muscle fatigability, further highlighting the importance of evaluating the RFD with the adoption of time-locked intervals instead of only RFDpeak. As expected, lower muscle strength and explosive capacity were observed in para-athletes with spinal cord injury compared to those with lower limb amputation; however, the two groups of para-athletes showed an equal decrease in strength despite starting from lower initial strength levels.

Author Contributions: Conceptualization, G.B., P.R.B., T.S. and A.R. (Alberto Rainoldi); methodology, G.B., T.S. and A.R. (Alberto Rainoldi); formal analysis, G.B.; investigation, G.B., L.B., P.R.B., I.P., R.F., D.M., A.R. (Anna Raguzzini), E.T. and T.S.; resources, G.B. and L.B.; data curation, G.B. and I.P.; writing—original draft preparation, G.B.; writing—review and editing, G.B., L.B., P.R.B., I.P., R.F., D.M., A.R. (Anna Raguzzini), E.T., T.S. and A.R. (Alberto Rainoldi); visualization, G.B.; supervision, G.B., T.S. and A.R. (Alberto Rainoldi); project administration, T.S. and A.R. (Alberto Rainoldi); funding acquisition, T.S., I.P. and A.R. (Alberto Rainoldi). All authors have read and agreed to the published version of the manuscript.

Funding: This research was funded by MINISTERO DELLA DIFESA grant number M_D E13985 REG2021 0032116 28-07-2021 (Project AMAMP).

Institutional Review Board Statement: The study was conducted in accordance with the Declaration of Helsinki and approved by the Ethics Committee of the Italian Army Medical Hospital, Rome, Italy (protocol code CE/2021u/03/a-31/03/2021-09.a and 31 March 2021).

Informed Consent Statement: Written informed consent was obtained from all subjects involved in the study.

Data Availability Statement: Data are unavailable due to privacy and ethical restrictions.

Conflicts of Interest: The authors declare no conflicts of interest.

References

1. Qi, L.; Zhang, L.; Lin, X.-B.; Ferguson-Pell, M. Wheelchair propulsion fatigue thresholds in electromyographic and ventilatory testing. *Spinal Cord* **2020**, *58*, 1104–1111. [CrossRef]
2. Van der Woude, L.H.; de Groot, S.; Janssen, T.W. Manual wheelchairs: Research and innovation in rehabilitation, sports, daily life and health. *Med. Eng. Phys.* **2006**, *28*, 905–915. [CrossRef] [PubMed]
3. Rodgers, M.M.; McQuade, K.J.; Rasch, E.K.; Keyser, R.E.; Finley, M.A. Upper-limb fatigue-related joint power shifts in experienced wheelchair users and nonwheelchair users. *J. Rehabil. Res. Dev.* **2003**, *40*, 27–38. [CrossRef] [PubMed]
4. Gandevia, S.C. Spinal and supraspinal factors in human muscle fatigue. *Physiol. Rev.* **2001**, *81*, 1725–1789. [CrossRef] [PubMed]
5. Maffiuletti, N.A.; Aagaard, P.; Blazevich, A.J.; Folland, J.; Tillin, N.; Duchateau, J. Rate of force development: Physiological and methodological considerations. *Eur. J. Appl. Physiol.* **2016**, *116*, 1091–1116. [CrossRef] [PubMed]
6. Rodriguez-Rosell, D.; Pareja-Blanco, F.; Aagaard, P.; Gonzalez-Badillo, J.J. Physiological and methodological aspects of rate of force development assessment in human skeletal muscle. *Clin. Physiol. Funct. Imaging* **2018**, *38*, 743–762. [CrossRef] [PubMed]
7. Tillin, N.A.; Jimenez-Reyes, P.; Pain, M.T.; Folland, J.P. Neuromuscular performance of explosive power athletes versus untrained individuals. *Med. Sci. Sports. Exerc.* **2010**, *42*, 781–790. [CrossRef]
8. McLellan, C.P.; Lovell, D.I.; Gass, G.C. The role of rate of force development on vertical jump performance. *J. Strength Cond. Res.* **2011**, *25*, 379–385. [CrossRef] [PubMed]
9. de Boer, M.D.; Maganaris, C.N.; Seynnes, O.R.; Rennie, M.J.; Narici, M.V. Time course of muscular, neural and tendinous adaptations to 23 day unilateral lower-limb suspension in young men. *J. Physiol.* **2007**, *583*, 1079–1091. [CrossRef]
10. Andersen, L.L.; Andersen, C.H.; Mortensen, O.S.; Poulsen, O.M.; Bjornlund, I.B.; Zebis, M.K. Muscle activation and perceived loading during rehabilitation exercises: Comparison of dumbbells and elastic resistance. *Phys. Ther.* **2010**, *90*, 538–549. [CrossRef]
11. Angelozzi, M.; Madama, M.; Corsica, C.; Calvisi, V.; Properzi, G.; Mccaw, S.T.; Cacchio, A. Rate of Force Development as an Adjunctive Outcome Measure for Return-to-Sport Decisions After Anterior Cruciate Ligament Reconstruction. *J. Orthop. Sports Phys.* **2012**, *42*, 772–780. [CrossRef] [PubMed]
12. Buckthorpe, M.; Pain, M.T.; Folland, J.P. Central fatigue contributes to the greater reductions in explosive than maximal strength with high-intensity fatigue. *Exp. Physiol.* **2014**, *99*, 964–973. [CrossRef]
13. Peñailillo, L.; Blazevich, A.; Numazawa, H.; Nosaka, K. Rate of force development as a measure of muscle damage. *Scand. J. Med. Sci. Sports* **2015**, *25*, 417–427. [CrossRef]
14. Rice, D.A.; Mannion, J.; Lewis, G.N.; McNair, P.J.; Fort, L. Experimental knee pain impairs joint torque and rate of force development in isometric and isokinetic muscle activation. *Eur. J. Appl. Physiol.* **2019**, *119*, 2065–2073. [CrossRef]
15. Del Vecchio, A. Neuromechanics of the Rate of Force Development. *Exerc. Sport Sci. Rev.* **2023**, *51*, 34–42. [CrossRef] [PubMed]
16. D'Emanuele, S.; Maffiuletti, N.A.; Tarperi, C.; Rainoldi, A.; Schena, F.; Boccia, G. Rate of Force Development as an Indicator of Neuromuscular Fatigue: A Scoping Review. *Front. Hum. Neurosci.* **2021**, *15*, 701916. [CrossRef]
17. Boccia, G.; D'Emanuele, S.; Brustio, P.R.; Rainoldi, A.; Schena, F.; Tarperi, C. Decreased neural drive affects the early rate of force development after repeated burst-like isometric contractions. *Scand. J. Med. Sci. Sports* **2024**, *34*, e14528. [CrossRef] [PubMed]

18. D'Emanuele, S.; Tarperi, C.; Rainoldi, A.; Schena, F.; Boccia, G. Neural and contractile determinants of burst-like explosive isometric contractions of the knee extensors. *Scand. J. Med. Sci. Sports* **2023**, *33*, 127–135. [CrossRef]
19. Cossich, V.; Maffiuletti, N. Early vs. late rate of torque development: Relation with maximal strength and influencing factors. *J. Electromyogr. Kinesiol.* **2020**, *55*, 102486. [CrossRef]
20. Bellumori, M.; Jaric, S.; Knight, C.A. The rate of force development scaling factor (RFD-SF): Protocol, reliability, and muscle comparisons. *Exp. Brain Res.* **2011**, *212*, 359–369. [CrossRef]
21. Brustio, P.R.; Casale, R.; Buttacchio, G.; Calabrese, M.; Bruzzone, M.; Rainoldi, A.; Boccia, G. Relevance of evaluating the rate of torque development in ballistic contractions of submaximal amplitude. *Physiol. Meas.* **2019**, *40*, 025002. [CrossRef] [PubMed]
22. Casartelli, N.C.; Lepers, R.; Maffiuletti, N.A. Assessment of the rate of force development scaling factor for the hip muscles. *Muscle Nerve* **2014**, *50*, 932–938. [CrossRef] [PubMed]
23. Djordjevic, D.; Uygur, M. Methodological considerations in the calculation of the rate of force development scaling factor. *Physiol. Meas.* **2017**, *39*, 015001. [CrossRef] [PubMed]
24. Freund, H.J.; Budingen, H.J. The relationship between speed and amplitude of the fastest voluntary contractions of human arm muscles. *Exp. Brain Res.* **1978**, *31*, 1–12. [CrossRef] [PubMed]
25. Klass, M.; Baudry, S.; Duchateau, J. Age-related decline in rate of torque development is accompanied by lower maximal motor unit discharge frequency during fast contractions. *J. Appl. Physiol.* **2008**, *104*, 739–746. [CrossRef] [PubMed]
26. Wierzbicka, M.M.; Wiegner, A.W.; Logigian, E.L.; Young, R.R. Abnormal most-rapid isometric contractions in patients with Parkinson's disease. *J. Neurol. Neurosurg. Psychiatry* **1991**, *54*, 210–216. [CrossRef] [PubMed]
27. Ivanenko, Y.P.; Poppele, R.E.; Lacquaniti, F. Spinal cord maps of spatiotemporal alpha-motoneuron activation in humans walking at different speeds. *J. Neurophysiol.* **2006**, *95*, 602–618. [CrossRef] [PubMed]
28. Gizzi, L.; Nielsen, J.F.; Felici, F.; Ivanenko, Y.P.; Farina, D. Impulses of activation but not motor modules are preserved in the locomotion of subacute stroke patients. *J. Neurophysiol.* **2011**, *106*, 202–210. [CrossRef] [PubMed]
29. Bellumori, M.; Jaric, S.; Knight, C.A. Age-related decline in the rate of force development scaling factor. *Motor Control* **2013**, *17*, 370–381. [CrossRef]
30. Corrêa, T.G.; Donato, S.V.; Lima, K.C.; Pereira, R.V.; Uygur, M.; de Freitas, P.B. Age-and Sex-Related Differences in the Maximum Muscle Performance and Rate of Force Development Scaling Factor of Precision Grip Muscles. *Motor Control* **2020**, *24*, 274–290. [CrossRef]
31. Kim, J.J.; Delmas, S.; Choi, Y.J.; Hubbard, J.C.; Weintraub, M.; Arabatzi, F.; Yacoubi, B.; Christou, E.A. Unique Neural Mechanisms Underlying Speed Control of Low-Force Ballistic Contractions. *J. Hum. Kinet.* **2024**, *90*, 29–44. [CrossRef] [PubMed]
32. Boccia, G.; Dardanello, D.; Brustio, P.R.; Tarperi, C.; Festa, L.; Zoppirolli, C.; Pellegrini, B.; Schena, F.; Rainoldi, A. Neuromuscular Fatigue Does Not Impair the Rate of Force Development in Ballistic Contractions of Submaximal Amplitudes. *Front. Physiol.* **2018**, *9*, 1503. [CrossRef] [PubMed]
33. Toti, E.; Cavedon, V.; Raguzzini, A.; Fedullo, A.L.; Milanese, C.; Bernardi, E.; Bellito, S.; Bernardi, M.; Sciarra, T.; Peluso, I. Dietary intakes and food habits of wheelchair basketball athletes compared to gym attendees and individuals who do not practice sport activity. *Endocr. Metab. Immune Disord.-Drug Targets (Former. Curr. Drug Targets-Immune Endocr. Metab. Disord.)* **2022**, *22*, 38–48. [CrossRef] [PubMed]
34. Boccia, G.; D'Emanuele, S.; Brustio, P.R.; Beratto, L.; Tarperi, C.; Casale, R.; Sciarra, T.; Rainoldi, A. Strength Asymmetries Are Muscle-Specific and Metric-Dependent. *Int. J. Environ. Res. Public Health* **2022**, *19*, 8495. [CrossRef] [PubMed]
35. Beretta Piccoli, M.; Rainoldi, A.; Heitz, C.; Wuthrich, M.; Boccia, G.; Tomasoni, E.; Spirolazzi, C.; Egloff, M.; Barbero, M. Innervation zone locations in 43 superficial muscles: Toward a standardization of electrode positioning. *Muscle Nerve* **2014**, *49*, 413–421. [CrossRef] [PubMed]
36. Merletti, R.; Muceli, S. Tutorial. Surface EMG detection in space and time: Best practices. *J. Electromyogr. Kinesiol.* **2019**, *49*, 102363. [CrossRef] [PubMed]
37. Smajla, D.; Žitnik, J.; Šarabon, N. Advancements in the Protocol for Rate of Force Development/Relaxation Scaling Factor Evaluation. *Front. Hum. Neurosci.* **2021**, *15*, 159. [CrossRef] [PubMed]
38. Crotty, E.D.; Furlong, L.M.; Hayes, K.; Harrison, A.J. Onset detection in surface electromyographic signals across isometric explosive and ramped contractions: A comparison of computer-based methods. *Physiol. Meas.* **2021**, *42*, 035010. [CrossRef] [PubMed]
39. Haff, G.G.; Ruben, R.P.; Lider, J.; Twine, C.; Cormie, P. A Comparison of Methods for Determining the Rate of Force Development During Isometric Midthigh Clean Pulls. *J. Strength Cond. Res.* **2015**, *29*, 386–395. [CrossRef]
40. Ditroilo, M.; Forte, R.; Benelli, P.; Gambarara, D.; De Vito, G. Effects of age and limb dominance on upper and lower limb muscle function in healthy males and females aged 40–80 years. *J. Sport Sci.* **2010**, *28*, 667–677. [CrossRef]
41. Cook, R.D. Detection of influential observation in linear regression. *Technometrics* **1977**, *19*, 15–18.
42. Balshaw, T.G.; Fry, A.; Maden-Wilkinson, T.M.; Kong, P.W.; Folland, J.P. Reliability of quadriceps surface electromyography measurements is improved by two vs. single site recordings. *Eur. J. Appl. Physiol.* **2017**, *117*, 1085–1094. [CrossRef] [PubMed]
43. Boccia, G.; Dardanello, D.; Tarperi, C.; Festa, L.; La Torre, A.; Pellegrini, B.; Schena, F.; Rainoldi, A. Fatigue-induced dissociation between rate of force development and maximal force across repeated rapid contractions. *Hum. Mov. Sci.* **2017**, *54*, 267–275. [CrossRef] [PubMed]

44. Boccia, G.; Dardanello, D.; Zoppirolli, C.; Bortolan, L.; Cescon, C.; Schneebeli, A.; Vernillo, G.; Schena, F.; Rainoldi, A.; Pellegrini, B. Central and peripheral fatigue in knee and elbow extensor muscles after a long-distance cross-country ski race. *Scand. J. Med. Sci. Sports* **2016**, *27*, 945–955. [CrossRef] [PubMed]
45. Del Vecchio, A.; Negro, F.; Holobar, A.; Casolo, A.; Folland, J.P.; Felici, F.; Farina, D. You are as fast as your motor neurons: Speed of recruitment and maximal discharge of motor neurons determine the maximal rate of force development in humans. *J. Physiol.* **2019**, *597*, 2445–2456. [CrossRef] [PubMed]
46. Kozinc, Z.; Smajla, D.; Sarabon, N. The rate of force development scaling factor: A review of underlying factors, assessment methods and potential for practical applications. *Eur. J. Appl. Physiol.* **2022**, *122*, 861–873. [CrossRef]
47. Kozinc, Ž.; Šarabon, N. Inter-Limb Asymmetries in Volleyball Players: Differences between Testing Approaches and Association with Performance. *J. Sports Sci. Med.* **2020**, *19*, 745–752. [PubMed]
48. Smajla, D.; Žitnik, J.; Sarabon, N. Quantification of inter-limb symmetries with rate of force development and relaxation scaling factor. *Front. Physiol.* **2021**, *12*, 871. [CrossRef]
49. Bellumori, M.; Uygur, M.; Knight, C.A. High-Speed Cycling Intervention Improves Rate-Dependent Mobility in Older Adults. *Med. Sci. Sports Exerc.* **2017**, *49*, 106–114. [CrossRef]
50. Uygur, M.; Barone, D.A.; Dankel, S.J.; DeStefano, N. Isometric tests to evaluate upper and lower extremity functioning in people with multiple sclerosis: Reliability and validity. *Mult. Scler. Relat. Disord.* **2022**, *63*, 103817. [CrossRef]

Disclaimer/Publisher's Note: The statements, opinions and data contained in all publications are solely those of the individual author(s) and contributor(s) and not of MDPI and/or the editor(s). MDPI and/or the editor(s) disclaim responsibility for any injury to people or property resulting from any ideas, methods, instructions or products referred to in the content.

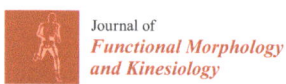
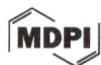

Article

Handgrip Strength and Upper Limb Anthropometric Characteristics among Latin American Female Volleyball Players

María Alejandra Camacho-Villa [1,2,†], Jhon Hurtado-Alcoser [3], Andrés Santiago Jerez [3], Juan Carlos Saavedra [1], Erika Tatiana Paredes Prada [1], Jeimy Andrea Merchán [1], Fernando Millan-Domingo [1,4], Carlos Silva-Polanía [5] and Adrián De la Rosa [1,*,†]

1. Laboratory of Exercise Physiology, Sports Science and Innovation Research Group (GICED), Unidades Tecnológicas de Santander (UTS), Bucaramanga 680006, Colombia; mcamacho@correo.uts.edu.co (M.A.C.-V.); jsaavedra@correo.uts.edu.co (J.C.S.); eparedes@correo.uts.edu.co (E.T.P.P.); jandreamerchan@correo.uts.edu.co (J.A.M.); fernando.millan-domingo@uv.es (F.M.-D.)
2. Pain Study Group (GED), Physical Therapy School, Universidad Industrial de Santander, Bucaramanga 680002, Colombia
3. Physical Activity and Sport Program, Sports Science and Innovation Research Group (GICED), Unidades Tecnológicas de Santander (UTS), Bucaramanga 680006, Colombia; jandersonhurtado@uts.edu.co (J.H.-A.); asjerez@uts.edu.co (A.S.J.)
4. Freshage Research Group, Department of Physiology, Faculty of Medicine, University of Valencia, CIBERFES, Fundación Investigación Hospital Clínico Universitario/INCLIVA, 46010 Valencia, Spain
5. Body, Physical Activity and Sport Study Group (GECAFD), Sports Department, Universidad Industrial de Santander, Bucaramanga 680002, Colombia; carlos2248261@correo.uis.edu.co
* Correspondence: adelarosa@correo.uts.edu.co
† These authors contributed equally to this work.

Citation: Camacho-Villa, M.A.; Hurtado-Alcoser, J.; Jerez, A.S.; Saavedra, J.C.; Paredes Prada, E.T.; Merchán, J.A.; Millan-Domingo, F.; Silva-Polanía, C.; De la Rosa, A. Handgrip Strength and Upper Limb Anthropometric Characteristics among Latin American Female Volleyball Players. *J. Funct. Morphol. Kinesiol.* **2024**, *9*, 168. https://doi.org/10.3390/jfmk9030168

Academic Editors: Roland Van den Tillaar and Pedro Miguel Forte

Received: 20 July 2024
Revised: 24 August 2024
Accepted: 1 September 2024
Published: 18 September 2024

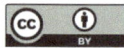

Copyright: © 2024 by the authors. Licensee MDPI, Basel, Switzerland. This article is an open access article distributed under the terms and conditions of the Creative Commons Attribution (CC BY) license (https://creativecommons.org/licenses/by/4.0/).

Abstract: Background: In volleyball, the upper limb dimensions and grip strength greatly influence offensive and defensive movements during a match. However, the relationship between these parameters remains underexplored in elite female volleyball players. **Objective:** This study aimed to contrast the upper limb anthropometric characteristics and handgrip strength (HGS) of female elite volleyball players against a control group. **Methods:** Selected upper limb anthropometric parameters and maximal HGS of 42 female volleyball players and 40 non-athletes were measured. **Results:** Players exhibited higher values in almost all variables studied than non-athletes. The differences were statistically significant ($p < 0.001$) except for body mass index and elbow and wrist diameters. Players showed a moderate correlation between dominant HGS and hand parameters (length $r = 0.43$ and breadth $r = 0.63$; $p < 0.05$). Weak correlations were identified with height, upper arm length, elbow diameter, and hand shape index ($r = 0.32$ to 0.38; $p < 0.05$). In the non-dominant hand, a moderate correlation with handbreadth ($r = 0.55$, $p \leq 0.01$) and weak correlations with upper arm length, wrist diameter, hand length, and hand shape index ($r = 0.32$ to 0.35; $p \leq 0.05$) was found. **Conclusions:** These findings underscore the importance of the upper limb anthropometric parameters as predictors of HGS and their utility in athlete selection. Future research should investigate biomechanical factors influencing HGS and injury prevention.

Keywords: grip strength; female athletes; hand dimensions; talent selection

1. Introduction

Volleyball sport requires several high-intensity and high-velocity actions combined with explosive exertions interspersed with short resting intervals [1]. During the game, success largely depends on motor abilities, particularly muscle strength conditioning, both in the lower and upper limbs. In elite female matches, technical actions that produce the highest score rely on the continuous engagement of the wrist and digit flexor, including attack (76.8–80%), block (14.5–15.6%), and serve (4.4–8.1%) [2,3]. Consequently, upper extremity and grip strength are fundamental to the sport, being the primary physical factors influencing these specific movements.

Additionally, some anthropometric measurements and morphological characteristics (e.g., height, weight, body composition, arm, and hand dimensions) impact the player's performance across this game, making all shots and passes work more efficiently when there is a larger hand surface and longer, stronger fingers [4,5]. For this reason, handgrip strength (HGS) and anthropometric dimensions have been investigated in other popular sports, such as basketball, softball, and handball, where the relationship between hand and ball is fundamental [6]. Nevertheless, in female volleyball players, research has extensively reported on the relationship between the strength of the lower limbs and volleyball success [7,8], with few authors investigating anthropometric and muscle strength in the upper limbs. For instance, Khanna and Koley found higher values in HGS, height, hand, and arm anthropometrics compared to the reference group ($p < 0.05$) [4]. Additionally, Koley and Kaur reported weak to moderate positive correlations ($r = 0.28$ to 0.48) between upper limb anthropometric variables (i.e., arm length, hand breadth, and hand length) and HGS among Indian inter-university female volleyball players [9].

HGS test has been extensively used to assess upper limb strength across various sports, with high levels of HGS identified as a critical factor for success. Recently, the relationship between HGS and serve reception efficiency has been reported in volleyball players, indicating that HGS is a key element in achieving success during games. Similarly, moderate correlations have also been reported between HGS and both the velocity of serving and spike [10,11]. These findings indicate that HGS assessment is a valuable tool for identifying talent, strengths, and weaknesses in the physical condition of volleyball players. Moreover, it is considered a non-invasive and cost-effective method for collecting extensive data [12].

Several anthropometric characteristics of the upper limbs are different across sports in female athletes. Thus, while hand breath and hand length were greater in basketball collegiate athletes as compared to the handball ones [6], these measurements, along with the forearm length and forearm circumference, were reported to be greater in a group of athletes as compared to non-athletes (national basketball players, collegian handball players, collegian volleyball players, and collegian wrestlers) [13]. Similarly, when comparing anthropometric measurements of elite volleyball players and non-athletes, researchers found that an athlete's hand measurements, such as hand length and hand finger length, but not hand width, were greater in the dominant hand [14]. Therefore, hand dimensions, including the aforementioned, are interrelated and have been described to significantly contribute to the techniques applied in grappling sports such as volleyball [13].

Although several studies have emphasized the link between upper limb anthropometric variables, HGS, and the specific skills required for volleyball players [9,11,14], the interplay between hand, forearm, and arm-anthropometric variables with HGS in elite female volleyball players remains largely unreported. Moreover, the influence of the practice of volleyball in HGS and some upper limbs anthropometric variables is unknown.

Hence, this study has two aims: (i) To contrast the upper limb anthropometric characteristics and HGS of female Latin American elite volleyball players against a control group, and (ii) To determine the relationship between these variables in female volleyball players. The present study has two hypotheses: (i) Latin American female volleyball players will have greater upper limb dimensions and HGS than the controls, and (ii) HGS will correlate with upper limb anthropometric variables.

2. Materials and Methods
2.1. Participants

A cross-sectional analytical study was conducted during the "International Cup Ciudad de Bucaramanga", which took place in July 2022 in Bucaramanga-Colombia. Forty-two female volleyball players belonging to the national teams of Chile ($n = 13$), Colombia

(n = 17), and Mexico (n = 13) were examined (age: 24.63 ± 5.31 yrs; height: 1.68 ± 0.04 m; weight: 67.26 ± 8.46 kg; years of volleyball experience: 10.45 ± 5.14 yrs). The control group was comprised of forty non-athlete young females (age 22.81 ± 2.27; body height 158 ± 0.06 cm; body weight 57.61 ± 5.99 kg). These participants were physically inactive university students from Unidades Tecnológicas de Santander in Bucaramanga, Colombia.

All the participants were informed of the purposes and content of the study; written informed consents were obtained from each player and woman in the control group. The research complied with the Helsinki Declaration and the protocol was approved by the Ethics Committee for Human Beings from the Unidades Tecnológicas de Santander, no. 0010-2022/02.05.2022.

2.2. Selection Criteria

The inclusion criteria were as follows: (a) for the control group, do not report more than 150 weekly minutes of moderate-intensity physical exercise (<600 METS-min/week) in the short version of the International Physical Activity Questionnaire (IPAQ); (b) free of any neuromuscular, orthopedic, or neurological conditions that might interfere with their sports performance, hand function, anthropometric characteristics and activities of daily living.

2.3. Procedures

For volleyball players, all data were collected before training in a private room in the Bicentenario Volleyball Coliseum under natural environmental conditions in the morning (between 8:00–11:00 a.m.).

Regarding the control group, data were collected throughout the same month at the sports science laboratory of the Unidades Tecnológicas de Santander under the same conditions as volleyball players. The entire sampling was assessed by the same two researchers with nine years of experience in sports research. Evaluations were conducted in the following order: body composition, upper limb anthropometric variables and finally the Handgrip strength assessment. Finally, to standardize the measurement technique of HGS, the investigator underwent training which included the participant's position and verbal encouragement.

2.4. Body Composition and Anthropometric Parameters

All the assessments were conducted by a level 2 anthropometrist, following the international standards for anthropometric assessment published by the International Society for the Advancement of Kinanthropometry—ISAK. For data analysis, the averages of two measurements of each anthropometric variable were calculated and processed.

Height was measured with the participants in bare feet using a mechanical stadiometer platform (Seca® 274, Hamburg, Germany; TEM = 0.019%). The movable headpiece was brought down to touch the top of their heads during deep inhalation, and the measurements were recorded in centimeters and rounded to the nearest 0.5 cm.

For body composition evaluation, a bioelectrical impedance device was used (TANITA BC 240, Tokyo, Japan), with measurements rounded to the nearest 0.1. Before the measurement, athletes were required not to carry metal objects, not to consume any caffeine or diuretics in the previous 3 h, and to urinate within 30 min before the test. The data collected included body mass (BM), body fat percentage (BF%), and total body water (BW%). Body mass index (BMI) was calculated as the ratio between weight and the square of height (kg/m^2), representing the easiest method to calculate any state of underweight (<18.5 kg/m^2), normal weight (18.5 to 24.9 kg/m^2), overweight (25 to 29.9 kg/m^2), or obesity (≥30 kg/m^2) [15].

2.5. Measurements of Upper Limbs Anthropometric Parameters

All the anthropometric measurements were taken, with the participants wearing minimal clothing and no shoes. For each upper limb, arm and forearm length, along with three parameters related to hand dimensions, were evaluated (handbreadth, hand length, and hand shape index) [4] as shown in Figure 1. A segmometer and a small bone anthropometer (Cescorf, Porto Alegre, Brazil) were used to measure lengths and diameters, respectively. All the upper limb measurements were taken to the nearest 0.1 cm.

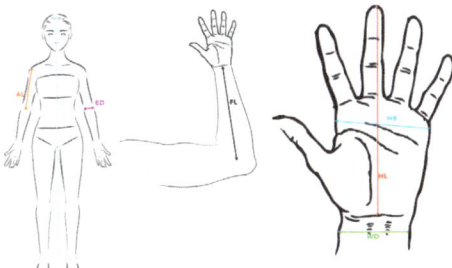

Figure 1. (AL) Arm Length. (H) Height. (ED) Elbow Length. (FL) Forearm Length. (WD) Wrist Diameter. (HL) Hand Length. (HB) Hand Breadth.

The anatomical references of selected anthropometric upper limb parameters were as follows:

- **Arm length:** the distance from the marked acromial to the marked radiale. The subject stands erect with the arms at the sides and palms against the thighs.
- **Forearm length:** the distance from the marked radiale to the marked stylion. The elbow is flexed, and the orientation of the tape is such that it parallels the long axis of the radius.
- **Elbow diameter:** this is the distance between the medial and lateral epicondyles of the humerus.
- **Wrist diameter:** the distance between the outer borders of the radial and ulnar styloid processes.
- **Hand length:** the measurement is taken as the shortest distance from the marked mid-stylion line to the Dactylion.
- **Handbreadth:** the distance between the radial side of the second metacarpal joint to the ulnar side of the fifth metacarpal joint.
- **Hand Shape index:** the handbreadth and length ratio multiplied by a hundred.

2.6. Measurements of Handgrip Strength

The maximal HGS was measured in both hands with a portable digital hand dynamometer (Takei 5401; Tokyo, Japan) with a precision of 0.1 kg. During the hand strength testing protocol, the participants maintained an upright posture with the shoulder of the test arm adducted and the elbow flexed at 90°. The forearm and wrist were kept in a neutral position, and the hand was aligned with the forearm holding the instrument. The dynamometer was adapted to each subject, fitting the hand and allowing flexion at the metacarpophalangeal joints. Specific verbal instructions were provided to the subjects before the evaluations, and verbal encouragement was given during the experiments [16,17].

The participants performed three maximum voluntary contractions for 5 s on each side, with a 60 s rest break between each trial. The subjects were instructed to squeeze the dynamometer as hard as possible. The scale of the dynamometer indicated HGS in kilograms (kg). For statistical analyses, the highest strength value from the three tests of each hand was used [18,19].

2.7. Statistical Analysis

All data were examined for normality of distribution using the Shapiro–Wilk and Ladder of Powers test. Descriptive, parametric, and non-parametric statistical analyses were performed with Stata 13 (StataCorp 2013). Depending on their distribution, sample descriptive values are presented as mean ± standard deviation or median ± interquartile range (IQR).

Comparisons between two independent samples (controls vs. volleyball players) in all variables were performed with the Student's *t*-test or Mann-Whitney test [20]. Cohen's d value was used to evaluate effect size (ES) for the independent nonparametric and parametric analyses. The effect size was interpreted using the following conventions: small effect (d ≥ 0.20), medium effect (d ≥ 0.50), and large effect (d ≥ 0.80) [21].

Pearson's and Spearman's correlation coefficients were used to establish the magnitude of the correlations between dominant and non-dominant HGS and anthropometric variables in volleyball players [22]. According to Schober et al. (2018) [22], the conventional approach to interpreting a correlation coefficient is to categorize it as "negligible" (r = 0.00–0.10), "weak" (r = 0.10–0.39), "moderate" (r = 0.40–0.69), "strong" (r = 0.70–0.89) and "very strong" (0.90–1.00).

In all analyses, a *p*-value of less than 0.05 was considered a statistically significant result.

3. Results

The right hand was identified as the dominant hand in 81.70% (*n* = 67) of the 82 participants. Table 1 shows the descriptive statistics of the sample, including anthropometric characteristics and HGS in both upper limbs. Latin-American female volleyball players exhibited higher values in almost all variables studied, except for body fat, than their control counterparts. These differences were statistically significant (*p* < 0.001) except for BMI and elbow and wrist diameter in both upper limbs.

Table 1. Descriptive statistics of HGS and some selected anthropometric characteristics in female volleyball players and controls.

Variables	Controls (*n* = 40)	Volleyball Players (*n* = 42)	Effect Size
Height (cm) [+]	158.02 (6.02)	179.04 (12.0) [†]	2.46
Body weight (kg)	57.21 (7.62)	71.12 (9.8) [†]	1.57
Body mass index (kg/m^2)	22.81 (2.91)	22.73 (2.3)	
Body fat (%)	25.23 (5.82)	22.22 (4.3) *	0.61
Body water (%) [+]	52.01 (2.71)	53.11 (3.0) *	0.01
Dominant upper limb			
Upper arm length (cm)	30.01 (1.21)	34.51 (2.21) [†]	2.40
Forearm length (cm)	23.44 (1.22)	25.84 (1.91) [†]	1.49
Elbow diameter (cm)	6.21 (0.32)	6.21 (0.42)	
Wrist diameter (cm)	5.35 (0.31)	5.23 (0.33)	
Hand length (cm) [+]	17.01 (1.02)	19.01 (1.52) [†]	1.29
Hand breadth (cm) [+]	7.32 (0.53)	7.53 (0.33) *	0.43
Hand length-breadth ratio [+]	9.22 (0.52)	9.34 (0.52)	
Hand shape index [+]	38.92 (3.54)	43.54 (2.63) [†]	2.0
Handgrip strength (kg)	26.11 (3.92)	32.21 (6.31) [†]	1.13
Non-dominant upper limb			
Upper arm length (cm)	29.81 (1.23)	33.61 (2.72) [†]	1.76
Forearm length (cm) [+]	23.02 (1.05)	25.63 (2.52) [†]	1.31
Elbow diameter (cm)	6.01 (0.43)	6.03 (0.51)	
Wrist diameter (cm)	5.34 (0.24)	5.24 (0.32)	
Hand length (cm) [+]	17.0 (0.53)	19.01 (1.84) [†]	1.35
Hand breadth (cm) [+]	7.31 (0.85)	7.31 (0.33)	
Hand length-breadth ratio [+]	9.32 (0.34)	9.42 (0.54)	
Hand shape index [+]	38.91 (3.62)	43.53 (2.64) [†]	1.79
Handgrip strength (kg)	24.51 (4.32)	31.32 (5.91) [†]	1.31

[+] Data presented as median ± IQR; SD: standard deviation; * Significant at ≤0.05 level; [†] Significant at ≤0.01 level; Effect size is shown for statistically significance differences.

Table 2 presents the correlations between anthropometric variables and dominant HGS in controls and Latin-American volleyball players. The control group showed a moderate positive correlation with forearm length and elbow and wrist diameter (r = 0.44 to 0.47; $p \leq 0.05$). Additionally, weak positive correlations were demonstrated for upper arm length, hand length, and hand breadth (r = 0.34 to 0.39; $p \leq 0.05$). Interestingly, only the female volleyball players showed a moderate positive correlation between dominant HGS and hand parameters (length r = 0.43 and breadth r = 0.63; $p \leq 0.05$). Furthermore, weak positive correlations were identified with height, upper arm length, elbow diameter, and hand shape index (r = 0.32 to 0.38; $p \leq 0.05$).

Table 2. Pearson's correlation coefficients between anthropometric variables and dominant HGS in controls and Latin-American female volleyball players.

Dominant Handgrip Strength	Controls	Volleyball Players
Height (cm)	0.24	0.38 *
Dominant upper arm length (cm)	0.39 †	0.38 *
Dominant forearm length (cm)	0.47 †	0.26
Dominant elbow diameter (cm)	0.45 †	0.32 *
Dominant wrist diameter (cm)	0.44 †	0.22
Dominant hand length (cm)	0.38 *	0.43 *
Dominant hand breadth (cm)	0.34 *	0.63 †
Hand length-breadth ratio	−0.15	−0.19
Hand shape index	−0.07	0.36 *

* Significant at ≤ 0.05 level; † Significant at ≤ 0.01 level.

In addition, Table 3 presents the correlations between anthropometric variables and non-dominant HGS in controls and volleyball players. In the control group, only weak correlations were observed with upper arm length, elbow diameter, and hand breadth (r = 0.35 to 0.38; $p \leq 0.05$). In contrast, volleyball players exhibited a moderate positive correlation with handbreadth (r = 0.55, $p \leq 0.01$) and weak positive correlations with upper arm length, wrist diameter, hand length, and hand shape index (r = 0.32 to 0.35; $p \leq 0.05$).

Table 3. Pearson's correlation coefficients between upper limb anthropometric variables and non-dominant HGS in Latin American female volleyball players and controls.

Non-Dominant Handgrip Strength	Controls	Volleyball Players
Height (cm)	0.07	0.29
Non-dominant upper arm length (cm)	0.35 *	0.34 *
Non-dominant forearm length (cm)	0.29	0.11
Non-dominant elbow diameter (cm)	0.38 †	0.16
Non-dominant wrist diameter (cm)	0.29	0.34 *
Non-dominant hand length (cm)	0.26	0.32 *
Non-dominant hand breadth (cm)	0.36 †	0.55 †
Hand length-breadth ratio	−0.09	0.13
Hand shape index	0.11	0.35 *

* Significant at ≤ 0.05 level; † Significant at ≤ 0.01 level.

4. Discussion

In this study, we have provided an overview of upper limb anthropometric characteristics and HGS of female volleyball players belonging to different National Teams in Latin America. Among the main findings, significant differences ($p < 0.05$) were found in all the lengths and breadths of both dominant and non-dominant upper limbs between volleyball players and non-athletes, with athletes exhibiting the largest measurements. In addition, we found an association between most of the hand, forearm, and arm dimensions with HGS.

Volleyball players are required to constantly develop their muscle strength, technique, and tactics to improve their performance during a match. Most researchers have mainly focused on the analysis of lower limb strength and body composition of male athletes. In this sense, the study of anthropometric and muscle strength in the upper limbs of female volleyball players has received less attention.

Several studies have described the importance of anthropometric profiles and HGS across sports [23–28]. In the present study, elite volleyball players were taller, had a lower body fat percentage, and exhibited higher values in most of the selected upper limb variables than the control group (Table 1). In addition, statistical differences were also found in HGS performance on both sides, with players being stronger than controls (Table 1). Greater height, larger body dimensions, and enhanced HGS have been previously identified as key factors contributing to success in volleyball [29–33].

Recent research on female university students in Poland, with at least five years of volleyball training experience, revealed similar results in wrist diameter, height, and BMI. However, they reported lower values in some upper limb anthropometric variables compared to our study, suggesting that this may be a differentiating factor related to the level of expertise in this sport [34].

In a study conducted by Fallahi and Jadidian [13], the authors compared different anthropometric upper limb dimensions and HGS in a group of athletes (national basketball players, collegian handball players, collegian volleyball players, and collegian wrestlers) and non-athletes. The researchers found greater HGS values in players, which were accompanied by higher measurements in hand length, palm length, palm width, forearm length, forearm circumference, and wrist circumference. In addition, most of the upper limb dimensions were positively correlated with HGS [13]. Despite the analysis not considering each sport separately, these results show that athletes who have handgrip movements with an object or opponent have specific characteristics that deserve to be trained or considered in talent identification.

Likewise, in female volleyball players of the Turkish league, Öcal et al. [14] reported higher hand dimensions when those were compared with non-athletes. Interestingly, researchers found statistical differences in only two of three selected hand measurements (hand length and hand finger length) and no differences in height. Despite the level of the athletes described in this research, these partial differences could have been due to a non-strict control group selection, as the authors did not report it.

Similar results to those reported in our study have been found by other researchers [9,29]. These studies compared upper limb dimensions and HGS between inter-university female volleyball players and a control group with no particular athletic background. Statistical differences were evidenced in the left-hand width and the lengths of the hand, forearm, and arm on both sides, with volleyball players exhibiting higher values. Moreover, volleyball players displayed higher HGS scores on both hands. Despite differences in the athletic level of the population as compared to those evaluated in our study, the results were similar and suggest an overall tendency for greater upper limb dimensions in volleyball players.

In our study, athletes were also stronger and taller, and they showed the largest measurements in hand length, hand breadth, and arm length as compared to those reported in Koyle's studies [9,29]. These differences could be explained, in part, by the fact that athletes in our study were the result of an exhaustive selection by national team coaches.

The latest findings from Sarafyniuk et al. [35] in 108 female volleyball players aged 16 to 20 found larger girth sizes in the upper limbs of athletes compared to the control group. Nevertheless, the authors did not report the years of training and level of expertise of the volleyball players, which may be crucial variables to explain the plausible differences between groups.

HGS scores in our study were also higher than those reported in other studies on volleyball players [4,6] and different sports in female athletes, ranging from 24.7 to 26.5 kg. These differences could be attributed to the specific characteristics of the participants in our study, who are elite volleyball players. Building on that point, it is important to note that a greater amount of strength in both hands is crucial for many offensive and defensive actions during a match, such as serving, passing, spiking, and blocking. For instance, while Pawlik et al. [11] reported moderated and large correlations between HGS in both hands and serve reception efficiency, and Novianingsih and Irianto [36] studied the influence of the hand's muscle strength on the volleyball float serve skill, in adolescent volleyball players. After the assessment, researchers reported more accuracy ($p < 0.05$) in the float serve in those who had higher hand strength.

With respect to correlations, in our study, anthropometric variables such as height, upper arm length, elbow diameter, and hand dimensions (length, breadth, and shape index) showed weak to moderate correlations with dominant HGS values in volleyball players. Similarly, in non-dominant HGS, upper arm length, wrist diameter, and hand dimension showed the same range of magnitude of correlation. Our findings underline that although height is considered one of the most important physical characteristics in volleyball players, this anthropometric measurement showed only a weak positive correlation with dominant HGS (Table 2). Similar findings have been reported by Pizzigally L. et al. [16] in Italian female basketball players, where the correlation reported between height and HGS was also weak ($r = 0.38$, $p < 0.05$).

In addition to height, arm length, hand length, hand breadth, and hand shape index should also be considered important parameters in the process of talent identification for female volleyball players. These anthropometric characteristics are crucial for increasing HGS and enhancing sports performance, given the numerous specific movements in volleyball, where the hand is the only point of physical contact between the athlete and the ball [16,32,37].

Regarding hand dimensions, in ball sports such as volleyball, players with larger hands and longer fingers have greater performance and accuracy in the blocking, spiking, and service techniques during the match [13]. Considering the positive association between hand measurements and HGS in both upper limbs found in our study, athletes with these features may possess the ability to apply greater force to the ball and perform a combination of finely controlled movements in defensive and offensive maneuvers that contribute to competitive success [13,32].

Additionally, the timing and sequencing of the force applied to an object (i.e., ball) by the hand depends on several factors including technique, strength, flexibility, and anthropometry [32]. Our results confirm that athletes with specific body anthropometric values such as height, arm length, and hand dimension, may have biomechanical advantages to achieve higher values of HGS.

Grip strength is produced by the joint contraction of the flexor and extensor muscles of the wrist (maintaining its dynamic stability during the test), and the predominant influence stems from the muscle strength of the fingers, specifically when the assessment is conducted with the elbow flexed at 90° [11,28]. Understanding the specific muscles engaged in the HGS test and its protocol among athletes is essential to potentially explain the relationship between hand anthropometric variables and HGS from a biomechanical approach.

As mentioned before, finger muscles play a pivotal role during the execution of the HGS test [13,32]. For this reason, some authors [16] have suggested that athletes with longer fingers and greater hand surfaces exhibit higher HGS. However, these studies have primarily involved handball and basketball players, with the majority being male [13,16]. To our knowledge, there is a lack of evidence addressing this relationship in female volleyball players, making this study the first to elucidate it. Further research may provide more relevant evidence on this topic among female volleyball players across different competitive levels.

Finally, hand length, breadth, and hand shape index in both upper limbs demonstrated the strongest correlation with HGS ($r = 0.32$ to 0.66). These findings underscore the potential significance of these anthropometric parameters as a valuable predictor of HGS, demonstrating their practical applications of these variables as an essential, feasible, and cost-effective tool for helping coaches select athletes. Additionally, the HGS could be considered a measurement of preventing upper limb injuries, particularly in wrist and fingers, due to the specific actions during a match (i.e., blocking, serving, spiking)

This study has some strengths and limitations. Our sample of Latin American female volleyball players may not be considered representative of the entire population, even though it has proved sufficient to draw relevant conclusions. Furthermore, our sample consisted only of Latin American players. For that reason, additional studies could be developed in different populations to generate reference values that consider ethnicity and age characteristics. Some of the strengths of our study include the measurements of numerous anthropometric variables collected by an expert, the utilization of accurate and adequate tools, the adherence to a standardized HGS protocol based on consensus recommendations, and measurements of HGS conducted by an experienced researcher.

5. Conclusions

This study presents, for the first time, anthropometric and HGS parameters in Latin American female volleyball players. Particularly, this study provides evidence about the influence of anthropometric body and upper limbs (height, arm length, and hand dimension) on HGS and performance outcomes in sports requiring precise gripping and manipulative actions. Furthermore, this evidence highlights the importance of arm length and hand dimensions as basic and reliable measurements when HGS evaluation is not possible during the talent search process or characterization of female volleyball players. Future studies should explore the biomechanical parameters affecting HGS and consider their influences on athletic training and injury prevention strategies in female elite sports settings.

Author Contributions: Conceptualization, A.D.l.R., M.A.C.-V. and J.C.S.; methodology, A.D.l.R., M.A.C.-V. and J.A.M.; validation, J.A.M., J.H.-A., A.S.J. and J.C.S.; formal analysis, M.A.C.-V., E.T.P.P. and C.S.-P.; investigation, A.D.l.R., M.A.C.-V., J.A.M., J.C.S. and C.S.-P.; data curation, J.A.M., J.H.-A., A.S.J., J.C.S. and F.M.-D.; writing—original draft preparation, A.D.l.R., M.A.C.-V., E.T.P.P., J.A.M. and F.M.-D.; writing—review and editing, A.D.l.R., M.A.C.-V., F.M.-D. and C.S.-P.; visualization, A.D.l.R. and M.A.C.-V.; supervision, A.D.l.R. and M.A.C.-V.; funding acquisition, A.D.l.R., M.A.C.-V. and J.C.S. All authors have read and agreed to the published version of the manuscript.

Funding: This research received no external funding.

Institutional Review Board Statement: The study was conducted in accordance with the Declaration of Helsinki and approved by the Ethics Committee for Human Beings from the Unidades Tecnológicas de Santander (no. 0010-2022/02.05.2022).

Informed Consent Statement: Informed consent was obtained from all subjects involved in the study.

Data Availability Statement: The datasets used and/or analyzed during the current study are available from the corresponding author upon reasonable request.

Acknowledgments: The authors are thankful to the coaches and players of the Colombian, Mexican, and Chilean national female volleyball teams.

Conflicts of Interest: The authors declare no conflicts of interest.

References

1. Gabbett, T.; Georgieff, B. Physiological and Anthropometric Characteristics of Australian Junior National, State, and Novice Volleyball Players. *J. Strength. Cond. Res.* **2007**, *21*, 902–908. [CrossRef]
2. Quiroga, M.E.; García-Manso, J.M.; Rodríguez-Ruiz, D.; Sarmiento, S.; De Saa, Y.; Moreno, M.P. Relation between In-Game Role and Service Characteristics in Elite Women's Volleyball. *J. Strength. Cond. Res.* **2010**, *24*, 2316–2321. [CrossRef] [PubMed]
3. Reeser, J.C.; Fleisig, G.S.; Bolt, B.; Ruan, M. Upper Limb Biomechanics During the Volleyball Serve and Spike. *Sports Health* **2010**, *2*, 368. [CrossRef] [PubMed]
4. Khanna, A.; Koley, S. Comparison of Anthropometric Profile and Handgrip Strength between Inter-University Volleyball Players and a Reference Group. *Biomed. Hum. Kinet.* **2020**, *12*, 82–90. [CrossRef]
5. Carvalho, A.; Roriz, P.; Duarte, D. Comparison of Morphological Profiles and Performance Variables between Female Volleyball Players of the First and Second Division in Portugal. *J. Hum. Kinet.* **2020**, *71*, 109–117. [CrossRef]

6. Barut, Ç.; Demirel, P.; K›ran, S. Introduction Evaluation of Hand Anthropometric Measurements and Grip Strength in Basketball, Volleyball, and Handball Players. *Anatomy* **2008**, *2*, 55–59. [CrossRef]
7. Buśko, K. Power–Velocity Relationship and Muscular Strength in Female Volleyball Players during Preparatory Period and Competition Season. *Acta Bioeng. Biomech.* **2019**, *21*, 31–36. [CrossRef]
8. Pereira, A.; Costa, A.M.; Santos, P.; Figueiredo, T.; João, P.V. Training Strategy of Explosive Strength in Young Female Volleyball Players. *Medicina (Lithuania)* **2015**, *51*, 126–131. [CrossRef]
9. Koley, S.; Kaur, S.P. Correlations of Handgrip Strength with Selected Hand-Arm-Anthropometric Variables in Indian Inter-University Female Volleyball Players. *Asian J. Sports Med.* **2011**, *2*, 220. [CrossRef]
10. Das, M.; Roy, B.; Let, B.; Chatterjee, K. Investigation of Relationship of Strength and Size of Different Body Parts to Velocity of Volleyball Serve and Spike. *IOSR J. Sports Phys. Educ. (IOSR-JSPE).* **2015**, *2*, 18–22. [CrossRef]
11. Pawlik, D.; Dziubek, W.; Rogowski, Ł.; Struzik, A.; Rokita, A. Strength Abilities and Serve Reception Efficiency of Youth Female Volleyball Players. *Appl. Bionics Biomech.* **2022**, *2022*, 4328761. [CrossRef]
12. Malina, R.M.; Meleski, B.W.; Shoup, R.F. Anthropometric, Body Composition, and Maturity Characteristics of Selected School-Age Athletes. *Pediatr. Clin. N. Am.* **1982**, *29*, 1305–1323. [CrossRef] [PubMed]
13. Fallahi, A.A.; Jadidian, A.A. The Effect of Hand Dimensions, Hand Shape and Some Anthropometric Characteristics on Handgrip Strength in Male Grip Athletes and Non-Athletes. *J. Hum. Kinet.* **2011**, *29*, 151. [CrossRef]
14. Defne, Ö.; Bilgehan, B.; Tuba, M. Comparison of Anthropometric Measurements of Dominant Hands between Adult Elite Volleyball Players and Sedentaries. *Ovidius Univ. Ann. Ser. Phys. Educ. Sport/Sci. Mov. Health* **2010**, *10*, 546–549.
15. Nickerson, B.S. Evaluation of Obesity Cutoff Values in Hispanic Adults: Derivation of New Standards. *J. Clin. Densitom.* **2021**, *24*, 388–396. [CrossRef]
16. Pizzigalli, L.; Cremasco, M.M.; Torre, A.L.; Rainoldi, A.; Benis, R. Hand Grip Strength and Anthropometric Characteristics in Italian Female National Basketball Teams. *J. Sports Med. Phys. Fit.* **2017**, *57*, 521–528. [CrossRef] [PubMed]
17. Richards, L.G.; Olson, B.; Palmiter-Thomas, P. How Forearm Position Affects Grip Strength. *Am. J. Occup. Ther.* **1996**, *50*, 133–138. [CrossRef] [PubMed]
18. Mathiowetz, V.; Wiemer, D.M.; Federman, S.M. Grip and Pinch Strength: Norms for 6- to 19-Year-Olds. *Am. J. Occup. Ther.* **1986**, *40*, 705–711. [CrossRef]
19. Pereira, H.M.; De Oliveira Menacho, M.; Takahashi, R.H.; Cardoso, J.R.; Paulo -Sp, S. Handgrip Strength Evaluation on Tennis Players Using Different Recommendations. *Rev. Bras. Med. Esporte* **2011**, *17*, 184–188. [CrossRef]
20. Fay, M.P.; Proschan, M.A. Wilcoxon-Mann-Whitney or T-Test? On Assumptions for Hypothesis Tests and Multiple Interpretations of Decision Rules. *Stat. Surv.* **2010**, *4*, 1–39. [CrossRef]
21. Fritz, C.O.; Morris, P.E.; Richler, J.J. Effect Size Estimates: Current Use, Calculations, and Interpretation. *J. Exp. Psychol. Gen.* **2012**, *141*, 2–18. [CrossRef]
22. Schober, P.; Schwarte, L.A. Correlation Coefficients: Appropriate Use and Interpretation. *Anesth. Analg.* **2018**, *126*, 1763–1768. [CrossRef]
23. Gualdi-Russo, E.; Zaccagni, L. Somatotype, Role and Performance in Elite Volleyball Players. *J. Sports Med. Phys. Fit.* **2001**, *2*, 256.
24. Leão, C.; Camões, M.; Clemente, F.M.; Nikolaidis, P.T.; Lima, R.; Bezerra, P.; Rosemann, T.; Knechtle, B. Anthropometric Profile of Soccer Players as a Determinant of Position Specificity and Methodological Issues of Body Composition Estimation. *Int. J. Environ. Res. Public Health* **2019**, *16*, 2386. [CrossRef]
25. D'Anastasio, R.; Milivojevic, A.; Cilli, J.; Icaro, I.; Viciano, J.; D'Anastasio, R.; Milivojevic, A.; Cilli, J.; Icaro, I.; Viciano, J. Perfiles Antropométricos y Somatotipos de Jugadoras de Voleibol Femenino y Voleibol de Playa. *Int. J. Morphol.* **2019**, *37*, 1480–1485. [CrossRef]
26. Quintero, A.M.; Fonseca, S.; Chagnaud, C.A.; De la Rosa, A. Comparison between Plethysmography and Body Fat Equations in Elite Taekwondo Athletes. *Ido Mov. Cult. J. Martial Arts Anthropol.* **2022**, *22*, 14–22. [CrossRef]
27. Monterrosa Quintero, A.; Fuentes-Garcia, J.P.; Poblete-Valderrama, F.; Pereira de Andrade, G.A.; De la Rosa, A. Body Composition, Power Muscle, and Baropodometric Assessment in Elite Muay Thai Athletes. *Ido Mov. Cult. J. Martial Arts Anthropol.* **2024**, *24*, 12–22. [CrossRef]
28. Monterrosa Quintero, A.; De La Rosa, A.; Arc-Chagnaud, C.; Quintero Gómez, J.M.; Pereira Moro, A.R. Morphology, Lower Limbs Performance and Baropodometric Characteristics of Elite Brazilian Jiu-Jitsu Athletes. *Ido Mov. Cult.* **2023**, *23*, 58–69. [CrossRef]
29. Koley, S.; Singh, J.; Sandhu, J.S. Anthropometric and Physiological characteristics on Indian Inter-University Volleyball Players. *J. Hum. Sport Exerc.* **2010**, *5*, 389–399. [CrossRef]
30. Vishaw Gaurav, S.; Kumar, R.; Singh, M.; Bhanot, P. Anthropometric Measurement of Volleyball Players at Different Level of Competition. *Int. J. Multidiscip. Curr. Res.* **2015**, *3*, 999–1002.
31. Joksimovic, M.; Goranovic, K.; Petkovic, J.; Badau, D.; Hantanu, C.G.; Joksimovic, M.; Goranovic, K.; Petkovic, J.; Badau, D.; Hantanu, C.G. Características Morfológicas de Jugadoras de Voleibol de Élite Menores de 19 Años. *Int. J. Morphol.* **2023**, *41*, 1203–1208. [CrossRef]
32. Cronin, J.; Lawton, T.; Harris, N.; Kilding, A.; Mcmaster, D.T. A Brief Review of Handgrip Strength and Sport Performance. *J. Strength. Cond. Res.* **2017**, *31*, 3187–3217. [CrossRef] [PubMed]
33. Spence, D.W.; Disch, J.G.; Fred, H.L.; Coleman, A.E. Descriptive Profiles of Highly Skilled Women Volleyball Players. *Med. Sci. Sports Exerc.* **1980**, *12*, 299–302. [CrossRef] [PubMed]

34. Kutseryb, T.; Hrynkiv, M.; Vovkanych, L.; Muzyka, F.; Melnyk, V. Anthropometric Characteristic and Body Composition of Female Students Involved in Volleyball Training. *Anthropol. Rev.* **2022**, *85*, 31–42. [CrossRef]
35. Sarafyniuk, L.; Stepanenko, I.; Khapitska, O.; Lezhnova, O.; Vlasenko, R. Anthropometric Features of Limbs in Volleyball Players of Different Somatotypes. *Bull. Med. Biol. Res.* **2024**, *6*, 52–63. [CrossRef]
36. Novianingsih, B.; Pekik Irianto, D. The Effect of Training Method and Strength of the Hand Muscles towards Float Serve in Volleyball Extracurricular. *Pedagog. Psychol. Sport* **2019**, *5*, 2391–8306. [CrossRef]
37. Wu, T.-C.; Pearsall, D.; Hodges, A.; Turcotte, R.; Lefebvre, R.; Montgomery, D.; Bateni, H. The Performance of the Ice Hockey Slap and Wrist Shots: The Effects of Stick Construction and Player Skill. *Sports Eng.* **2003**, *6*, 31–39. [CrossRef]

Disclaimer/Publisher's Note: The statements, opinions and data contained in all publications are solely those of the individual author(s) and contributor(s) and not of MDPI and/or the editor(s). MDPI and/or the editor(s) disclaim responsibility for any injury to people or property resulting from any ideas, methods, instructions or products referred to in the content.

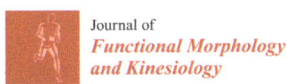

Article

Post-Arthroplasty Spatiotemporal Gait Parameters in Patients with Hip Osteoarthritis or Developmental Dysplasia of the Hip: An Observational Study

Sophia Stasi [1,2,*], Georgios Papagiannis [2], Athanasios Triantafyllou [1,2], Panayiotis Papagelopoulos [2] and Panagiotis Koulouvaris [2]

[1] 1st Department of Orthopaedic Surgery, National and Kapodistrian University of Athens, 12462 Athens, Greece; athanat@gmail.com

[2] Biomechanics Laboratory, Department of Physiotherapy, University of the Peloponnese, 23100 Sparta, Greece; grpapagiannis@yahoo.gr (G.P.); pjportho@med.uoa.gr (P.P.); info@drkoulouvaris.gr (P.K.)

* Correspondence: stasis@go.uop.gr

Abstract: Total hip arthroplasty (THA) is a preferred treatment for primary osteoarthritis (OA) or secondary degenerative arthropathy due to developmental hip dysplasia (DDH). Gait analysis is considered a gold standard for evaluating post-arthroplasty walking patterns. This study compared post-THA spatiotemporal gait parameters (SGPs) between OA and DDH patients and explored correlations with demographic and clinical variables. Thirty patients (15 per group) were recorded during gait and their SGPs were analyzed. Functionality was evaluated with the Oxford Hip Score (OHS). The OA patients were significantly older than DDH patients ($p < 0.005$). Significant and moderate to strong were the correlations between SGPs, age, and four items of the OHS concerning hip pain and activities of daily life ($0.31 <$ Pearson's r < 0.51 all $p < 0.05$). Following THA, both groups exhibited similar levels of the examined gait parameters. Post-arthroplasty SGPs and OHS correlations indicate limitations in certain activities. Given the absence of pre-operative data and the correlation between age and SGPs and OHS, ANCOVA testing revealed that age adjusts OHS and SGP values, while pre-operative diagnosis has no main effect. These findings indicate that hip OA or DDH do not affect postoperative SGPs and patients' functionality. Future studies should examine both kinematic and kinetic data to better evaluate the post-THA gait patterns of OA and DDH patients.

Keywords: orthopedics biomechanics; spatiotemporal gait parameters; functionality; total hip arthroplasty; hip osteoarthritis; developmental hip dysplasia

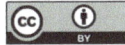

1. Introduction

Total hip arthroplasty (THA) is the treatment of choice for end-stage arthritic hip conditions that cause chronic pain, discomfort, and significant functional impairment [1]. Among the pathological conditions that lead to THA are primary osteoarthritis and secondary degenerative arthropathy due to developmental dysplasia of the hip (DDH) [1].

Osteoarthritis (OA) is the most common type of primary degenerative arthropathy and is a major cause of chronic disability [2]. OA is the clinical and pathological outcome of a sequence of biological and metabolic processes of joint components/tissues, and is associated with structural alterations, such as degeneration of articular cartilage and changes in the subchondral bone. It ultimately leads to the limitation or abolition of the functionality joint as a kinetic and—in the case of the hip joint—supporting skeleton unit [3]. On the other hand, in DDH, the acetabulum and femur are underdeveloped, the femur adapts to an abnormal position, and the soft tissues of the area are shortened [4]. Leg-length discrepancy (LLD), decreased hip abduction range of motion, positive Trendelenburg sign, and shortened iliopsoas and hip adductor muscles are often seen in patients with DDH, while usually they walk with plantar flexion (toe support) [4]. These patients develop symptomatic secondary OA in their fourth or fifth decade of life, and a large number of them are forced to resort to THA at a younger age than patients with primary OA [5,6].

Gait assessment is an essential measure of postoperative outcomes after THA, as gait is a crucial indicator of the level of functional recovery [7,8]. Gait analysis is used to assess gait patterns in different groups of patients [9]. Specifically, spatiotemporal gait parameters are a way to objectively assess dysfunctional gait and monitor treatment progress in a clinical setting [10]. They are also considered a valuable adjunct to clinical and radiological assessment [9].

In the gait analysis of hip OA patients, several non-physiological features can be observed that result from the main symptoms of osteoarthritis. The most characteristic change is reduced gait speed with the gait pattern, including LLD [11]. A systematic meta-analysis, which included 30 studies that studied spatiotemporal characteristics in hip OA patients, reported that the selected walking speed and the average walking pace were slower compared to healthy individuals. At the same time, the step and stride lengths were shorter, the double support phase was shorter, and the step width was larger than those of their healthy peers [10]. Similarly, in gait analysis studies where the gait pattern of DDH patients has been studied, it has been reported that in relation to healthy peers, they walk with a reduced gait speed [12–14], have a shorter step length [12,14], and the affected limb shows a longer double support time and a shorter single leg support time [12,13]. Postoperatively, gait pattern improves significantly in all patients regardless of preoperative diagnosis [15]. Nevertheless, even ten years after undergoing THA surgery, it has been reported that patients' walking ability does not reach the same levels as their peers of the same age [16].

However, the literature review revealed that in most gait analysis studies concerning the post-THA gait, either in patients with hip OA or DDH patients, the comparison was carried out with non-operated [17,18] or with healthy peers [16,19]. Up to our knowledge, only one study compares post-arthroplasty gait parameters between patients with primary OA and DDH patients [20]. Therefore, the present study aims to compare the post-arthroplasty gait spatiotemporal parameters in patients with primary OA and patients with DDH. The primary study hypothesis is that the distinct pathomechanics associated with each condition contribute to the preoperative adaptations in gait. Consequently, it is thought that there may be variations in the improvement of postoperative spatiotemporal characteristics. Secondary outcomes included potential correlations between postoperative spatiotemporal and demographic/clinical characteristics relating to patients' functionality. Based on previous relevant studies on post-THA patients [21,22], we hypothesized that postoperative spatiotemporal characteristics have the same trend with patient-reported outcomes. Biomechanists and rehabilitation experts could utilize such evidence to advance the development of targeted rehabilitation programs that ultimately improve the functional capacity of patients.

2. Materials and Methods

2.1. Trial Design

This research was conducted in a biomechanics laboratory (Ethics Approval No: 42609/05-05-2022). Patients who agreed to participate in the study were given written informed consent according to the principles of the Declaration of Helsinki and its later amendments [23]. The present study conformed to the "Strengthening the Reporting of Observational Studies in Epidemiology" (STROBE) statement for reporting observational studies [24] (Supplementary File).

2.2. Participants

Patients over 45 were included in the present study, as it has been reported that one in four arthroplasties performed before age fifty are due to hip dysplasia [25]. The patients were required to have undergone primary THA three to five years prior to their enrollment in the present study; namely, the THA surgery must have been performed from January 2019 to December 2021. This postoperative time was chosen as a sufficient period to allow all patients to adopt a stable gait pattern [26]. All participants underwent a cementless THA through a posterior approach [27,28] performed by the same team of orthopaedic surgeons and all patients followed the same postoperative physiotherapy program. Information was obtained by reviewing the registry data from their admission for THA surgery and by conducting telephone interviews. After the first screening, the enrolled patients were divided into two groups according to their preoperative diagnosis. The first group (OA group) included patients who underwent THA due to unilateral hip OA and the second group (DDH group) included patients who underwent THA due to secondary degenerative arthropathy due to unilateral DDH. Patients were excluded from the study if they had had previous hip joint-preserving procedures or acquired post-THA a leg-length discrepancy (LLD) greater than 2 cm, a nerve injury, a history of other orthopedic surgery on the lower limbs or spine, declared that they suffered from a severe balance disorder, any neurological and musculoskeletal diseases that prevented them from performing free walking, or used a walking aid.

2.3. Outcomes

Initially, the demographic characteristics (age, gender, height, weight, and body mass index) of the two groups' populations were recorded. The preoperative grade of hip OA was recorded according to the Kellgren–Lawrence classification system [29] and the grade of DDH according to the Crowe classification system [30]. Anthropometric data were collected using a Seca scale (model 803) and a height meter. The knee and ankle joints' diameters, anterior superior iliac spine (ASIS) distance, and pelvic depth were measured with a caliper.

Patients' functionality was measured using the Oxford Hip Score (OHS), which consisted of 12 questions assessing pain and function during activities of daily living (ADLs). The OHS questionnaire was designed and developed to assess patients undergoing THA [31]. Items' response scores range from 0 points (most severe symptoms) to 4 points (least symptoms), with a total score between 40 and 48 indicating satisfactory joint function [32].

2.4. Instrumentation and Procedure

A motion recording system with six Vicon MCam optoelectronic cameras (Oxford MetricsGroup Ltd., Oxford, UK) was used to record the patients' spatiotemporal parameters, which were recorded during walking.

The equipment was calibrated every morning by the same biomechanist before the measurements, according to the applicable local protocols, to ensure accuracy and enable the calculation of each marker's three-dimensional (3D) coordinates. The mean error in calculating the difference between the measured and actual distance of two markers fixed to the ends of a rigid rod 600 mm apart was within 0.3 mm. The calibrated volume for this application was 10 m in length (x-axis of the laboratory reference system), 3 m in height (y-axis of the laboratory reference system), and 3 m along the z-axis of the laboratory reference system. Records of these checks and associated calibrations were saved along with all session data.

All six optoelectronic cameras also used a frequency of 120 Hz for data acquisition, while the motion analysis system error was <0.1 mm in a $10 \times 3 \times 3$ m laboratory space volume (Figure 1). These calibration parameters also ensured the accuracy of the recorded data.

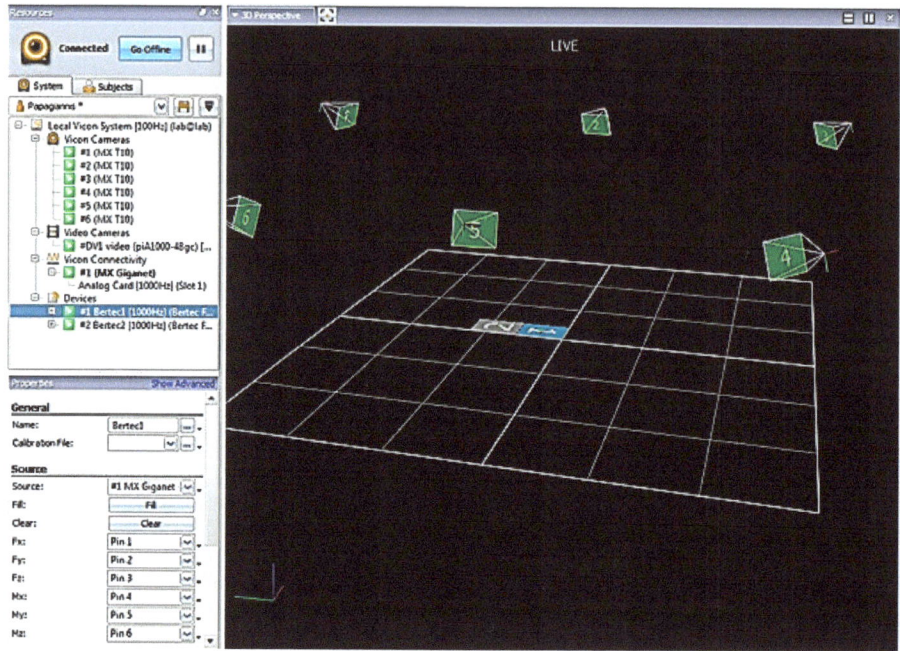

Figure 1. The ViconNexus software version 2.3 figure of data acquisition procedure, depicting laboratory dimensions, six optoelectronic cameras, and two force plates).

2.5. Modeling—Placement of Markers

Motion modeling is an essential concept in the field of biomechanical data recording. The Plug-in Gait marker fitting procedure was employed due to this rationale [33]. Markers were strategically positioned in the anatomical areas of the pelvis and lower extremities. The pelvic markers were placed at the anatomical landmarks of the left anterior superior iliac spine (LASI marker), the right anterior superior iliac spine (RASI marker), the left posterior superior iliac spine (LPSI marker), and the right posterior superior iliac spine (RPSI marker). As for the lower extremities, both the left and right, the following markers were positioned: on the upper lateral 1/3 area of the left and right thigh (LTHI/RTHI markers), on the flexion-extension axis of the left and right knee (LKNE/RKNE markers), and on the lower 1/3 area of the left/right shank (LTIB/RTIB markers). To reconstruct the foot section, markers were positioned on the left/right lateral malleolus, passing along an imaginary line across the left/right transmalleolar axis (LANK/RANK markers), on the left/right calcaneus bone (LHEE/RHEE markers), and on the left/right second metatarsal head, on the mid-foot side of the equinus break between the fore-foot and mid-foot (LTOE/RTOE markers).

To achieve precise localization and positioning of knee markers (LKNE and RKNE), a slight passive flexion and extension of the knee were performed while carefully observing the lateral knee joint skin area. The location where the knee joint's axis intersects the knee's outer surface was identified by locating the layer of skin on the thigh that moved the least. This landmark was designated with a pen as the focal point for the rotational movement of the foot's bottom.

Thigh markers (LTHI and RTHI) are utilized to identify the location of the knee flexion axis. The LTHI marker was positioned on the lower one-third of the outside lateral area of the thigh, while the RTHI marker was put on the upper one-third of the outer lateral surface of the thigh, slightly under the arm's reach point. However, the exact height of the markers is not an essential factor in this measurement. Proper identification of the knee flexion axis relies on the reflectors' anteroposterior location. The thigh marker's location was modified to align with the plane, including the hip and knee joints center and the axis representing knee flexion and extension.

The alignment of the plantar flexion axis is determined using tibial markers, namely the LTIB and RTIB. The LTIB marker was positioned on the lower one-third of the tibial surface, while the RTIB marker was placed on the upper one-third of the tibial surface, like the thigh markers. The tibial marker was positioned inside the plane, including the center of the knee and ankle joints and the axis representing ankle flexion and extension.

The participants conducted the walking process during a single laboratory session. They were instructed to walk in a manner that closely resembled their usual walking style, with occasional cues given, for a distance of approximately 6 m at a self-chosen tempo. A preliminary static trial was conducted to establish the orientations of the markers before processing the model. Subsequently, participants performed two dynamic trials to familiarize themselves with the testing processes. Ultimately, they completed three additional trials that were considered sufficient and were then analyzed to obtain the representative values of the spatiotemporal parameters [19].

2.6. Data Synthesis

Anthropometric measurements were combined with data from markers' deflections. All markers' location data were captured using Nexus 2.3 software. The spatiotemporal parameters measured in this study were walking speed, cadence, double support time, single support, step time and length, and stride time and length.

The above spatiotemporal parameters were included in the statistical analysis and were calculated using inverse dynamics and normalization in terms of body mass and length [34].

2.7. Statistical Analysis

Data were expressed for continuous variables as mean ± standard deviation (SD) and for categorical variables as frequencies (percentages).

Normality was assessed by Q-Q plot inspection. Pearson's r correlation index assessed correlations between continuous variables (demographic, clinical, and spatiotemporal parameters' data) of all patients. Group differences assessed using ANVOVA.

All tests were two-sided, with the significance level being $p = 0.05$. All tests were performed using SPSS v.29 (IBM Corporation, Somers, NY, USA).

3. Results

3.1. Participants

A total of 50 patients were enrolled in the present study (the minimum required total sample after Power Analysis was found to be 29 subjects). Of the 50 patients, 25 were diagnosed with hip OA before THA and 25 had unilateral DDH. Ten did not meet the inclusion criteria, nine refused to participate, and one hip OA patient had passed away because of a cause unrelated to THA. Finally, 30 patients (15 in each group) were included. The detailed procedure of the participants' selection is presented in a flow diagram (Figure 2).

3.2. Demographic and Clinical Characteristics

The Q-Q plot inspection revealed that variables had normal distribution; hence, parametric testing was performed. The mean ± SD of the demographic and clinical characteristics of the study's sample are presented in Table 1. There were no significant demographic or clinical differences between the groups, except for age ($p < 0.005$). When the THA was performed, the mean age of the OA group was 60.1 years (min = 53, max = 68), and the mean age of the DDH group was 46.13 years (min = 36, max = 55 years). The OA group included five men and ten women, while the DDH group consisted of three men and 12 women. Eight patients of the OA group underwent THA due to grade III and seven due to grade IV hip OA, according to the Kellgren–Lawrence classification system. According to the Crowe classification system, the DDH group included four patients with Crowe II, six with Crowe III, and four with Crowe IV dysplastic hip. The greater preoperative LLD of the DDH group was 5 cm, while the hip OA preoperative LLD was not reported in the record files. The means of the post-THA time period were for the hip OA group 3.91 years (min = 3.3, max = 5) and for the DDH group 3.69 years (min = 3.1, max = 4.8).

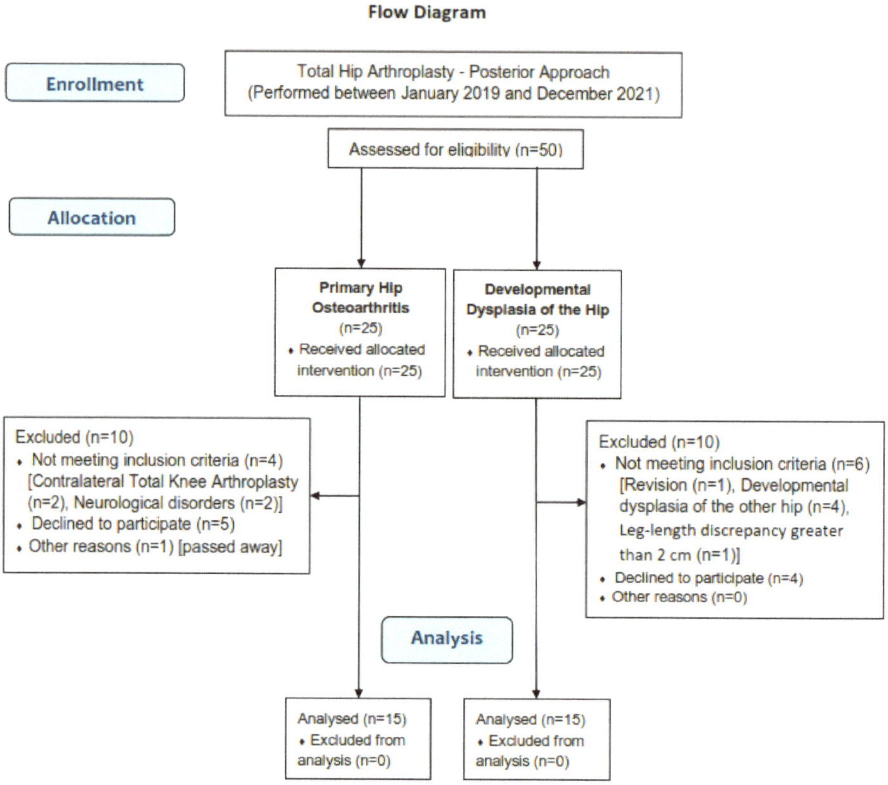

Figure 2. This study's flow diagram.

Table 1. Demographic and clinical characteristics of the study's sample (N = 30).

Characteristics	OA Group (N = 15)	DDH Group (N = 15)	p-Value
Age (years)	60.1 ± 3.82	46.13 ± 5.93	<0.005
Sex (Men/Women) [N (%)]	5(33.3%)/10(66.7%)	3(20%)/12(80%)	0.409
Height (cm)	163.95 ± 3.6	164.42 ± 3.1	0.181
Weight (kg)	69.35 ± 5.6	68.41 ± 4.5	0.135
Body Mass Index (kg/m^2)	25.78 ± 2.6	25.30 ± 2.07	0.289
Years post-THA	3.91 ± 0.52	3.69 ± 0.52	0.123

The values for continuous variables are expressed as mean ± standard deviation (SD) and for categorical variables as frequencies (percentages).

3.3. Correlation Analysis

The correlation analysis revealed significant moderate to strong correlations. Specifically, moderate and positive were the correlations between age and walking speed, step length, and total OHS score (r = 0.31, p = 0.00, r = 0.34, p = 0.00, and r = 0.36, p = 0.04.

respectively), while negative and strong was the correlation between age and step time (r = −0.51, p = 0.04). Positive and moderate correlations were found between walking speed and item 5 of the OHS ("Could you do the household shopping on your own?") (r = 0.40, p = 0.02) and between cadence and item 11 of the OHS ("How much has pain from your hip interfered with your usual work, including housework?") (r = 0.38, p = 0.03). The single support time positively and moderately correlated with item 5 of the OHS (r = 0.46, p = 0.01). Strong and negative was the correlation between step time and item 5 of the OHS (r = −0.51, p = 0.00). The step length was moderately and negatively correlated with item 4 of the OHS ("Have you been able to put on a pair of socks, stockings or tights?") (r = −0.41, p = 0.02), while the stride length was moderately and negatively correlated with item 6 ("For how long have you been able to walk before the pain in your hip becomes severe (with or without a walking aid)?") (r = −0.36, p = 0.04) and with item 4 (r = −0.44, p = 0.01) of the OHS.

3.4. Group Differences

Given the absence of pre-THA data, the correlations between age and SGPS and OHS group differences were assessed using analysis of covariance (ANCOVA).

After controlling for age revealed (Pillai's trace = 0.05, Wilk's Lamba = 0.05) the ANCOVA showed that age adjusts the values of the outcomes (SPGs and OHS). Additionally, the multivariate test for the OA and DDH groups (Pillai's trace = 0.651, Wilk's Lamba = 0.651) indicated no significant main effect amongst the independent groups of the outcome mentioned above when controlling for age. The above indicates that age does indeed adjust the results, but there are no statistically significant main effects between the two groups, which is a significant finding.

3.5. Outcomes

The OHS total score ranged from 38 to 42 in the OA group and 37 to 42 in the DDH group. The mean ± SD of the item scores and the total Oxford Hip Score of both groups are included in Table 2. No significant statistical differences were also observed between the two groups regarding their spatiotemporal parameters. The mean ± SD of SGPs of both groups are presented in Table 3.

Table 2. Item scores and overall Oxford Hip Scores (N = 30).

Items	OA Group (N = 15)	DDH Group (N = 15)
1. How would you describe the pain you usually have in your hip?	3.40 ± 0.74	3.33 ± 0.72
2. Have you had any trouble with washing and drying yourself (all over) because of your hip?	4.00 ± 0.00	3.93 ± 0.26
3. Have you had any trouble getting in and out of a car or using public transportation because of your hip? (whichever you tend to use)	3.66 ± 0.5	3.60 ± 0.49
4. Have you been able to put on a pair of socks, stockings or tights?	2.33 ± 0.47	2.47 ± 0.51
5. Could you do the household shopping on your own?	4.00 ± 0.00	3.86 ± 0.26
6. For how long have you been able to walk before the pain in your hip becomes severe? (with or without a walking aid)	3.60 ± 0.51	3.13 ± 0.77
7. Have you been able to climb a flight of stairs?	3.20 ± 0.40	3.07 ± 0.26
8. After a meal (sat at a table), how painful has it been for you to stand up from a chair because of your hip?	3.36 ± 0.49	3.53 ± 0.52
9. Have you been limping when walking, because of your hip?	3.13 ± 0.61	3.00 ± 0.55
10. Have you had any sudden, severe pain—"shooting", "stabbing", or "spasms"—from your affected hip?	3.40 ± 0.52	3.20 ± 0.91
11. How much has pain from your hip interfered with your usual work (including housework)?	3.8 ± 0.47	3.53 ± 0.75
12. Have you been troubled by pain from your hip in bed at night?	3.47 ± 0.72	3.06 ± 0.72
Oxford Hip Score (total score)	41.67 ± 2.19	39.73 ± 1.58

The values are expressed as mean ± standard deviation (SD).

Table 3. Spatiotemporal parameters of the study's sample (N = 30).

Parameters	OA Group (N= 15)	DDH Group (N= 15)
Walking speed (cm/s)	77.26 ± 4.83	74.75 ± 3.24
Cadence (steps/min)	94.69 ± 2.73	92.93 ± 3.17
Double support time (% cycle)	33.18 ± 2.13	31.78 ± 3.81
Single support (% cycle)	37.09 ± 3.8	35.12 ± 5.57
Step time (s)	0.66 ± 0.08	0.72 ± 0.11
Step length (cm)	48.62 ± 2.84	47.18 ± 2.87
Stride time (s)	1.23 ± 0.20	1.27 ± 0.11
Stride length (cm)	97.83 ± 5.45	95.45 ± 5.65

The values are expressed as mean ± standard deviation (SD).

4. Discussion

Our observational study aimed to compare postoperative SGPs in patients who received THA due to either primary hip OA or DDH and to explore any possible correlations with demographic or clinical variables. Our results showed that the values of SGPs of the OA group were slightly better than those of the DDH group without revealing a statistically significant difference. The distinct pathomechanics of OA or DDH associated with preoperative alterations in gait improved after THA to similar levels in both groups. As expressed by the OHS results, the OA group reported a better overall trend of the scores than the DDH group regarding self-estimated functionality. Significant correlations were found between the sample's SGPs with age, the total OHS score, and four items of the OHS concerning hip pain and ADLs.

In the present study, the patients of the OA group were significantly older than the DDH group. This finding was expected since it is well-known that hip OA is a chronic disorder resulting from several distinct etiologic factors, including aging. Hip OA affects 7–25% of people older than 55 years [35] and demonstrates an increase in mean prevalence with advancing age [36]. On the other hand, DDH is the most common cause of secondary osteoarthritis in adults under 40 years of age, since abnormal hip biomechanics resulting in contact stresses predispose patients with DDH to arthritic changes earlier than the normal population and require THA at an early age [37]. Also expected was the fact that our groups consisted of more women than men, in line with studies reporting that hip OA prevalence is higher among women [38], while DDH is more common among girls [37]. Regarding age and sex, our groups were relatively representative of both populations studied [35–38].

The correlation analysis revealed statistically significant correlations between participants' age, OHS scores (total and items), and the SGPs. Specifically, severe pain during long-time walking (item 5) was correlated with shorter stride length. Similarly, shorter step and stride length correlated with difficulty putting on socks, stockings, or tights (item 7). Additionally, the patient's ability to perform household shopping independently (item 11) was correlated with faster walking speed, longer single support time, and shorter step time. On the other hand, a lower level of hip pain interference in usual work/housework (item 12) was linked to a slower cadence. Our findings support previous studies in which self-reported outcomes and biomechanical parameters were correlated in post-THA patients 12 months post-THA [21,22]. In the study of John et al. [21], the Hip Disability and Osteoarthritis Outcome Score (HOOS) correlated strongly with hip strength, while the correlations with step length asymmetry and contact time asymmetry were not significant and relatively weak (r < 0.32). In the study of Bolink et al. [22], moderate to strong significant correlations were found between the Western Ontario and McMaster Universities Osteoarthritis Index (WOMAC) and walking speed, cadence, and step time (0.31 < Pearson's r < 0.51). Unfortunately, it is not possible to directly compare our OHS item results with the findings of the studies mentioned earlier, since the WOMAC and HOOS evaluate different aspects of pain and functionality than the OHS, which records experienced difficulty during a specific activity. However, correlations between self-reported outcomes and gait parameters may provide additional information showing how the latter affects post-THA-specific ADLs. These correlations can be used to develop personalized exercise programs for patients. By analyzing the data, healthcare professionals can identify specific areas of deficits and weaknesses in patients and create tailored exercise programs that target those areas. This approach helps reduce the deficits and improves the patient's overall independence and quality of life.

No statistically significant differences between the two groups were observed in the SGPs. This can be explained by the effect of age as well as the lack of pre-operative data. However, our findings are consistent with the study conducted by Marangoz et al. [20], the only biomechanical study that directly compared the gait of post-THA OA and DDH patients [20]. Upon studying their results, we noticed that the average values of the SGPs of their groups were quite comparable to our findings. However, we did identify a difference in the walking speed and cadence of their DDH group, which were lower than the corresponding values we obtained in our study [20]. These differences might be due to the fact that their study's gait analysis was carried out 12.5 months after THA, while in our study, the participants were measured after a three-and-a-half-year period. Studies have reported that after THA, the gait pattern generally improved significantly in all patients. However, patients with DDH tend to experience a more persistent pathological gait pattern, which subsides slowly over a more extended period [1,18]. This is due to the distorted hip anatomy (underdeveloped acetabulum and femur), LLD, decreased hip abduction range of motion, positive Trendelenburg sign, shortened iliopsoas, and hip adductors muscles that lead to asymmetrical gait than that of healthy controls. Patients tend to protect their DDH limb from childhood, and this compensation mechanism for the unaffected side in protecting the affected side remains after THA [19]. Therefore, it is suggested that a follow-up period longer than one year is necessary to obtain relevant results [39]. Extending the follow-up period beyond one year is essential to yield meaningful and insightful results. Thus, it is highly recommended that researchers extend their follow-up periods to achieve significant and relevant results [39].

Postoperative gait analysis is generally accepted as an objective measurement of surgical success since it effectively quantifies SGPs [20]. In addition to the objective gait assessment, the use of self-reported outcomes like OHS can provide unique information on the impact of treatment from the patient's perspective [40], and it is complementary to the overall assessment of patients' recovery; this is essential in clinical research and practice involving THA patients [40]. In our study, although the OA group had better outcome values (SGPs and OHS) than the DDH group, this was not reflected in the statistical analysis results, due to the lack of pre-THA data and the potential effect of age. However, these findings suggest that the pathological anatomy of DDH might be responsible for the observed phenomenon. Although the hip joint was reconstructed after THA, patients may continue to experience pain and discomfort on the affected side [19]. The possible reason is that in most DDH cases, widened intraoperative articular capsule release and tenotomies of the shortened hip muscles are advocated [28]. These necessary intraoperative soft tissue releases, combined with the aforementioned compensation mechanism of the unaffected side protecting the affected side, may impact the performance of daily activities in DDH patients, even after THA [19]. In order to minimize the soft tissue releases' effects, studies suggest that patients with developmental dysplasia of the hip (DDH) can benefit from individualized exercise programs that prioritize strengthening the intact muscles in the lower limb. Specifically, exercises targeting hip flexors, hip abductors, and knee extensors have been effective [15,19].

To our knowledge, this is the second study that directly compares post-arthroplasty gait parameters between patients with primary OA and DDH patients. Our study supports the previous study's findings [20], indicating that the distinct pathomechanics of OA or DDH, associated with pre-operative alterations in gait, improved after THA to similar levels in both groups. In addition, this is one of the very few studies [21,22] in which objective gait assessment via SGPs was correlated with patient-reported outcomes. These correlations can be utilized as a valuable tool for closely monitoring the progress of treatments within a clinical setting. Furthermore, they can significantly contribute to the advancement of tailored and personalized rehabilitation programs, ultimately enhancing the functional capacity and overall well-being of patients.

On the other hand, some limitations have to be mentioned. The main limitation is that this is a retrospective study of post-THA patients. Pre-operative data such as SGPs, LLD, Trendelenburg signs, possible muscle atrophies, or patient-reported outcomes were unavailable. Furthermore, the lack of pre-operative data regarding the correlations between age, SGPs, and OHS, as well as the lack of matching regarding age, prohibit us from conducting a more in-depth statistical analysis to explore group differences. It is important to note that the results of correlation analysis cannot be generalized due to the small sample size. Therefore, it is essential to interpret them with caution. Being mindful of this will lead to more accurate conclusions and better decision-making. More comparative and longitudinal biomechanical studies should be performed to improve the power of the current results and further investigate the postoperative gait of OA and DDH patients.

Reflective surface markers are commonly used in traditional motion capture to assess joint kinematics. However, using skin markers on human tissue for motion analysis can introduce a possible source of measurement inaccuracy due to artifacts caused by the skin's relative mobility compared to the underlying bone structures. Nonetheless, the literature strongly indicates that accurate and thorough tracking of gait analysis techniques minimizes any possible influence of errors on data collection when measuring kinetic and kinematic parameters with such equipment [41].

Future studies should be conducted while taking into account the potential effect of age when designing experimental protocols since, based on our results, age as a variable may influence the outcomes. Furthermore, combining kinematic and kinetic analysis with electromyography data studies can help evaluate the post-THA gait patterns of OA and DDH patients and optimize specific rehabilitation protocols.

5. Conclusions

In our study, postoperative spatiotemporal parameter analysis after THA of OA patients and DDH patients revealed no significant statistical differences between groups, despite gait being slightly better in the OA group than the DDH group. Notably, there were significant correlations between post-arthroplasty SGPs and specific ADLs, suggesting that there may be a potential impact on the ability to perform specific activities. These findings should be correlated with kinetic gait analysis data to fully evaluate the differences in gait and functionality improvement after THA in these patient groups.

Supplementary Materials: The following supporting information can be downloaded at: https://www.mdpi.com/article/10.3390/jfmk9030110/s1.

Author Contributions: Conceptualization, S.S.; methodology, S.S., G.P., and A.T.; software, G.P.; validation, A.T.; formal analysis, G.P., and A.T.; investigation, S.S., and A.T.; resources, P.P., and P.K.; data curation, G.P., and A.T.; writing—original draft preparation, S.S.; writing—review and editing, S.S., G.P., A.T., P.P., and P.K.; visualization, S.S., G.P., and A.T.; supervision, P.P., and P.K.; project administration, P.P., and P.K. All authors have read and agreed to the published version of the manuscript.

Funding: This research received no external funding.

Institutional Review Board Statement: This study was conducted in accordance with the Declaration of Helsinki and approved by the Institutional Review Board (or Ethics Committee) of University Hospital ATTIKON, National and Kapodistrian University of Athens, Greece (protocol code: 42609/5 May 2022).

Informed Consent Statement: Informed consent was obtained from all subjects involved in the study.

Data Availability Statement: The data that support the findings of this study are available from the corresponding author, S.S., upon reasonable request. Data are available only on request due to privacy and ethical issues.

Conflicts of Interest: The authors declare no conflicts of interest.

References

1. Pivec, R.; Johnson, A.J.; Mears, S.C.; Mont, M.A. Hip arthroplasty. *Lancet* **2012**, *380*, 1768–1777. [CrossRef]
2. Chen, D.; Shen, J.; Zhao, W.; Wang, T.; Han, L.; Hamilton, J.L.; Im, H.J. Osteoarthritis: Toward a comprehensive understanding of pathological mechanism. *Bone Res.* **2017**, *5*, 16044. [CrossRef]
3. Altman, R.D.; Hochberg, M.C.; Moskowitz, R.W.; Schnitzer, T.J. American College of Rheumatology Subcommittee on Osteoarthritis Guidelines. Recommendations for the medical management of osteoarthritis of the hip and knee: 2000 update. *Arthritis Rheum* **2000**, *43*, 1905–1915. [CrossRef]
4. Moura, D.L.; Figueiredo, A. High congenital hip dislocation in adults—Arthroplasty and functional results. *Rev. Bras. Ortop.* **2018**, *53*, 226–235. [CrossRef]
5. Hartofilakidis, G.; Stamos, K.; Ioannidis, T.T. Low friction arthroplasty for old untreated congenital dislocation of the hip. *J. Bone Jt. Surg. Br. Vol.* **1988**, *70*, 182–186. [CrossRef]
6. Erdemli, B.; Yilmaz, C.; Atalar, H.; Güzel, B.; Cetin, I. Total hip arthroplasty in developmental high dislocation of the hip. *J. Arthroplast.* **2005**, *20*, 1021–1028. [CrossRef]
7. Bennett, D.; Humphreys, L.; O'brien, S.; Kelly, C.; Orr, J.F.; Beverland, D.E. Gait kinematics of age-stratified hip replacement patients—A large scale, long-term follow-up study. *Gait Posture* **2008**, *28*, 194–200. [CrossRef]
8. van den Akker-Scheek, I.; Stevens, M.; Bulstra, S.K.; Groothoff, J.W.; van Horn, J.R.; Zijlstra, W. Recovery of gait after short-stay total hip arthroplasty. *Arch. Phys. Med. Rehabil.* **2007**, *88*, 361–367. [CrossRef]
9. Xu, C.; Wen, X.; Wei, W.; Huang, L.; Wang, J.; Yan, Y.; Lei, W. Gait parameters associated with untreated developmental dysplasia of the hip: A systematic review. *Int. J. Clin. Exp. Med.* **2017**, *10*, 13037–13047.
10. Constantinou, M.; Barrett, R.; Brown, M.; Mills, P. Spatial-temporal gait characteristics in individuals with hip osteoarthritis: A systematic literature review and meta-analysis. *J. Orthop. Sports Phys. Ther.* **2014**, *44*, 291-B7. [CrossRef]
11. Cichy, B.; Wilk, M. Gait analysis in osteoarthritis of the hip. *Med. Sci. Monit.* **2006**, *12*, CR507–CR513.
12. Romano, C.L.; Frigo, C.; Randelli, G.; Pedotti, A. Analysis of the gait of adults who had residual of congenital dysplasia of the hip. *J. Bone Jt. Surg. Am.* **1996**, *78*, 1468–1479. [CrossRef]
13. Jacobsen, J.S.; Nielsen, D.B.; Sorensen, H.; Soballe, K.; Mechlenburg, I. Changes in walking and running in patients with hip dysplasia. *Acta Orthop.* **2013**, *84*, 265–270. [CrossRef]
14. Lai, K.A.; Lin, C.J.; Su, F.C. Gait analysis of adult patients with complete congenital dislocation of the hip. *J. Formos. Med. Assoc.* **1997**, *96*, 740–744.
15. Cho, S.H.; Lee, S.H.; Kim, K.H.; Yu, J.Y. Gait analysis before and after total hip arthroplasty in hip dysplasia and osteonecrosis of the femoral head. *J. Korean Orthop. Assoc.* **2004**, *39*, 482–488. [CrossRef]
16. Bennett, D.; Humphreys, L.; O'Brien, S.; Beverland, D.E. Temporospatial parameters of hip replacement patients ten years post-operatively. *Int. Orthop.* **2009**, *33*, 1203–1207. [CrossRef]
17. Guedes, R.C.; Dias, J.M.; Dias, R.C.; Borges, V.S.; Lustosa, L.P.; Rosa, N.M. Total hip arthroplasty in the elderly: Impact on functional performance. *Braz. J. Phys. Ther.* **2011**, *15*, 123–130. [CrossRef]
18. Lai, K.A.; Lin, C.J.; Jou, I.M.; Su, F.C. Gait analysis after total hip arthroplasty with leg-length equalization in women with unilateral congenital complete dislocation of the hip—Comparison with untreated patients. *J. Orthop. Res.* **2001**, *19*, 1147–1152. [CrossRef]
19. Nie, Y.; Ning, N.; Pei, F.; Shen, B.; Zhou, Z.; Li, Z. Gait kinematic deviations in patients with developmental dysplasia of the hip treated with total hip arthroplasty. *Orthopedics* **2017**, *40*, e425–e431. [CrossRef]
20. Marangoz, S.; Atilla, B.; Gök, H.; Yavuzer, G.; Ergin, S.; Tokgözoğlu, A.M.; Alpaslan, M. Gait analysis in adults with severe hip dysplasia before and after total hip arthroplasty. *Hip Int.* **2010**, *20*, 466–472. [CrossRef]
21. John, S.; Esch, M.; Steinert, M.; Witte, K. Relationship between self-reported function, functional tests and biomechanical parameters in patients 12 months after total hip arthroplasty: A preliminary cross-sectional study. *Indian J. Orthop.* **2023**, *57*, 1032–1040. [CrossRef]
22. Bolink, S.A.; Lenguerrand, E.; Brunton, L.R.; Wylde, V.; Gooberman-Hill, R.; Heyligers, I.C.; Blom, A.W.; Grimm, B. Assessment of physical function following total hip arthroplasty: Inertial sensor based gait analysis is supplementary to patient-reported outcome measures. *Clin. Biomech.* **2016**, *32*, 171–179. [CrossRef]
23. World Medical Association (WMA). Declaration of Helsinki—Ethical principles for medical research involving human subjects. 2013. Available online: https://www.wma.net/policies-post/wma-declaration-of-helsinki-ethical-principles-for-medical-research-involving-human-subjects/ (accessed on 2 October 2021).
24. von Elm, E.; Altman, D.G.; Egger, M.; Pocock, S.J.; Gotzsche, P.C.; Vandenbroucke, J.P. The strengthening of the reporting of observational studies in epidemiology (STROBE) statement: Guidelines for reporting observational studies. *Lancet* **2007**, *370*, 1453–1457. [CrossRef]

25. Prosser, G.H.; Yates, P.J.; Wood, D.J.; Graves, S.E.; de Steiger, R.N.; Miller, L.N. Outcome of primary resurfacing hip replacement: Evaluation of risk factors for early revision. *Acta Orthop.* **2010**, *81*, 66–71. [CrossRef]
26. Huch, K.; Müller, K.A.C.; Stürmer, T.; Brenner, H.; Puhl, W.; Günther, K.-P. Sports activities 5 years after total knee or hip arthroplasty: The Ulm Osteoarthritis Study. *Ann. Rheum. Dis.* **2005**, *64*, 1715–1720. [CrossRef]
27. Hoppenfeld, S.; DeBoer, P.; Buckley, R. *Surgical Exposures in Orthopaedics: The Anatomic Approach*, 5th ed.; Wolters Kluwer: Philadelphia, PA, USA, 2017; pp. 800–820.
28. Papachristou, G.C.; Pappa, E.; Chytas, D.; Masouros, P.T.; Nikolaou, V.S. Total Hip Replacement in Developmental Hip Dysplasia: A narrative review. *Cureus* **2021**, *13*, e14763. [CrossRef]
29. Kellgren, J.H. Atlas of standard radiographs of arthritis. In *The Epidemiology of Chronic Rheumatism*; Ball, J.R., Jeffrey, M.R., Kellgren, J.H., Eds.; Blackwell: London, UK, 1963; Volume 2, pp. 22–23.
30. Crowe, J.F.; Mani, V.J.; Ranawat, C.S. Total hip replacement in congenital dislocation and dysplasia of the hip. *J. Bone Jt. Surg. Am.* **1979**, *61*, 15–23. [CrossRef]
31. Dawson, J.; Fitzpatrick, R.; Carr, A.; Murray, D. Questionnaire on the perceptions of patients about total hip replacement. *J. Bone Jt. Surg. Br.* **1996**, *78*, 185–190. [CrossRef]
32. Murray, D.W.; Fitzpatrick, R.; Rogers, K.; Pandit, H.; Beard, D.J.; Carr, A.J.; Dawson, J. The use of the Oxford hip and knee scores. *J. Bone Jt. Surg. Br.* **2007**, *89*, 1010–1014. [CrossRef] [PubMed]
33. Vicon Motion Systems Ltd. Vicon Plug-in Gait Reference Guide. Available online: https://help.vicon.com/space/Nexus216/116 07059/Plug-in+Gait+Reference+Guide (accessed on 6 May 2022).
34. Hof, A.L. Scaling gait data to body size. *Gait Posture* **1996**, *4*, 222–223. [CrossRef]
35. van Berkel, A.C.; Schiphof, D.; Waarsing, J.H.; Runhaar, J.; van Ochten, J.M.; Bindels, P.J.E.; Bierma-Zeinstra, S.M.A. 10-Year natural course of early hip osteoarthritis in middle-aged persons with hip pain: A CHECK study. *Ann. Rheum. Dis.* **2021**, *80*, 487–493. [CrossRef]
36. Lespasio, M.J.; Sultan, A.A.; Piuzzi, N.S.; Khlopas, A.; Husni, M.E.; Muschler, G.F.; Mont, M.A. Hip osteoarthritis: A Primer. *Perm. J.* **2018**, *22*, 17–084. [CrossRef]
37. Wang, Y. Current concepts in developmental dysplasia of the hip and Total hip arthroplasty. *Arthroplasty* **2019**, *1*, 2. [CrossRef]
38. Murphy, L.B.; Helmick, C.G.; Schwartz, T.A.; Renner, J.B.; Tudor, G.; Koch, G.G.; Dragomir, A.D.; Kalsbeek, W.D.; Luta, G.; Jordan, J.M. One in four people may develop symptomatic hip osteoarthritis in his or her lifetime. *Osteoarthr. Cartil.* **2010**, *18*, 1372–1379. [CrossRef]
39. Kadaba, M.P.; Ramakrishnan, H.K.; Wootten, M.E. Measurement of lower extremity kinematics during level walking. *J. Orthop. Res.* **1990**, *8*, 383–392. [CrossRef]
40. Mercieca-Bebber, R.; King, M.T.; Calvert, M.J.; Stockler, M.R.; Friedlander, M. The importance of patient-reported outcomes in clinical trials and strategies for future optimization. *Patient Relat. Outcome Meas.* **2018**, *9*, 353–367. [CrossRef]
41. Triantafyllou, A.; Papagiannis, G.; Nikolaou, V.S.; Papageloupoulos, P.J.; Babis, G.C. Similar biomechanical behavior in gait analysis between Ceramic-on-Ceramic and Ceramic-on-XLPE Total Hip Arthroplasties. *Life* **2021**, *11*, 1366. [CrossRef]

Disclaimer/Publisher's Note: The statements, opinions and data contained in all publications are solely those of the individual author(s) and contributor(s) and not of MDPI and/or the editor(s). MDPI and/or the editor(s) disclaim responsibility for any injury to people or property resulting from any ideas, methods, instructions or products referred to in the content.

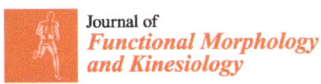
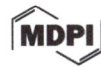

Article

Assessing the Test-Retest Reliability of MyotonPRO for Measuring Achilles Tendon Stiffness

Krystof Volesky [1], Jan Novak [1], Michael Janek [1], Jakub Katolicky [2], James J. Tufano [1], Michal Steffl [1], Javier Courel-Ibáñez [3] and Tomas Vetrovsky [1,*]

[1] Faculty of Physical Education and Sport, Charles University, 162 52 Prague, Czech Republic; k.volesk@gmail.com (K.V.)
[2] Department of Rehabilitation and Sports Medicine, Second Faculty of Medicine, University Hospital in Motol, Charles University, 150 06 Prague, Czech Republic
[3] Department of Physical Education and Sport, Faculty of Sport Sciences, University of Granada, 520 71 Melilla, Spain
* Correspondence: tomas.vetrovsky@gmail.com

Abstract: Objectives: This study evaluates the test-retest reliability and inter-rater reliability of the MyotonPRO for measuring Achilles tendon stiffness at two standardized sites over various time frames and settings. **Methods**: Eight healthy participants underwent assessments by three raters over six visits. Tendon stiffness was measured at proximal (mid-portion) and distal (insertional) regions of the Achilles tendon at various time frames (10–15 s, 10–15 min, 24 h, and 14 days apart). Measurements included participant repositioning and two activity stimuli (daily living and sport). Reliability was calculated using the intraclass correlation coefficient (ICC), its 95% confidence interval, coefficient of variation, standard error of measurement, and minimal detectable change. **Results**: Short-term reliability (10–15 min) was excellent, with an ICC of 0.956 (0.929–0.974). Between days reliability (24 h) was good, with an ICC of 0.889 (0.802–0.938). Between weeks reliability (2 weeks) was good with an ICC of 0.886 (0.811–0.931). Short-term reliability with the simulation of activity of daily living was good, with an ICC of 0.917 (0.875–0.945). Short-term reliability with the simulation of sport was good with an ICC of 0.933 (0.891–0.96). Between days reliability with the simulation of sport was good, with an ICC of 0.920 (0.859–0.955). **Conclusions**: When used in a standardized position, the MyotonPRO demonstrates reliable repeated measurements of Achilles tendon stiffness. This protocol provides a foundation for clinical research and rehabilitation by clarifying expected reliability across minutes, days, and weeks, thus aiding clinicians and researchers in monitoring tendon adaptations and making evidence-based decisions.

Keywords: Achilles tendon; stiffness; reliability; MyotonPRO; tendon

1. Introduction

The Achilles tendon transmits force and absorbs energy during activities such as walking, running, and jumping [1] and is subject to extremely high mechanical loads, often up to ten times the body weight [2]. In athletes, excessive mechanical loading can lead to Achilles tendinopathy, a condition characterized by tendon pain and loss of function [3]. Its prevalence among athletes stands at 6%, affecting both men and women equally [4]. Although Achilles tendinopathy can be an acute injury, it often evolves into a chronic condition that can impair quality of life and work productivity [5]. A significant number of affected individuals experience persistent symptoms for years, resulting in reduced physical activity levels [6].

Considering the prevalence and consequences of Achilles tendinopathy, understanding the biomechanical properties of the Achilles tendon, namely its elasticity and stiffness, is essential for assessing its functional dynamics and vulnerability to injury. Elasticity enables the tendon to store energy in a spring-like manner, while stiffness reduces the extent of elongation, protecting collagen fibers against damage. In general, tendons can elongate by up to 4% of their length without sustaining any damage. However, if the resistance to elongation is inadequate, elongation between 4 and 8% may lead to the breakdown of collagen cross-links [7]. This can lead to structural changes that contribute to the development of tendinopathy. When elongation exceeds a critical threshold (above 8%), collagen fibers may undergo macroscopic failure, potentially leading to Achilles tendon rupture and complete loss of function. Thus, the stiffness of the tendon, in conjunction with the strength of the triceps surae muscle, is critical in determining the level of resistance to elongation and in preventing excessive elongation that could damage collagen fibers [8].

There are several methods for measuring Achilles tendon stiffness. For example, research involving healthy subjects has often relied on calculations that quantify tendon displacement (Δmm) during maximal voluntary contraction of plantar flexor muscles [9]. However, this approach may not be suitable for tendinopathy cases, as central inhibition of plantar flexors can limit true maximal voluntary contraction. Thus, to assess stiffness in individuals who present tendinopathy, shear wave ultrasound elastography (SWUE) has been commonly employed [10]. Despite studies showing good reliability of SWUE, its reliability is highly dependent on the operator and requires extensive ultrasound expertise to accurately identify the structures and artifacts being assessed [11]. Consequently, there is a need for more accessible techniques that can reliably measure tendon stiffness in tendinopathy patients in both research and clinical settings [12].

The MyotonPRO is a promising tool for quantifying the stiffness of the Achilles tendon in patients with tendinopathy, where a force is applied transversely to the tendon fiber axis, and the resultant displacement of the tendon tissue is measured. Originally designed for assessing skeletal muscles, the MyotonPRO is a portable device that employs a controlled preload of 0.18 N to compress the subcutaneous tissue, followed by a 15 ms impulse of 0.40 N of mechanical force, which elicits a damped or decaying natural oscillation within the tissue, enabling the measurement of tendon stiffness [13]. Compared to more operator-dependent modalities (e.g., ultrasound elastography), the MyotonPRO requires less specialized training and reduces user-dependent variability. Its portability and straightforward setup make it a convenient tool for researchers and clinicians to measure soft-tissue stiffness quickly and accurately. To determine a device's reliability, it is critical to consider the magnitude of measurement errors in absolute values after repeated conditions. In practical terms, absolute errors are essential to identify whether the changes in tendon stiffness observed after a given intervention are due to the actual changes in the functional dynamics of the athletes (adaptations) [14].

Several key factors influence the reliability of measuring tendon stiffness via the MyotonPRO. First, the accuracy of the results is highly contingent on the precise location of the measurement and the participant's positioning [15]. Therefore, standardizing both the device's position and the participant's posture is essential for ensuring consistent, repeatable measurements in research and clinical practice. However, existing studies evaluating the MyotonPRO's reliability lack straightforward recommendations for standardized positioning. Second, temporal fluctuations in Achilles stiffness are particularly relevant in clinical settings and in monitoring patients with tendinopathy [16]. Moreover, physical activity stimuli like walking, biking, or sports practice often precede or occur between measurements, making the understanding of their impact vital for interpreting clinical stiffness measurements. Yet, studies reporting on MyotonPRO's reliability have neither standardized device and patient positioning [17–19] nor accounted for various time intervals and stimuli between measurements [20,21].

Considering the lack of established reliability data, the objective of this study was to (1) assess the test-retest reliability of the MyotonPRO in measuring Achilles tendon stiffness using a newly established standardized position, (2) determine whether different time intervals (ranging from seconds to weeks) influence measurement reliability, and (3) evaluate how physical activity stimuli (activities of daily living and sport-like exercises) affect short-term reliability. Furthermore, (4) we explored the inter-rater reliability of the MyotonPRO in this context.

We hypothesized that, under standardized conditions, the MyotonPRO would demonstrate good to excellent test-retest reliability (intraclass correlation coefficient > 0.75) across all assessed intervals and activity stimuli.

Regarding the time frames specifically, immediate measurements at 10–15 s apart allowed us to capture consecutive trials without any repositioning of the participant. The 10–15 min interval served as a short-term retest period, encompassing practical requirements such as repositioning participants, marking the measurement site, and, in some cases, performing a quick activity stimulus or rest. This slight variability (i.e., sometimes closer to 10 min, sometimes 15 min) reflects realistic conditions in clinical and research settings, where minor procedural or participant-related delays commonly occur.

By providing both a clear hypothesis and a rationale for the time intervals used, this study addresses a gap in the literature and offers a reproducible methodology for reliably assessing Achilles tendon stiffness in healthy and potentially clinical populations.

2. Materials and Methods

2.1. Sample

Eight healthy young adults were recruited for this study through convenience sampling at the Charles University campus between March and July 2022. The sample comprised six males and two females, with a median age of 27.5 years (IQR 3.5), median body mass of 75 kg (IQR 15.5), and median height of 178 cm (IQR 5.8). On average, they engaged in 5.5 h (IQR 3) of sports training per week.

To calculate the sample size required to estimate the ICC of 0.9 with the lower bound of 95% confidence interval greater than 0.5 (the threshold for moderate reliability), we used Zou's formula, as implemented in ICC.Sample.Size package (version 1.0) in R. Assuming three ratings per participant, a desired power of 80%, and using a two-sided 0.05 significance level, the required sample size is 8 [22]. Because this was a focused reliability study, we did not perform a separate power analysis for each subset of reliability measures.

Eligibility criteria included being under the age of 30 years, engaging in regular physical activity, and having no history of lower limb injuries within the previous six months. Participants also had to be free from any neurological, vascular, or systemic diseases and possess a valid sports permit from a medical doctor.

These criteria yielded a relatively narrow age range (median: 27.5 years), which may limit generalizability to a broader population. Furthermore, although the MyotonPRO may be used in tendinopathy cases, our sample included only healthy participants.

This study was approved by the Ethics Committee of the Faculty of Physical Education and Sport of Charles University (ID: 255/2021), and written informed consent was provided by the participants.

2.2. Experimental Approach

This study comprised 3 waves of data collection, each spaced 14 days apart (Figure 1). Each wave consisted of 2 visits on 2 consecutive days. The 1st visit involved 3 sessions (session 1 to session 3), and the 2nd visit consisted of 2 sessions (session 4 and session 5). A set of standardized measurements (SM) was taken during each session, consisting of 3 measurements at two different points (proximal and distal) on each leg, resulting in 12 measurements per SM. Between session 1 and session 2, a protocol mimicking vigorous sports activities—simulation of sport activity (SP) was introduced, while a protocol—simulation of activities of daily living (ADL) was applied between session 4 and session 5. In summary, each participant underwent 180 measurements: 3 waves × 5 sessions × 2 legs × 2 points × 3 measurements each. Figure 1 illustrates the measurement timeline for an individual participant. These measurements were used to calculate test-retest reliability across various time frames (10–15 s, 10–15 min, 24 h, and 14 days apart), repositioning of the subject (standardized measurements consistency), and physical activity stimuli (ADL and SP; Table 1).

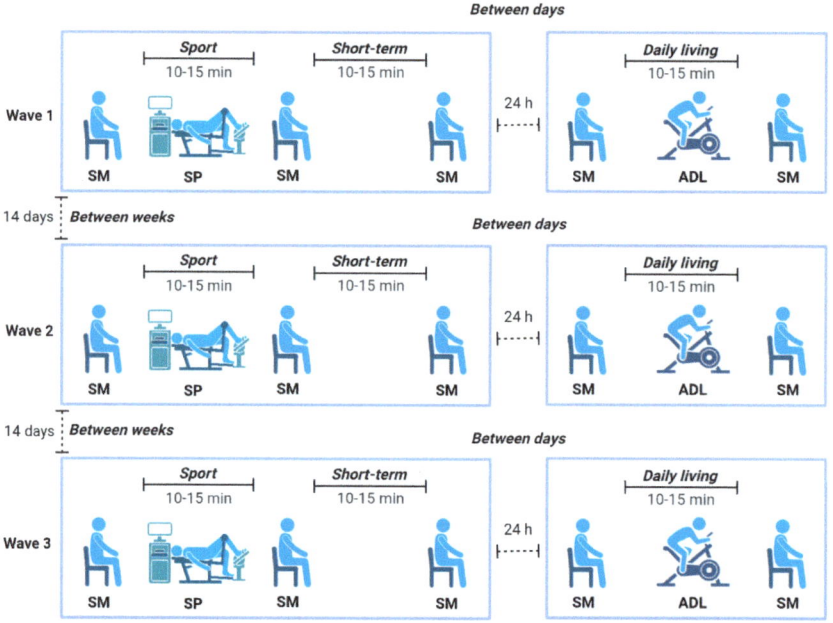

SM: Set of standardized measurement. Involves 12 measures: x3 distal and x3 proximal for each leg, 10-15 s between.
ADL: Simulation of activities of daily living: ergometer cycling, 5 min, 100 W, 80 rpm.
SP: Simulation of sport activity: eccentric, concentric and isometric plantar flexion in dynamometer, 12 sets, 15 s work, 30 s rest.

Figure 1. Scheme of measurements-time intervals and different settings.

Table 1. Overview of time frames, repositioning, and stimuli.

	Time Interval Between Measurements	In-Between Repositioning	In-Between Stimulus	Purpose
Immediate SM	10–15 s	NO	NO	Consistency of measurement
Short-term SM	10–15 min	YES	NO	Test-retest reliability
Short-term ADL	10–15 min	YES	ADL	Impact of low-intensity loading
Short-term SP	10–15 min	YES	SP	Impact of high-intensity loading
Between days SM	24 h	YES	NO	Test-retest reliability between days
Between days SP	24 h	YES	SP	Impact of high-intensity loading
Between weeks SM	14 days	YES	NO	Test-retest reliability between weeks
Inter-rater reliability	24 h	YES	NO	Operator influence on reliability

SM: Set of standardized measurement. Involves 12 measures: ×3 distal and ×3 proximal for each leg, 10–15 s between. ADL: Simulation of activities of daily living: ergometer cycling, 5 min, 100 W, 80 rpm. SP: Simulation of sport activity: eccentric, concentric, and isometric plantar flexion in dynamometer, 12 sets, 15 s work, 30 s rest.

2.3. Rationale for Time Intervals

The 10–15 s interval enabled immediate consecutive measurements without repositioning, reflecting direct repeatability. The 10–15 min interval accounted for practical short-term repositioning and minor procedural tasks. The 24 h interval represented next-day follow-up, commonly employed in clinical check-ups. Finally, the 14-day interval allowed the assessment of stability over a longer period, relevant for monitoring rehabilitation programs.

2.4. Achilles Tendon Stiffness

The MyotonPRO (Muomeetria, Tallinn, Estonia; Model 000607) was used to collect data from the tendon stiffness (Supplementary Photo S1). The device applies a controlled preload of 0.18 N to compress the subcutaneous tissue, followed by a 15 ms impulse of 0.40 N of mechanical force, which elicits a damped or decaying natural oscillation within the tissue, enabling the measurement of tendon stiffness [13].

2.5. Standardized Measurement

Standardized measurement started with participants sitting on a box with their buttocks fixed using a wedge (Figure 2A). The height of the box was set so that the angle at the ankle and knee was 90° as controlled by a goniometer, and the line connecting the medial side of the heel and big toe was adjusted to be perpendicular to the box. Achilles tendon stiffness (N/m) was measured at two specific points (Figure 2B): the distal point, situated 1 cm proximally to the tuber calcanei, and the proximal point, located 6 cm proximally to the tuber calcanei [23]. The MyotonPRO device was placed on the adjustable rack during measurement (Supplementary Photo S2). These points were marked with a permanent marker lasting until the next day but not until the next wave of measurements. In this position, the distance between the big toe and the box, as well as the distance between the first metatarsi of the left and right feet, were recorded (Figure 2C). Finally, the MyotonPRO was underlaid by an adjustable rack, and the height of the rack for both distal and proximal measurement points was also recorded (Figure 2D).

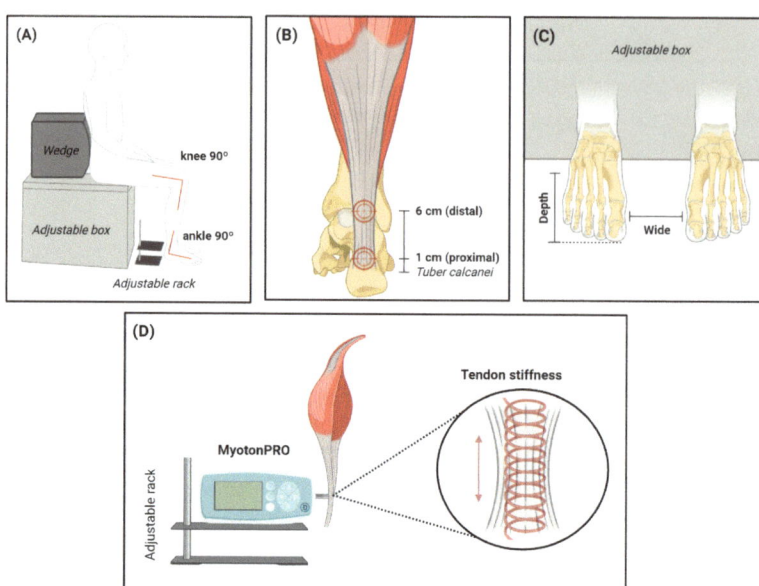

Figure 2. Standardized measurement of Achilles tendon stiffness. (**A**) Sitting position; (**B**) Measured sites; (**C**) Foot positioning; (**D**) MyotonPRO positioning.

2.6. Simulation of Sports and Activities of Daily Living

The simulation of the sports activities (SP) targeted a single leg using the HumacNorm dynamometer (Cybex 770 NORM ®, Humac, CA, USA). The targeted leg was chosen randomly for each participant, and this selection was maintained for all three waves. The simulation involved loading the Achilles tendon by performing plantar flexion with maximum effort and consisted of 12 sets, each set including 15 s under tension; the sets were interspersed with 30 s rest periods. Three different loading types were used to simulate various conditions during sports: eccentric, isometric, and combined concentric/eccentric loading (Supplementary Table S1). The plantar flexion was performed with the knee flexed at 90° while lying down on the back. The range of motion in the angle for eccentric and concentric/eccentric loading was from 30° of plantar flexion to 15° of dorsiflexion; the isometric loading was performed at 0° (Supplementary Table S1) [24,25].

The simulation of the ADL included a five-minute session on an ergometer at 100 watts and 80 revolutions per minute, followed by 20 heel raises. Its aim was to simulate conditions typically preceding assessments in clinical and research practice, such as cycling or walking to the lab and climbing up the stairs [26].

2.7. Procedures

Approximately one week before the first wave of measurement, participants underwent a familiarization session. During this session, participants practiced the simulation of daily living (ADL) and sports activities (SP). Furthermore, the setup of the standardized position was recorded (height of the rack, toe-to-box and inter-metatarsal distances) so that the standardized position (Figure 2) could be replicated across all measurement sessions. Finally, participants were instructed to refrain from engaging in any physically strenuous activity 3 days prior to each wave of measurement.

For each of the three waves separated by 14 days (Figure 1), the participants followed the same procedure: at the start of the 1st visit, participants rested in the lying position for 5 min. Then, they assumed the predetermined seated position as established during the familiarization session, the points of measurement were marked, and the first set of standardized measurements (SM) was taken. After the first SM, the participants underwent the SP protocol simulating the sports activities (Supplemental Table S1). Then, immediately, they re-assumed the standardized position, and the second SM was taken. After 15 min of rest, the participants re-assumed the standardized position once more, and the third SM of the first visit was taken. The 2nd visit was conducted 24 h after the 1st visit and also began with a 5 min period of rest. Following the rest, participants assumed the standardized position, and the first SM was taken. After that, the simulation of ADL conducted. After completing the simulation, participants re-assumed the standardized position and the second SM of the 2nd visit was taken.

Sessions 1 to 3 were measured by Operator 1, while sessions 4 and 5 were measured by Operator 2 or 3, randomly assigned. All operators were doctoral students in kinesiology with prior training in identifying the distal and proximal Achilles tendon landmarks. Before data collection, they practiced marking and measuring at least 20 trials on pilot participants to ensure consistency in identification and device handling.

2.8. Statistical Analysis

The intraclass correlation coefficients (ICC) and their 95% confidence intervals were calculated using the irr package (version 0.84.1) in R statistical software. The analysis was conducted using the "two-way" model, "agreement" type, and "single" or "average" unit of analysis [27,28]. The magnitude of the intraclass correlation coefficient was interpreted based on its lower-bound of the 95% confidence interval (LCI), as follows: <0.50, poor reliability; 0.50 to 0.75, moderate reliability; 0.75 to 0.90, good reliability; and >0.90, excellent reliability [27].

We initially screened all the data for extreme outliers (values exceeding the mean $\pm$ 3SD), but none met our predefined exclusion criteria. To assess potential systematic bias between repeated measurements for immediate reliability, we compared exactly two measurements at a time (i.e., measurements 1 and 2, 2 and 3, and 1 and 3) using a Bland–Altman analysis (Supplementary Materials). For each pair, the mean difference (bias) and 95% limits of agreement were calculated, and a paired t-test was performed to determine whether the bias was statistically significant. The magnitude of the observed bias was then compared to the minimal detectable change (MDC) to evaluate its clinical relevance.

The immediate reliability was calculated as a comparison between 3 single measurements within each SM for both legs. The short-term reliability was calculated as a comparison between 3 averages (of the 3 single measurements) from sessions 1, 2, and 3 only for an unloaded leg. The short-term reliability with simulation of activities of daily living was calculated as a comparison between 2 averages from sessions 4 and 5 (with the ADL protocol in between) for both legs. The short-term reliability with simulation of sport was calculated as a comparison between averages from session 1, 2, and 3 only for a loaded leg. The between-day reliability with and without simulation of sports was calculated as a comparison between 2 averages from sessions 1 and 4 for an unloaded and a loaded leg, respectively. The between-week reliability was calculated as a comparison between 2 averages from waves 1, 2, and 3 for sessions 1, 2, and 3 and only for an unloaded leg. The inter-rater reliability was calculated as a comparison between 2 averages from sessions 1 and 5 for an unloaded leg. The data used for the calculation of individual ICCs are summarized in Table 2.

Table 2. Data used for calculation of the intraclass correlation coefficients.

	Number of Measurements Compared	Unit of Analysis	Sessions Included	Legs Included	Total Number of Measurements Included
Immediate SM	3	single	1 to 5	both	1440
Short-term SM	3	mean	1 to 3	unloaded	144
Short-term ADL	2	mean	4 and 5	both	192
Short-term SP	3	mean	1 to 3	loaded	144
Between days SM	2	mean	1 and 4	unloaded	96
Between days SP	2	mean	1 and 4	loaded	96
Between weeks SM	2	mean	1 and 2	unloaded	128
Inter-rater reliability	2	mean	1 and 5	unloaded	96

SM: Set of standardized measurement. Involves 12 measures: ×3 distal and ×3 proximal for each leg, 10–15 s between. ADL: Simulation of activities of daily living: ergometer cycling, 5 min, 100 W, 80 rpm. SP: Simulation of sport activity: eccentric, concentric, and isometric plantar flexion in dynamometer, 12 sets, 15 s work, 30 s rest.

The coefficient of variation (CV) was calculated by formula in R statistical software: (standard deviation/mean) × 100. The standard error of measurement (SEM) was calculated using plotrix package (version 3.8-4) package in R statistical software. The minimal detectable change (MDC) was calculated by formula in R statistical software: $1.96 \times SEM \times 2$. All valid data points were analyzed, and no outliers were excluded.

3. Results

The median stiffness at the proximal point of the Achilles tendon was 852.5 N/m (IQR 194.5) and at the distal point, 1019.3 N/m (IQR 129.5). The reliability of the MyotonPRO measurement of Achilles tendon stiffness across different time frames and settings ranged from good to excellent (Table 3). The test-retest reliability, both with and without subject repositioning, was excellent with the lower bound of 95% confidence interval exceeding 0.9. The test-retest reliability, including effect of time (1 day to 2 weeks) and physical activity stimuli (ADLs, SPs), was good with the lower bound of 95% confidence interval exceeding 0.75 (Figure 3).

Table 3. Results from reliability analyses for the different testing conditions.

Testing Condition	ICC (95% CI)	CV (%)	SEM (N/m)	MDC (N/m)	Median (IQR) (N/m)
Immediate SM	0.973 (0.968 to 0.978)	15.99	3.95	15.46	951 (238.25)
Short-term SM	0.956 (0.929 to 0.974)	16.14	12.50	49.01	948 (232)
Short-term ADL	0.917 (0.875 to 0.945)	16.00	10.88	42.63	955.5 (236.5)
Short-term SP	0.933 (0.891 to 0.96)	15.74	12.26	48.07	944 (237.5)
Between days SM	0.889 (0.802 to 0.938)	16.51	15.65	61.34	945.5 (254.75)
Between days SP	0.920 (0.859 to 0.955)	16.67	15.91	62.35	956.5 (234.75)
Between weeks SM	0.886 (0.811 to 0.931)	15.82	13.05	51.17	953 (219)
Inter-rater reliability	0.887 (0.798 to 0.937)	16.48	15.61	61.21	942 (252.5)

ICC: Intraclass correlation coefficient. CV: Coefficient of variation. SEM: Standard error of measurement. MDC: Minimal detectable change.

Subgoup and Systemic Bias Analysis

In addition to the overall reliability analyses, we performed subgroup analyses comparing the two measurement sites on the Achilles tendon. The proximal measurement point yielded an intraclass correlation coefficient (ICC) of 0.966 (0.958–0.973), while the distal measurement point yielded an ICC of 0.956 (0.944–0.966) for immediate SM. These high and comparable ICC values at both sites further support the robustness and consistency of our standardized measurement protocol. Formal analysis of potential systematic bias was performed. The Bland–Altman analysis revealed statistically significant negative systematic biases ranging from −5.43 to −11.52 N/m (all $p < 0.001$) (Supplementary Materials). However, in all cases, the bias remained within the range of minimal detectable change (MDC = ~15–~62 N/m), indicating that the observed differences are unlikely to be clinically meaningful.

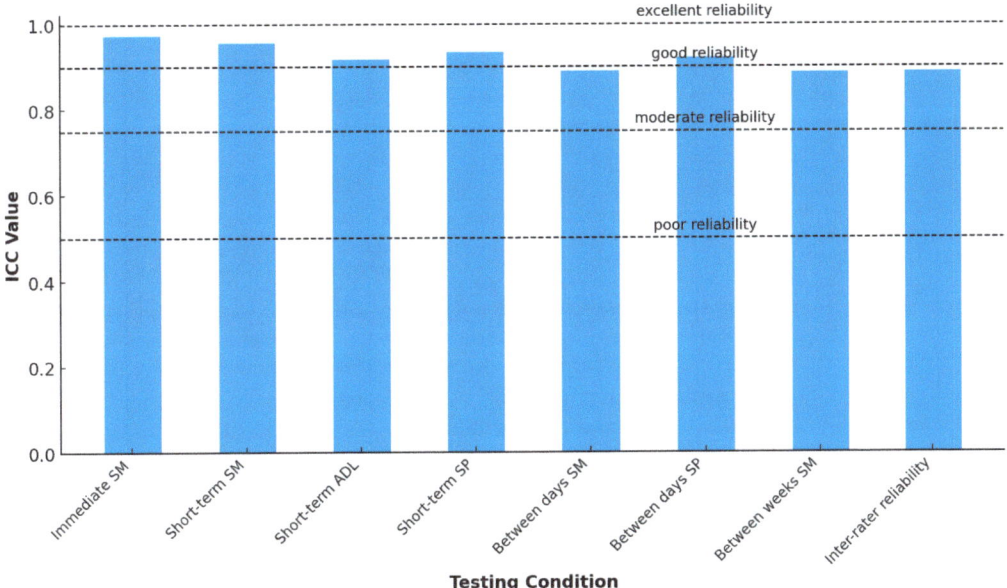

Figure 3. Graph of reliability analysis for different testing conditions.

4. Discussion

This study brings novel insights into the reliability of the MyotonPRO and provides standardized procedures for measuring Achilles tendon stiffness in clinical trials with patients. The main findings are that (1) the proposed standardized seating position is highly reliable in measuring Achilles tendon stiffness; (2) the standardized seating position allowed for highly reliable readings after repositioning the participant; (3) the simulated ADL did not influence Achilles tendon stiffness; (4) the simulated SP also did not influence Achilles tendon stiffness; (5) the records were consistent between days and weeks in all testing conditions. However, a mild decrease in reliability was noted with longer testing intervals, potentially reflecting variations in tendon biomechanics over the longer periods (weeks). Collectively, these findings recommend following the proposed standardized procedures to measure Achilles tendon stiffness with the MyotonPRO, ensuring high reliability regardless of the time between measurements and physical activity.

Our additional subgroup analyses indicated that the proximal and distal measurement points provide similarly high reliability, with ICCs of 0.966 and 0.956, respectively. This finding confirms that both regions of the Achilles tendon can be reliably measured using the MyotonPRO in the standardized seated position. Although we did not perform formal sensitivity analyses, these subgroup results, in conjunction with our other reliability assessments, strongly support the validity and robustness of our measurement approach. We acknowledge that future studies may benefit from incorporating sensitivity analyses to further explore potential variability across different analytical models.

Previous studies have tested the MyotonPRO inter-session reliabilities (up to one week apart) for Achilles tendon stiffness in a relaxed prone, ankle-free position (i.e., with the foot hanging freely), finding ICCs from 0.80 to 0.90, SEMs from 24.7 to 58.8 N/m and MDCs from 58.8 to 69.0 N/m [17,29,30]. These outcomes can be improved by using a splint to maintain the same ankle range of motion, resulting in ICCs of 0.95, SEMs of 13.8 N/m and MDCs of 36.7 N/m [15]. Building on this, our study designed a standardized seated position and provided a comprehensive reliability report under different exercise stimuli and time intervals. Results showed comparable excellent outcomes in all settings (ICC from 0.89 to 0.97, SEM from 4.0 to 15.9 N/m, MDC from 15.5 to 62.4 N/m), thus recommending its implementation in future studies involving Achilles tendon stiffness measurement.

In comparison with other techniques, such as shear-wave ultrasound elastography (SWUE) or ultrasound-based displacement measurements during maximal voluntary contraction, the MyotonPRO offers several advantages. Most importantly, it is less operator-dependent, providing direct quantitative results for stiffness without the need for extensive ultrasound expertise or visual interpretation of tissue images. While SWUE can provide detailed tendon structure, it requires specialized training and reproducibility can vary widely. In contrast, our results suggest that the MyotonPRO provides a convenient and portable solution, particularly in situations where visual imaging is not essential but reliable numerical estimates of tendon stiffness are required. Nevertheless, future studies could compare seated measurements to prone or standing methods to determine whether the seated position confers additional benefits in terms of participant comfort, reduced muscle tension, or ease of landmark identification.

Not only does this study show superior reliability outcomes with a standardized seated position, it also demonstrated consistent outcomes between days and weeks. Although the inter-session reliability has been previously assessed at 7 days [17,29,30] and 5 days apart [15], to our knowledge, our study is the first to assess reliability over longer time intervals (14 days). Measurements between weeks are crucial for evaluating the clinical effect in tendinopathy patients, where initial improvements may take weeks or even months to occur [16,31]. Nonetheless, considering magnitude of errors in relation to the absolute tendon stiffness (i.e., 850 to 1000 N/m), the expected variability across days would represent less than 0.35% of the outcome, which is highly acceptable.

Muscle tension may also influence stiffness measurements, as any residual activation in the triceps surae could slightly alter the measured tendon properties. By seating participants with knees bent at 90° and encouraging full relaxation, we attempted to minimize this confounder. However, more sensitive electromyographic (EMG) monitoring might be employed in future work to ensure negligible muscle activation during testing. Additionally, our results revealed that both activities of daily living (ADL) and the simulation of sport had no notable immediate impact on Achilles tendon stiffness. While this suggests a certain resilience of tendon stiffness to single bouts of loading, it also provides practical insight for planning measurement schedules in clinical or research settings. Nonetheless, the cumulative effects of repetitive or prolonged loading over days or weeks remain an important area for further investigation.

The Achilles tendon stiffness showed no apparent changes after both exercise stimuli. Accordingly, researchers can expect that a low-to-moderate physical activity, such as walking or cycling, will have no effect on Achilles tendon stiffness. Similarly, a single high-impact effort (i.e., isometric maximal plantar flexion) seems not to evoke noticeable changes in the records. Because this is the first report detailing measurement errors under these specific exercise conditions, future research could expand upon this work by examining other forms of loading (e.g., plyometric jumps or sprint protocols) and longer bouts of repetitive stress. Future studies are encouraged to determine the reliability of Achilles tendon stiffness measurement under other stimuli (e.g., jumps or sprints). This information is essential for designing high-quality clinical trials capable of identifying real changes after a given intervention. All in all, the cumulative effect of loading during days or weeks should be considered by researchers, as tendon tissue can react after consistent loading over weeks to months [24].

Regarding clinical application, the minimal detectable change (MDC) values observed (ranging from ~15 to ~62 N/m) provide a frame of reference for interpreting "true" changes in tendon stiffness. For instance, if a treatment yields a stiffness alteration below the MDC, clinicians might question whether this shift is clinically meaningful or simply a random error. Thus, the absolute indices reported here serve as practical thresholds when monitoring rehabilitation or training outcomes.

In sum, this study provides background for assessing Achilles tendon stiffness in clinical studies and explains what to expect from a reliability standpoint when measuring with intervals of minutes, days, and weeks between measurements. The information herein lays the foundation for determining accurate, meaningful changes in Achilles tendon stiffness after a rehabilitation or training program. Based on the data, it is recommended to use a standardized position for each measurement to achieve excellent reliability of MyotonPRO in the Achilles tendon region over a time horizon between measurements ranging from 10–15 min to 2 weeks. The sitting position may be the best option as it causes less of a stretch in the plantar flexors compared to lying on the belly with a 90° angle in the ankle. This means that the tendon tissue is less affected by the muscle during measurements. Standardizing the ankle position, relaxing the plantar flexors, and fixing the position of MyotonPRO proved to be crucial in maintaining reliability, even with several weeks between measurements.

There are some limitations to this study that should be noted. Only healthy participants were recruited, so the results may be different in tendinopathy patients. This choice may introduce biases, as the stiffness, and any potential central inhibition in clinical populations could differ from those in healthy individuals. The stiffness measurement was only taken at two points, so there may be different results for different points on the Achilles tendon. However, we did not observe any significant differences between the proximal and distal locations in data analysis. The simulation of sport was conducted on a dynamometer, which may be different in comparison to real sport conditions. However, the dynamometer enabled a comparable and controlled environment for all participants. The ADL simulation involved an ergometer followed by heel rises, so the results for actual walking or stairs climbing may differ. However, this setup again provided a comparable and controlled environment.

5. Conclusions

Overall, the MyotonPRO has demonstrated good to excellent reliability when utilizing a standardized participant position and precise positioning of the measuring device on the rack to eliminate any deviations in the angle relative to the measured Achilles tendon. Nevertheless, these findings primarily apply to healthy young adults under controlled conditions, and must be interpreted with caution in clinical scenarios involving older or symptomatic populations. The reliability of the MyotonPRO has been confirmed for the same operator across different days and weeks, as well as between two operators using the same standardized measurement protocol. Within these parameters, the MyotonPRO can be confidently employed to capture tendon stiffness values in a consistent manner. However, additional research is warranted to determine the device's performance in diverse patient groups and real-world clinical settings.

In conclusion, while these findings underscore the reliability of MyotonPRO measurements for Achilles tendon stiffness in healthy young adults, they should be interpreted with caution when applying them to clinical populations. Future work might explore other sampling sites, employ alternative exercise stimuli, and include symptomatic individuals to better elucidate the MyotonPRO's full potential in rehabilitation and performance contexts.

Supplementary Materials: The following supporting information can be downloaded at https://www.mdpi.com/article/10.3390/jfmk10010083/s1, Supplementary Photo S1: MyotonPRO; Supplementary Photo S2: Adjustable rack for standardization; Table S1: Sport simulation loading protocol (SP); Supplementary—Systematic Bias Analysis.

Author Contributions: Conceptualization, K.V., J.J.T. and T.V.; methodology, J.J.T. and T.V.; software, K.V. and T.V.; validation, T.V.; formal analysis, K.V., J.J.T. and T.V.; investigation, K.V., J.N. and M.J.; resources, M.S.; data curation, T.V.; writing—original draft preparation, K.V.; writing—review and editing, J.K., J.J.T., M.S., J.C.-I. and T.V.; visualization, J.C.-I.; supervision, J.J.T., M.S., J.C.-I. and T.V.; project administration, J.N. and M.J.; funding acquisition, K.V. All authors have read and agreed to the published version of the manuscript.

Funding: This research was funded by the Grant Agency of Charles University grant number 94622 and the APC was funded by the Faculty of Physical Education and Sport—Charles University.

Institutional Review Board Statement: This study was conducted in accordance with the Declaration of Helsinki, and approved by the Institutional Ethics Committee of the Faculty of Physical Education and Sport of Charles University (protocol code 255/2021; date of approval—12 January 2022).

Informed Consent Statement: Informed consent was obtained from all subjects involved in this study.

Data Availability Statement: The data presented in this study are available on request from the corresponding author due to the need to protect participant privacy and confidentiality, as stipulated by ethical guidelines and data protection regulations.

Acknowledgments: The authors would like to express their gratitude to the Charles University—Faculty of Physical Education and Sport and for the invaluable support provided during this research. Access to exercise physiology laboratory facilities and resources significantly contributed to the successful completion of this study. We also acknowledge the dedicated efforts of the university's administrative and technical staff, whose assistance was instrumental in facilitating various aspects of this work.

Conflicts of Interest: The authors declare no conflicts of interest. The funders had no role in the design of this study; in the collection, analyses, or interpretation of data; in the writing of the manuscript; or in the decision to publish the results.

Abbreviations

The following abbreviations are used in this manuscript:

ICC	Intraclass correlation coefficient
Δmm	Tendon displacement
SWUE	Shear wave ultrasound elastography
SM	Standardized measurements
SP	Sports activities
ADL	Activities of daily living
IQR	Interquartile range
kg	Kilogram
R	R Studio
ID	Identification
N/m	Stiffness
CV	Coefficient of variation
SEM	Standard error of measurement
MDC	Minimal detectable change

References

1. Doral, M.N.; Alam, M.; Bozkurt, M.; Turhan, E.; Atay, O.A.; Dönmez, G.; Maffulli, N. Functional anatomy of the Achilles tendon. *Knee Surg. Sports Traumatol. Arthrosc.* **2010**, *18*, 638–643. [CrossRef] [PubMed]
2. Dederer, K.M.; Tennant, J.N. Anatomical and Functional Considerations in Achilles Tendon Lesions. *Foot Ankle Clin.* **2019**, *24*, 371–385. [CrossRef]
3. Scott, A.; Squier, K.; Alfredson, H.; Bahr, R.; Cook, J.L.; Coombes, B.; de Vos, R.J.; Fu, S.N.; Grimaldi, A.; Lewis, J.S.; et al. ICON 2019: International Scientific Tendinopathy Symposium Consensus: Clinical Terminology. *Br. J. Sports Med.* **2020**, *54*, 260–262. [CrossRef] [PubMed]
4. Wang, Y.; Zhou, H.; Nie, Z.; Cui, S. Prevalence of Achilles tendinopathy in physical exercise: A systematic review and meta-analysis. *Sports Med. Health Sci.* **2022**, *4*, 152–159. [CrossRef] [PubMed]
5. Visser, T.S.S.; van der Vlist, A.C.; van Oosterom, R.F.; van Veldhoven, P.; Verhaar, J.A.; de Vos, R.J. Impact of chronic Achilles tendinopathy on health-related quality of life, work performance, healthcare utilisation and costs. *BMJ Open Sport Exerc. Med.* **2021**, *7*, e001023. [CrossRef] [PubMed]
6. Van der Plas, A.; de Jonge, S.; de Vos, R.J.; Van Der Heide, H.J.L.; Verhaar, J.A.N.; Weir, A.; Tol, J.L. A 5-year follow-up study of Alfredson's heel-drop exercise programme in chronic midportion Achilles tendinopathy. *Br. J. Sports Med.* **2012**, *46*, 214–218. [CrossRef] [PubMed]
7. Wang, J.H.-C. Mechanobiology of tendon. *J. Biomech.* **2006**, *39*, 1563–1582. [CrossRef] [PubMed]
8. Hess, G.W. Achilles tendon rupture: A review of etiology, population, anatomy, risk factors, and injury prevention. *Foot Ankle Specialist* **2010**, *3*, 29–32. [CrossRef]
9. Peter Magnusson, S.; Aagaard, P.; Rosager, S.; Dyhre-Poulsen, P.; Kjaer, M. Load-displacement properties of the human triceps surae aponeurosis in vivo. *J. Physiol.* **2001**, *531*, 277–288. [CrossRef]
10. Zhang, Z.J.; Ng, G.Y.F.; Fu, S.N. Effects of habitual loading on patellar tendon mechanical and morphological properties in basketball and volleyball players. *Eur. J. Appl. Physiol.* **2015**, *115*, 2263–2269. [CrossRef] [PubMed]
11. Mifsud, T.; Gatt, A.; Micallef-Stafrace, K.; Chockalingam, N.; Padhiar, N. Elastography in the assessment of the Achilles tendon: A systematic review of measurement properties. *J. Foot Ankle Res.* **2023**, *16*, 23. [CrossRef] [PubMed]
12. Fernandes, G.L.; Orssatto, L.B.R.; Shield, A.J.; Trajano, G.S. Runners with mid-portion Achilles tendinopathy have greater triceps surae intracortical inhibition than healthy controls. *Scand. J. Med. Sci. Sports* **2022**, *32*, 728–736. [CrossRef] [PubMed]
13. Schneider, S.; Peipsi, A.; Stokes, M.; Knicker, A.; Abeln, V. Feasibility of monitoring muscle health in microgravity environments using Myoton technology. *Med. Biol. Eng. Comput.* **2015**, *53*, 57–66. [CrossRef] [PubMed]
14. Hopkins, W.G. Measures of Reliability in Sports Medicine and Science. *Sports Med.* **2000**, *30*, 1–15. [CrossRef] [PubMed]
15. Wang, X.Q. Quantifying the Stiffness of Achilles Tendon: Intra- and Inter-Operator Reliability and the Effect of Ankle Joint Motion. *Med. Sci. Monit.* **2018**, *24*, 4876–4881. [CrossRef]
16. Kubo, K.; Ikebukuro, T.; Yata, H.; Tsunoda, N.; Kanehisa, H. Time course of changes in muscle and tendon properties during strength training and detraining. *J. Strength. Cond. Res.* **2010**, *24*, 322–331. [CrossRef] [PubMed]
17. Finnamore, E.; Waugh, C.; Solomons, L.; Ryan, M.; West, C.; Scott, A. Transverse tendon stiffness is reduced in people with Achilles tendinopathy: A cross-sectional study. *PLoS ONE* **2019**, *14*, e0211863. [CrossRef]
18. Morgan, G.E.; Martin, R.; Williams, L.; Pearce, O.; Morris, K. Objective assessment of stiffness in Achilles tendinopathy: A novel approach using the MyotonPRO. *BMJ Open Sport Exerc. Med.* **2018**, *4*, e000446. [CrossRef] [PubMed]
19. Taş, S.; Salkın, Y. An investigation of the sex-related differences in the stiffness of the Achilles tendon and gastrocnemius muscle: Inter-observer reliability and inter-day repeatability and the effect of ankle joint motion. *Foot* **2019**, *41*, 44–50. [CrossRef]
20. Feng, Y.N.; Li, Y.P.; Liu, C.L.; Zhang, Z.J. Assessing the elastic properties of skeletal muscle and tendon using shearwave ultrasound elastography and MyotonPRO. *Sci. Rep.* **2018**, *8*, 17064. [CrossRef]
21. Chang, T.T.; Feng, Y.N.; Zhu, Y.; Liu, C.L.; Wang, X.Q.; Zhang, Z.J. Objective assessment of regional stiffness in achilles tendon in different ankle joint positions using the MyotonPRO. *Med. Sci. Monit.* **2020**, *26*, e926407. [CrossRef] [PubMed]
22. Zou, G.Y. Sample size formulas for estimating intraclass correlation coefficients with precision and assurance. *Stat. Med.* **2012**, *31*, 3972–3981. [CrossRef] [PubMed]
23. Winnicki, K.; Ochała-Kłos, A.; Rutowicz, B.; Pękala, P.A.; Tomaszewski, K.A. Functional anatomy, histology and biomechanics of the human Achilles tendon—A comprehensive review. *Ann. Anat.* **2020**, *229*, 151461. [CrossRef]
24. Kubo, K.; Ikebukuro, T.; Maki, A.; Yata, H.; Tsunoda, N. Time course of changes in the human Achilles tendon properties and metabolism during training and detraining in vivo. *Eur. J. Appl. Physiol.* **2012**, *112*, 2679–2691. [CrossRef] [PubMed]
25. Kelly, C.; Al-Uzri, M.; O'Neill, S. 49 Effect Of Eccentric Training On Isokinetic Endurance Of Calf With Reliability Testing. *Br. J. Sports Med.* **2014**, *48* (Suppl. 2), A32. [CrossRef]
26. Fujisawa, H.; Suzuki, H.; Nishiyama, T.; Suzuki, M. Comparison of ankle plantar flexor activity between double-leg heel raise and walking. *J. Phys. Ther. Sci.* **2015**, *27*, 1523–1526. [CrossRef]

27. Koo, T.K.; Li, M.Y. A Guideline of Selecting and Reporting Intraclass Correlation Coefficients for Reliability Research. *J. Chiropr. Med.* **2016**, *15*, 155–163. [CrossRef]
28. McGraw, K.O.; Wong, S.P. Forming Inferences about Some Intraclass Correlation Coefficients. *Psychol. Methods* **1996**, *1*, 30–46. [CrossRef]
29. Schneebeli, A.; Falla, D.; Clijsen, R.; Barbero, M. Myotonometry for the evaluation of Achilles tendon mechanical properties: A reliability and construct validity study. *BMJ Open Sport Exerc. Med.* **2020**, *6*, e000726. [CrossRef] [PubMed]
30. Muckelt, P.E.; Warner, M.B.; Cheliotis-James, T.; Muckelt, R.; Hastermann, M.; Schoenrock, B.; Martin, D.; MacGregor, R.; Blottner, D.; Stokes, M. Protocol and reference values for minimal detectable change of MyotonPRO and ultrasound imaging measurements of muscle and subcutaneous tissue. *Sci. Rep.* **2022**, *12*, 13654. [CrossRef]
31. Stevens, M.; Chee-Wee, T. Effectiveness of the Alfredson protocol compared with a lower repetition-volume protocol for midportion Achilles tendinopathy: A randomized controlled trial. *J. Orthop. Sports Phys. Ther.* **2014**, *44*, 59–67. [CrossRef] [PubMed]

Disclaimer/Publisher's Note: The statements, opinions and data contained in all publications are solely those of the individual author(s) and contributor(s) and not of MDPI and/or the editor(s). MDPI and/or the editor(s) disclaim responsibility for any injury to people or property resulting from any ideas, methods, instructions or products referred to in the content.

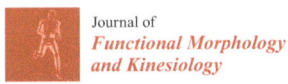

Article

A Comparison of Bioelectric and Biomechanical EMG Normalization Techniques in Healthy Older and Young Adults during Walking Gait

Drew Commandeur [1,2,†], Marc Klimstra [1,2,3,*,†], Ryan Brodie [3] and Sandra Hundza [1,2,4]

1. Motion and Mobility Laboratory, University of Victoria, Victoria, BC V8P 5C2, Canada
2. School of Exercise Science, Physical and Health Education, University of Victoria, Victoria, BC V8W 3P2, Canada
3. Canadian Sport Institute Pacific, Victoria, BC V9E 2C5, Canada; rbrodie@csipacific.ca
4. International Collaboration on Repair Discoveries (ICORD), Vancouver, BC V5Z 1M9, Canada
* Correspondence: klimstra@uvic.ca
† Co-first authors.

Abstract: This study compares biomechanical and bioelectric electromyography (EMG) normalization techniques across disparate age cohorts during walking to assess the impact of normalization methods on the functional interpretation of EMG data. The biomechanical method involved scaling EMG to a target absolute torque (EMG_{TS}) from a joint-specific task and the chosen bioelectric methods were peak and mean normalization taken from the EMG signal during gait, referred to as dynamic mean and dynamic peak normalization (EMG_{Mean} and EMG_{Peak}). The effects of normalization on EMG amplitude, activation pattern, and inter-subject variability were compared between disparate cohorts, including OLD (76.6 yrs N = 12) and YOUNG (26.6 yrs N = 12), in five lower-limb muscles. EMG_{Peak} normalization resulted in differences between YOUNG and OLD cohorts in Biceps Femoris (BF) and Medial Gastrocnemius (MG) that were not observed with EMG_{Mean} or EMG_{TS} normalization. EMG_{Peak} and EMG_{Mean} normalization also demonstrated interactions between age and the phase of gait in BF that were not seen with EMG_{TS}. Correlations showed that activation patterns across the gait cycle were similar between all methods for both age groups and the coefficient of variation comparisons found that EMG_{TS} produced the greatest inter-subject variability. We have shown that the normalization technique can influence the interpretation of findings when comparing disparate populations, highlighting the need to carefully interpret functional differences in EMG between disparate cohorts.

Citation: Commandeur, D.; Klimstra, M.; Brodie, R.; Hundza, S. A Comparison of Bioelectric and Biomechanical EMG Normalization Techniques in Healthy Older and Young Adults during Walking Gait. *J. Funct. Morphol. Kinesiol.* **2024**, *9*, 90. https://doi.org/10.3390/jfmk9020090

Academic Editor: Pedro Miguel Forte

Received: 12 April 2024
Revised: 15 May 2024
Accepted: 20 May 2024
Published: 22 May 2024

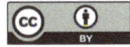

Copyright: © 2024 by the authors. Licensee MDPI, Basel, Switzerland. This article is an open access article distributed under the terms and conditions of the Creative Commons Attribution (CC BY) license (https://creativecommons.org/licenses/by/4.0/).

Keywords: EMG; EMG normalization; biomechanical normalization; bioelectric normalization; ageing; gait

1. Introduction

The amplitude of raw electromyography (EMG) can be greatly affected by conditions during collection including subcutaneous tissue thickness [1], electrode placement [2], joint angle and muscle movement [3], as well as cross talk from nearby muscles [4]. Therefore, it is not valid to make comparisons of raw EMG amplitude between subjects, muscles, tasks, or after changing the placement of electrodes. To enable comparisons of EMG between individuals, groups and conditions over time during walking gait, EMG is typically normalized using either bioelectric or biomechanical techniques [5]. Bioelectric methods normalize EMG to a level recorded during a task such as walking or an isolated normalization task. Commonly employed bioelectric techniques include maximum voluntary isometric contraction (MVIC), dynamic EMG peak (EMG_{Peak}) or dynamic EMG mean (EMG_{Mean}), among others [6]. For a detailed comparison of bioelectric methods, see [5]. EMG_{Peak} and EMG_{Mean} are the maximum and mean EMG amplitude achieved during a task, respectively. MVIC is the average maximum EMG amplitude achieved during an isometric contraction using an independent isometric task. One issue of using MVICs to normalize EMG is the lack of consistency between trials, as demonstrated by Yang and Winter (1984) [7], who found that within-day and between-day submaximal contractions are more reliable compared to MVIC. Further, for older individuals, there can be a hesitancy to perform a true MVIC due to discomfort or pain associated with this task [8], particularly if the patients have an age-related injury or pathology [9,10] such as arthritis [11]. Submaximal contractions for normalization of EMG_{Peak} and EMG_{Mean} are less physically strenuous and therefore address the issues of consistency and discomfort associated with the MVIC technique [7,12].

A limitation of bioelectric normalization techniques is that they could result in a misrepresentation of the absolute amplitude of force generated by the muscle and impede apposite comparison between functionally disparate groups [6]. For example, in clinical populations, during a task such as walking, the force generated by a muscle could be much lower than the controls, but this would not be adequately captured using MVIC, EMG_{Peak} and EMG_{Mean} normalization [13].

Bioelectric normalization methods are used to examine the relative differences between individuals or groups, but often an absolute comparison may provide more relevant information concerning force production during a task. Therefore, the use of a biomechanical EMG normalization technique based on torque-scaled values of EMG could enable functionally relevant comparisons between disparate populations [5,14]. This type of normalization technique has been previously employed [7,15,16]. For example, Ng et al. (2002) [15] assessed the difference in the EMG activity of trunk muscles between individuals with and without back pain using submaximal contractions to specific loads. To date, bioelectric and biomechanical methods of normalization have not been rigorously compared to determine the effect of the normalization technique on the capacity to detect differences between disparate cohorts during walking gait. While Yang and Winter (1984) [7] did compare bioelectric and biomechanical methods of normalization, the biomechanical normalization method used a subject relative load (50% MVIC), and thus this method did not incorporate EMG activation associated with an externally determined target absolute load. Therefore, there is a need to compare bioelectrical EMG normalization techniques to a biomechanical EMG normalization method that uses a common target absolute load to detect differences in EMG amplitude and activation pattern between disparate cohorts during walking gait.

This study compared EMG between OLD and YOUNG subjects using an EMG torque-scaled (EMG_{TS}) normalization technique and two popular methods of bioelectric EMG normalization, EMG_{Mean} and EMG_{Peak}. These methods were compared with respect to their ability to detect differences in EMG amplitude, activation pattern and inter-subject variability during walking gait. Having a better understanding of the limitations and benefits of each normalization technique facilitates a more informed choice that may impact the interpretation of findings. As the current literature provides little evidence to characterize the relationship of the amplitude and activation pattern differences between bioelectric and biomechanical normalization methods, we sought to determine whether the chosen normalization method impacts the functional interpretation of the data. We also expected that the inter-individual variability of EMG would be preserved with biomechanical normalization and reduced with bioelectrical methods.

2. Materials and Methods
2.1. Participants

Twelve healthy YOUNG (six males, six females, aged 26.6 ± 5.5 yrs) and twelve healthy OLD (eight males, four females, aged 76.6 ± 5.0 yrs) adults were convenience sampled and participated in the study with informed written consent. Subjects were screened using the Canadian PAR-Q+ questionnaire and medical clearance was requested for participants who answered Yes to any question. Inclusion criteria for the study required participants to be able to walk unassisted, have a mini-mental state exam score of 24 or greater, and older participants were aged 65 years or older. Participants were excluded if they were unable to walk at least 200 m or had a musculoskeletal or neurological disorder. The experimental protocol was approved by the University of Victoria Human Research Ethics Committee (12-272).

2.2. Protocol

2.2.1. Walking Trials

Subjects walked on a treadmill at a self-selected walking pace (OLD—3.57 +/− 0.58 km/h; YOUNG—4.14 +/− 0.74 km/h) while EMG was recorded from the right lower limb throughout the gait cycle.

2.2.2. Submaximal Isometric Contraction Trials and Load–EMG Relationship Determination

Subjects were seated in a chair with a padded cuff attached to their right lower leg for the knee flexion/extension task or the foot for ankle plantarflexion/dorsiflexion task. To determine the torque–EMG relationship for the muscles studied, four submaximal isometric contractions were performed with the force of each contraction measured via a load cell (model LC101-50, Omega Sensing Solutions ULC, St Eustache, QC, Canada). For knee flexion and extension, the knee was positioned at an angle of 120° with the cuff 20 cm distal to the knee joint centre; participants produced and maintained torque moments of 0.91 Nm (knee flexion) and 1.36 Nm (knee extension) corresponding to a load of 10 lbs and 15 lbs, respectively. For plantarflexion and dorsiflexion, the subject was standing and facing a padded chair, the knee was placed at 90 degrees on the seat with the ankle held at 90° and the cuff positioned on the foot 10 cm distal to the centre of medial malleolus; subjects produced and maintained torque moments of 0.682 Nm (plantarflexion) and 0.273 Nm (dorsiflexion) corresponding to loads of 15 lbs and 6 lbs, respectively. Knee and ankle joint angles were positioned and maintained by the researcher using a manual goniometer. Participants were instructed to gradually increase the force of contraction to the target force (± 0.05 kg) and maintain for 5 s. A digital oscilloscope was used to provide visual feedback to the participant. Familiarization trials were performed until the participant could reliably maintain the target force.

2.3. EMG Collection and Conditioning

Electromyographic (EMG) activity was collected using Ag-AgCl bi-polar disposable electrodes (model T3425, Thought Technology, Montreal, QC, Canada) spaced 2 cm from centre-to-centre. EMG electrode sites were prepared by removing body hair and thoroughly cleaning the area with alcohol swabs. EMG was recorded from tibialis anterior (TA), soleus (SOL), medial gastrocnemius (MG), vastus lateralis (VL), and biceps femoris (BF) on the right side. Common grounds were placed over the patellar surface. EMG for both the torque scaled and walking trials were pre-amplified at a gain of 5000 and filtered at 10–300 Hz by Grass Technologies P511 (model P511 Grass Instruments, AstroNova, Brossard, QC, Canada). Recorded EMG was full-wave rectified and then filtered using a 40 Hz fourth order Butterworth low pass-filter to create a linear envelope for further analysis.

EMG was sampled at 1000 Hz with a 16-bit A/D converter and collected and analyzed using custom-written LabView 2013 software (National Instruments Corp., Austin, TX, USA). EMG data for the walking trial were phase averaged into 16 equal phases across the gait cycle. Phases 1–10 correspond to stance, while phases 11–16 correspond to swing for the right leg (See Figure 1). EMG recording and processing methods follow the work of Hundza et al., 2018 [17].

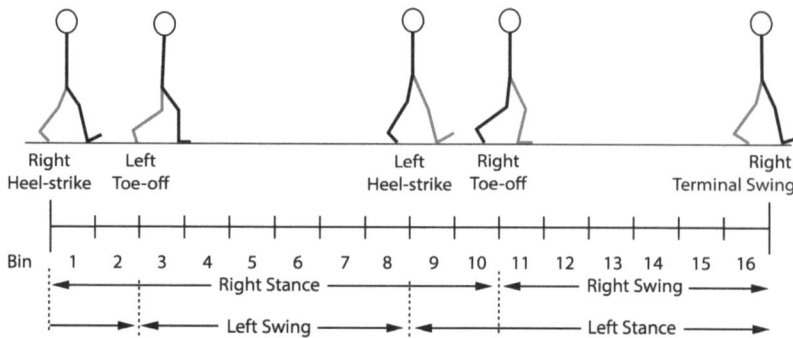

Figure 1. Adult gait cycle from right heel-strike to right termination of forward swing separated into sixteen equal phases.

2.4. Normalization of EMG Data

Averaged data for each phase were normalized using each of the three normalization techniques for each participant (see Section 2.5 for Formulae). Maximum EMG amplitude and mean EMG amplitude achieved across the phases during the walking task (EMG_{Task}) were used for the EMG_{Peak} and EMG_{Mean} normalization techniques, respectively. The background (at rest) EMG was calculated from the mean EMG during a 500 ms window of the isometric submaximal contraction trial before the contraction began. The average load during the window of the isometric contraction was then divided by the subtracted EMG to create a scaling factor in units of Nm. To calculate EMG_{TS}, each subject's EMG_{Task} was multiplied by the scaling factor for that participant.

2.5. Formulae

$$\text{Dynamic Peak Method}: EMG_{Peak} = \frac{EMG_{Task}}{EMG_{Task(Peak)}}$$

$$\text{Dynamic Mean Method}: EMG_{Mean} = \frac{EMG_{Task}}{EMG_{Task(Mean)}}$$

$$\text{Torque-scaled Method}: EMG_{TS} = EMG_{Task} \frac{Torque(Nm)}{EMG_{Load}}$$

2.6. Statistical Analysis

Phase averaged data for EMG_{Peak}, EMG_{Mean} and EMG_{TS} normalization techniques were compared. Separate repeated measures analysis of variance (ANOVA) tests for each of the 5 muscles and 3 normalization methods were conducted using a 2 (Age) × 16 (Phase) model with Tukey's HSD post-hoc analysis. The coefficient of variation (CV) was calculated for all normalization methods for each cohort as a measure of inter-individual variability across phases. CV was compared between ages, normalization methods, and age*normalization method interactions for each muscle using repeated measures ANOVA with Tukey's HSD post-hoc analysis. Pearson's product–moment correlations were performed between cohorts across all phases. Significance was set at $\alpha < 0.05$ for all comparisons and correlation coefficients were interpreted as <0.40 = weak, 0.40–0.69 = moderate, 0.70–0.89 = strong, and >0.90 very strong [18]. ANOVA effect sizes were reported as partial eta squared (np^2) with values of 0.02 considered small, 0.13 as medium, and 0.26 as large [19]. All data are presented as mean ± SEM except subjects' ages, which are presented as mean ± SD.

3. Results
3.1. Amplitude Differences

Normalized EMG activity values averaged across participants across the phases of the gait cycle for YOUNG and OLD cohorts for each normalization method are displayed in Figure 2. The main effects for age were observed with a medium effect size in BF ($F(1,22) = 6.266$; $p = 0.020$, $np^2 = 0.21$) and MG ($F(1,22) = 6.631$; $p = 0.017$, $np^2 = 0.14$) for EMG_{Peak} normalization with a greater EMG amplitude for OLD (BF = 47.96 +/− 7.02; MG = 51.36 +/− 8.21) than YOUNG (BF = 43.93 +/− 6.88; MG = 48.62 +/− 8.66) cohorts. Age*phase interactions were observed with EMG_{Mean} and EMG_{Peak} in VL, BF, and TA and for EMG_{TS} in BF and TA with small effects observed for all comparisons except EMG_{Mean} and EMG_{Peak} in BF, which had a medium effect size (see Table 1).

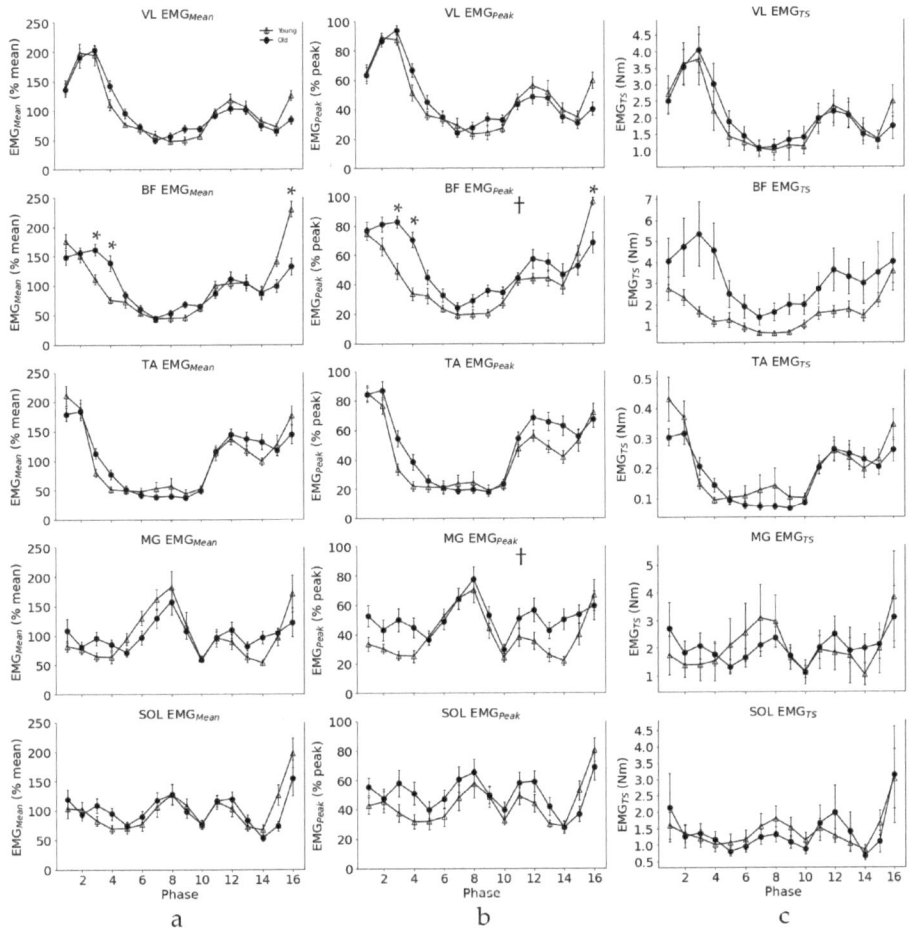

Figure 2. Normalized EMG averaged across YOUNG (N = 12) and OLD (N = 12) participants (+/− SEM) for EMG_{Peak} (**a**), EMG_{Mean} (**b**) and EMG_{TS} (**c**) for lower-limb muscles across the gait cycle during walking. Significant differences between cohorts at a given phase of movement are indicated by *, while † indicates a main effect for age.

Table 1. Significant age*phase interactions between OLD (N = 12) and YOUNG (N = 12) mean EMG across the gait cycle (16 phases) in five muscles involved in walking.

Muscle	Normalization	df	p	F	np^2
VL	EMG$_{Mean}$	15, 330	0.036	1.781	0.08
VL	EMG$_{Peak}$	15, 330	0.003	2.334	0.10
BF	EMG$_{Mean}$	15, 330	0.000	7.333	0.25
BF	EMG$_{Peak}$	15, 330	0.000	6.088	0.22
BF	EMG$_{TS}$	15, 330	0.001	2.592	0.11
TA	EMG$_{Mean}$	15, 330	0.046	1.721	0.07
TA	EMG$_{Peak}$	15, 330	0.007	2.170	0.09
TA	EMG$_{TS}$	15, 330	0.032	1.814	0.08

Post-hoc Tukey's test for age*phase interactions revealed that there were significant differences in the BF muscle with EMG$_{Mean}$ normalization in phases 3 ($p < 0.01$), 4 ($p < 0.001$), and 16 ($p < 0.05$). There were also differences in the BF muscle with EMG$_{Peak}$ normalization in phases 3 ($p < 0.05$), 4 ($p < 0.01$), and 16 ($p < 0.001$). With both normalization methods, the EMG amplitude was greater in OLD than YOUNG cohorts for phases 3 and 4 and greater in YOUNG than OLD cohorts for phase 16. Post-hoc analysis did not reveal differences between YOUNG and OLD cohorts for any other comparisons with interaction effects. The EMG amplitude for each age group can be seen for the five muscles across the phases of gait, including significant main and interaction effects, in Figure 2.

3.2. EMG Pattern

Normalized EMG activities for each cohort were compared for each muscle across the 16 phases of the gait cycle for each normalization method. There were very strong correlations observed for all comparisons between EMG$_{Mean}$ and EMG$_{Peak}$ for both cohorts with an average correlation across all muscles of r = 0.99 for OLD and r = 1.00 for YOUNG cohorts. EMG$_{Peak}$ vs. EMG$_{TS}$ were very strongly correlated for all muscles in the YOUNG cohort and for VL, BF, and TA in the OLD cohort with MG and SOL strongly correlated (average r = 0.88 for OLD and r = 0.98 for YOUNG). EMG$_{Mean}$ vs. EMG$_{TS}$ were very strongly correlated for all muscles in the YOUNG cohort and for VL, BF, and TA, and SOL in the OLD cohort with MG strongly correlated (average r = 0.90 for OLD and r = 0.98 for YOUNG). See Table 2 for all correlation results.

Table 2. Pearson's correlations between OLD (N = 12) and YOUNG (N = 12) mean EMG across the gait cycle (16 phases) in five muscles involved in walking.

Age	Correlation	VL	BF	TA	MG	SOL
OLD	EMG$_{Peak}$ vs. EMG$_{Mean}$	1.00	1.00	1.00	0.99	0.98
OLD	EMG$_{Peak}$ vs. EMG$_{TS}$	0.99	0.98	1.00	0.70	0.72
OLD	EMG$_{Mean}$ vs. EMG$_{TS}$	0.99	0.98	1.00	0.70	0.84
YOUNG	EMG$_{Peak}$ vs. EMG$_{Mean}$	1.00	1.00	1.00	1.00	0.99
YOUNG	EMG$_{Peak}$ vs. EMG$_{TS}$	1.00	1.00	0.99	0.93	0.97
YOUNG	EMG$_{Mean}$ vs. EMG$_{TS}$	1.00	1.00	0.99	0.92	0.98

3.3. Inter-Subject Variability

The coefficient of variation (CV) across phases of the gait cycle averaged for each cohort and normalization technique for each muscle is displayed in Figure 3. The main effects for age were observed in BF, TA, and MG with a moderate effect size for BF, small effect size for TA, and large effect size for MG. The main effects with large effect sizes were observed for all normalization methods except TA, which had a medium effect size. There were age*normalization interactions with large effect sizes in BF and MG, while SOL had an age*normalization interaction with a small effect. See Table 3 for all significant results.

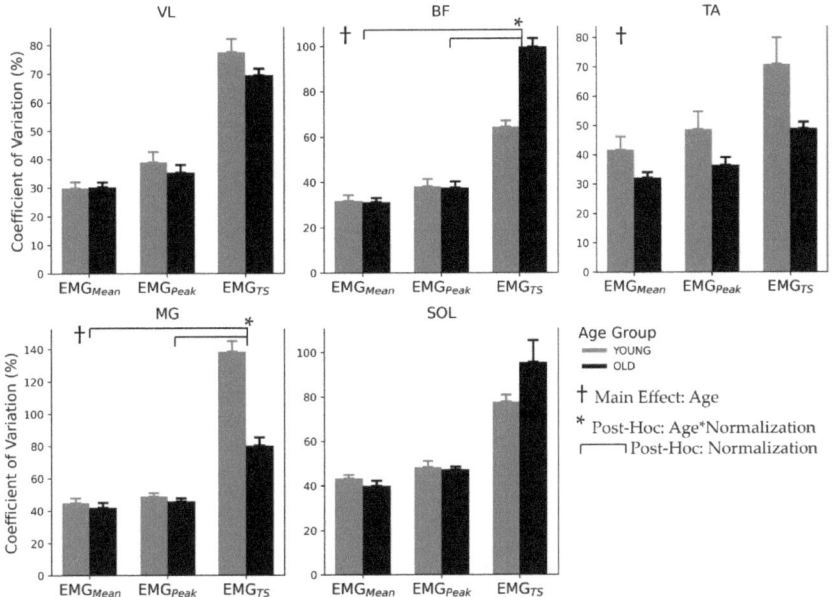

Figure 3. Mean coefficient of variation of three EMG normalization techniques for YOUNG (N = 12) and OLD (N = 12) participants in lower-limb muscles during walking. Significant main effect for age is indicated by †, significant age*normalization interactions by *, and significant post-hoc comparisons of normalization are indicated by horizontal bars.

Table 3. Significant age, normalization, and age*normalization interactions between OLD (N = 12) and YOUNG (N = 12) EMG coefficient of variation across the gait cycle (16 phases) in five muscles involved in walking.

Effect	Muscle	df	p	F	np2
Age	BF	1, 90	0.000	23.667	0.21
Age	TA	1, 90	0.001	12.470	0.12
Age	MG	1, 90	0.000	44.749	0.33
Normalization	VL	2, 90	0.000	119.460	0.73
Normalization	BF	2, 90	0.000	185.955	0.81
Normalization	TA	2, 90	0.000	11.348	0.20
Normalization	MG	2, 90	0.000	176.677	0.80
Normalization	SOL	2, 90	0.000	57.755	0.56
Age*Normalization	BF	2, 90	0.000	26.188	0.37
Age*Normalization	MG	2, 90	0.000	32.780	0.42
Age*Normalization	SOL	2, 90	0.043	0.821	0.02

Post-hoc Tukey's tests identified differences in CV between EMG_{Peak} vs. EMG_{TS} ($p < 0.001$) and EMG_{Mean} vs. EMG_{TS} ($p < 0.001$) with EMG_{TS} CV being higher in both cases, but with no difference between EMGMean and EMGPeak. Post-hoc analysis of the interaction between age and normalization effect between matched cases found that in BF, EMG_{TS} CV was greater in OLD than YOUNG ($p < 0.001$) cohorts and in MG, EMG_{TS} CV was greater in YOUNG than OLD ($p < 0.001$) cohorts.

4. Discussion

There were three main findings of this study comparing bioelectric (EMG_{Mean} and EMG_{Peak}) and biomechanical (EMG_{TS}) normalization techniques in older (OLD) and young

(YOUNG) adults. First, there was no agreement for the statistical interpretation of EMG amplitude differences between age groups with the three normalization techniques. The EMG_{Peak} method identified amplitude differences between the two age groups in two of the five muscles (BF and MG) that EMG_{Mean} and EMG_{TS} did not. Additionally, both EMG_{Peak} and EMG_{Mean} normalization resulted in age*phase interactions in the biceps femoris muscle. This highlights the fact that the interpretation of EMG is dependent on the normalization method used, and it is essential to consider the strengths and limitations of each method when making functional interpretations.

The second notable finding was that EMG activation patterns across the gait cycle were generally similar between the normalization methods. As mentioned, the normalization method did result in notable EMG amplitude differences between cohorts for some muscles at some phases of the gait cycle, but the activation pattern across the phases were generally not different and they were strongly correlated for both cohorts.

Finally, the coefficient of variation (CV), the representation of inter-individual variability, was much greater for EMG_{TS}, while EMG_{Mean} and EMG_{Peak} were alike for all muscles. This finding supports our hypothesis that EMG_{TS} normalization would retain more inter-individual variability, which in some cases may be highly desirable; however, it also emphasizes that even when large differences are expected, a larger sample size may be required to counteract the increase in variability.

Our findings clearly demonstrate that the normalization method can influence the results and thus the conclusions drawn from EMG interpretation and highlights the importance of choosing a normalization technique based on the specific research question with a full understanding of the limitations and bias of the normalization procedure.

4.1. Rationale for Normalization Protocols

The bioelectric techniques, EMG_{Mean} and EMG_{Peak}, were chosen for the present study as they are currently popular techniques [5]. Normalization to MVIC was excluded as a technique as it poses an injury, pain, or fear risk to an older cohort [20]. The biomechanical normalization method was designed to be easily performed across disparate populations (i.e., OLD and YOUNG cohorts) and include submaximal isometric contraction with absolute target torques at reproducible joint angles. Because the joint angle can influence force production and different populations may have different available ranges of motion, mid-range joint angles were chosen within an optimal force-joint angle range. Thus, this normalization method could be employed in any paradigm that was comparing EMG levels across disparate populations in different tasks. Isometric MVC is known to have equal inter-subject variability compared to dynamic submaximal contractions [6] and greater variability compared to isometric submaximal contractions [21]. Also, Burden et al. (2003) [6] reported that the use of dynamic (isokinetic) contraction methods does not decrease the intra-individual variability over isometric methods, while it does comparatively increase the complexity and duration of the normalization protocol. Thus, it is reasonable to infer that isometric submaximal contraction should have the lowest inter-subject variability. Finally, an absolute submaximal load for each muscle contraction was chosen to enable functionally relevant comparisons between disparate populations at the same absolute load [5,14].

While EMG_{TS} provides an individual scaling factor to normalize across subjects and populations, it does not account for the potential curvilinear relationship between muscle force and EMG during static contraction [22,23] and more complex relationships during dynamic contractions [24,25]. Importantly, the individual load scaling method presented in this study is a means to bring all subject-specific values to an approximate absolute load and is not meant to infer accurate measures of joint torques through EMG measurement. Therefore, as with all normalization techniques, functional interpretations of the results must account for these limitations.

4.2. EMG Activation Pattern and Amplitude

When comparing muscle activation across different populations, or before and after an intervention, it is valuable to evaluate both the amplitude and pattern of EMG activation as well as their interaction and consider the functional interpretation of the results. The differences observed between the OLD and YOUNG EMG amplitude across the phases of the gait cycle in the present study depend on the normalization technique used. Both EMG_{Peak} and EMG_{Mean} identified age*phase interactions in three muscles (VL, BF, and TA), while EMG_{TS} showed interactions in BF and TA, although following post-hoc analysis, significant age*phase interactions were only observed in BF for phases 3,4, and 16 with EMG_{Peak} and EMG_{Mean} normalization. These phases are critical transition points of the gait cycle in the BF muscle during weight acceptance in the stance phase (phases 3 and 4) and terminal swing (phase 16). In the stance phase, the pattern of EMG_{TS} generally agrees with both EMG_{Mean} and EMG_{Peak}; however, terminal swing displays large differences where OLD EMG amplitude was greater than YOUNG using EMG_{Peak} and EMG_{Mean} normalization, while EMG_{TS} showed no evidence of differences (see Figure 2). This discrepancy leads to the potential for incorrect functional interpretations of results. For instance, one could infer that older adults have insufficient activation of BF during terminal swing based on the results of EMG_{Peak} and EMG_{Mean} and over-activation during the early stance phase. This phenomena is more likely a result of the normalization technique rather than a true functional difference between groups [5]. Thus, the normalization technique can influence the conclusions that can be drawn, which may have critical implications for studies attempting to support clinical differences between groups.

Despite the potential differences in EMG amplitude with the three normalization techniques, the muscle activation patterns across the gait cycle were generally similar between the cohorts across the normalization methods as evidenced by the significant correlations between OLD and YOUNG for each muscle. This indicates that each method effectively characterises the inherent phase modulation during gait.

4.3. Inter-Subject Variability

While EMG_{Peak} remains a common normalization technique, EMG_{Mean} has been suggested as the preferred bioelectric normalization method because it has been reported to reduce inter-individual variability more than EMG_{Peak} while maintaining the characteristic activation profile [6,7,26]. In a review by Burden (2010) [5], it was identified that EMG normalization procedures that reduce inter-subject variability are viewed positively because they increase the power of statistical comparisons between groups. However, normalization techniques that allow the expression of variability may more accurately represent the "true" variability in the EMG amplitude related to absolute force production during a task by subjects within a group. Therefore, it is important to consider the effect of a normalization technique on the inter-subject variability inherent in the raw EMG as well as maintaining variability associated with "true" differences in EMG amplitude relative to absolute force production during task performance. This is aptly demonstrated when comparing the effect of normalization using EMG_{TS} compared to the EMG_{Mean} and EMG_{Peak}. This can be observed in the larger CV values for EMG_{TS} compared to EMG_{Mean} and EMG_{Peak} for all muscles (see Figure 3). The EMG_{TS} method takes into account the subjects' capacity relative to an absolute load when comparing EMG during the walking task, whereas EMG_{Mean} and EMG_{Peak} take into account the subjects' performance relative to a trial-specific EMG. However, greater variability with EMG_{TS} results in reduced statistical power and likely warrants larger sample sizes than either of the bioelectrical normalization techniques.

A potential source of error that could increase inter-individual variability in torque-scaled normalization is the accuracy of the force generated by the participant. Even small deviations from the target force could result in large changes in the $Nm/\mu V$ estimate. This phenomenon was also observed by Yang and Winter (1984) [7] who used 50% MVIC–moment relationships to normalize EMG and found that the accuracy of the submaximal contraction was important as small deviations from 50% resulted in large errors in their scaling factor, particularly if the EMG–moment relationship was not linear. Therefore, it remains to be confirmed if increased variability with load scale normalization truly represents actual differences among individuals or if methodological rigour contributes to this variability. The effects of age on variability of force production and motor unit discharge patterns imply that older individuals have intrinsically higher variability in force production [27]. This is supported by our finding that OLD CV was larger than YOUNG CV when normalized to EMG_{TS} for BF where OLD CV was greater than YOUNG CV, but our results observed the opposite in MG where YOUNG CV was greater than OLD CV. No age differences in CV were observed with EMG_{Mean} and EMG_{Peak} methods. Since the bioelectric normalization methods intentionally suppress inter-individual variability, this result is not unexpected [5]. This highlights the concerns raised by Hsu et al. (2006) [28] that normalizing EMG to the mean or peak of a task reduces inter-individual variability and dilutes the true variation in gait EMG and does not represent a subject's actual capacity, but rather the EMG activation relative to the task-specific EMG value.

5. Conclusions

The current findings demonstrate that depending on the normalization technique employed, different results emerge from the same raw EMG data, leading to the potential for different conclusions to be drawn. Thus, it is critical to have an in depth understanding of the influence of the normalization method used to make an informed choice of the most appropriate method to address the research question and accurately interpret the results. We noted the differing effect of the normalization method on EMG amplitude and inter-subject variability. Additionally, although the activation patterns across phases were generally similar between normalization methods, there were notable differences between cohorts in some muscles depending on the normalization technique used.

Author Contributions: Conceptualization, D.C., R.B., S.H. and M.K.; methodology, D.C., R.B., S.H. and M.K.; software, D.C., R.B. and M.K.; formal analysis, D.C., R.B. and M.K.; investigation, D.C. and R.B.; resources, D.C., R.B., S.H. and M.K.; data curation, D.C. and R.B.; writing—original draft preparation, D.C.; writing—review and editing D.C., R.B., S.H. and M.K.; visualization, D.C. All authors have read and agreed to the published version of the manuscript.

Funding: This research received no external funding.

Institutional Review Board Statement: This study was conducted in accordance with the Declaration of Helsinki and approved by the Institutional Review Board of the University of Victoria (12-272).

Informed Consent Statement: Informed consent was obtained from all subjects involved in the study.

Data Availability Statement: Data used in this study cannot be shared outside of the original research group.

Conflicts of Interest: The authors declare no conflicts of interest.

References

1. Hemingway, M.A.; Biedermann, H.J.; Inglis, J. Electromyographic Recordings of Paraspinal Muscles: Variations Related to Subcutaneous Tissue Thickness. *Biofeedback Self. Regul.* **1995**, *20*, 39–49. [CrossRef]
2. Beck, T.W.; Housh, T.J.; Mielke, M.; Cramer, J.T.; Weir, J.P.; Malek, M.H.; Johnson, G.O. The Influence of Electrode Placement over the Innervation Zone on Electromyographic Amplitude and Mean Power Frequency versus Isokinetic Torque Relationships. *J. Neurosci. Methods* **2007**, *162*, 72–83. [CrossRef]
3. Basmajian, J.V.; DeLuca, C.J. *Muscles Alive: Their Functions Revealed by Electromyography*, 5th ed.; Williams & Wilkins: Baltimore, MD, USA, 1985.
4. Koh, T.J.; Grabiner, M.D. Evaluation of Methods to Minimize Cross Talk in Surface Electromyography. *J. Biomech.* **1993**, *26* (Suppl. S1), 151–157. [CrossRef]
5. Burden, A. How Should We Normalize Electromyograms Obtained from Healthy Participants? What We Have Learned from over 25 Years of Research. *J. Electromyogr. Kinesiol.* **2010**, *20*, 1023–1035. [CrossRef]
6. Burden, A.M.; Trew, M.; Baltzopoulos, V. Normalisation of Gait EMGs: A Re-Examination. *J. Electromyogr. Kinesiol.* **2003**, *13*, 519–532. [CrossRef]

7. Yang, J.F.; Winter, D.A. Electromyographic Amplitude Normalization Methods: Improving Their Sensitivity as Diagnostic Tools in Gait Analysis. *Arch. Phys. Med. Rehabil.* **1984**, *65*, 517–521.
8. Marras, W.S.; Davis, K.G.; Maronitis, A.B. A Non-MVC EMG Normalization Technique for the Trunk Musculature: Part 2. Validation and Use to Predict Spinal Loads. *J. Electromyogr. Kinesiol.* **2001**, *11*, 11–18. [CrossRef]
9. Cholewicki, J.; van Dieën, J.; Lee, A.S.; Reeves, N.P. A Comparison of a Maximum Exertion Method and a Model-Based, Sub-Maximum Exertion Method for Normalizing Trunk EMG. *J. Electromyogr. Kinesiol.* **2011**, *21*, 767–773. [CrossRef]
10. Knauer, S.R.; Freburger, J.K.; Carey, T.S. Chronic Low Back Pain among Older Adults: A Population-Based Perspective. *J. Aging Health* **2010**, *22*, 1213–1234. [CrossRef]
11. Covinsky, K. Aging, Arthritis, and Disability. *Arthritis Rheum.* **2006**, *55*, 175–176. [CrossRef]
12. Lehman, G.J.; Mcgill, S.M. The Importance of Normalization in the Interpretation of Surface Electromyography: A proof of principle. *J. Manip. Physiol. Ther.* **1999**, *22*, 444–446. [CrossRef]
13. Zehr, E.P.; Loadman, P.M.; Hundza, S.R. Neural Control of Rhythmic Arm Cycling after Stroke. *J. Neurophysiol.* **2012**, *108*, 891–905. [CrossRef]
14. Mathiassen, S.E.; Winkel, J.; Hägg, G.M. Normalization of Surface EMG Amplitude from the Upper Trapezius Muscle in Ergonomic Studies—A Review. *J. Electromyogr. Kinesiol.* **1995**, *5*, 197–226. [CrossRef]
15. Ng, J.K.F.; Richardson, C.A.; Parnianpour, M.; Kippers, V. EMG Activity of Trunk Muscles and Torque Output during Isometric Axial Rotation Exertion: A Comparison between Back Pain Patients and Matched Controls. *J. Orthop. Res.* **2002**, *20*, 112–121. [CrossRef]
16. Allison, G.T.; Marshall, R.N.; Singer, K.P. EMG Signal Amplitude Normalization Technique in Stretch-Shortening Cycle Movements. *J. Electromyogr. Kinesiol.* **1993**, *3*, 236–244. [CrossRef]
17. Hundza, S.R.; Gaur, A.; Brodie, R.; Commandeur, D.; Klimstra, M.D. Age-Related Erosion of Obstacle Avoidance Reflexes Evoked with Electrical Stimulation of Tibial Nerve during Walking. *J. Neurophysiol.* **2018**, 1528–1537. [CrossRef]
18. Schober, P.; Schwarte, L.A. Correlation Coefficients: Appropriate Use and Interpretation. *Anesth. Analg.* **2018**, *126*, 1763–1768. [CrossRef]
19. Bakeman, R. Recommended Effect Size Statistic. *Behav. Res. Methods* **2005**, *37*, 379–384. [CrossRef]
20. Marras, W.S.; Davis, K.G. A Non-MVC EMG Normalization Technique for the Trunk Musculature: Part 1. Method Development. *J. Electromyogr. Kinesiol.* **2001**, *11*, 1–9. [CrossRef]
21. Hansson, G.Å.; Nordander, C.; Asterland, P.; Ohlsson, K.; Strömberg, U.; Skerfving, S.; Rempel, D. Sensitivity of Trapezius Electromyography to Differences between Work Tasks—Influence of Gap Definition and Normalisation Methods. *J. Electromyogr. Kinesiol.* **2000**, *10*, 103–115. [CrossRef]
22. Woods, J.J.; Bigland Ritchie, B. Linear and Non-Linear Surface EMG/Force Relationships in Human Muscles. An Anatomical/Functional Argument for the Existence of Both. *Am. J. Phys. Med.* **1983**, *62*, 287–299. [PubMed]
23. Alkner, B.A.; Tesch, P.A.; Berg, H.E. Quadriceps EMG/Force Relationship in Knee Extension and Leg Press. *Med. Sci. Sports Exerc.* **2000**, *32*, 459–463. [CrossRef] [PubMed]
24. Lawrence, J.H.; DeLuca, C.J. Myoelectric Signal versus Force Relationship in Different Human Muscles Myoelectric in Different Signal versus Force Relationship Human Muscles. *J. Appl. Physiol.* **1983**, *54*, 1653–1659. [CrossRef] [PubMed]
25. Earp, J.E.; Newton, R.U.; Cormie, P.; Blazevich, A.J. Knee Angle-Specific EMG Normalization: The Use of Polynomial Based EMG-Angle Relationships. *J. Electromyogr. Kinesiol.* **2013**, *23*, 238–244. [CrossRef] [PubMed]
26. Shiavi, R.; Bourne, J.; Holland, A. Automated Extraction of Activity Features in Linear Envelopes of Locomotor Electromyographic Patterns. *IEEE Trans. Biomed. Eng.* **1986**, *33*, 594–600. [CrossRef] [PubMed]
27. Vaillancourt, D.E.; Larsson, L.; Newell, K.M. Effects of Aging on Force Variability, Single Motor Unit Discharge Patterns, and the Structure of 10, 20, and 40 Hz EMG Activity. *Neurobiol. Aging* **2003**, *24*, 25–35. [CrossRef]
28. Hsu, W.-L.; Krishnamoorthy, V.; Scholz, J.P. An Alternative Test of Electromyographic Normalization in Patients. *Muscle Nerve* **2006**, *33*, 232–241. [CrossRef]

Disclaimer/Publisher's Note: The statements, opinions and data contained in all publications are solely those of the individual author(s) and contributor(s) and not of MDPI and/or the editor(s). MDPI and/or the editor(s) disclaim responsibility for any injury to people or property resulting from any ideas, methods, instructions or products referred to in the content.

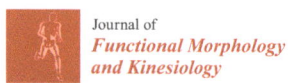 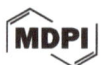

Brief Report

Changing the Mandibular Position in Rowing: A Brief Report of a World-Class Rower

Filipa Cardoso [1,2,*], Ricardo Cardoso [1,2], Pedro Fonseca [2], Manoel Rios [1,2], João Paulo Vilas-Boas [1,2], João C. Pinho [3,4], David B. Pyne [5] and Ricardo J. Fernandes [1,2]

[1] Centre of Research, Education, Innovation and Intervention in Sport (CIFI2D), Faculty of Sport, University of Porto, 4200-450 Porto, Portugal; up201200394@edu.fade.up.pt (R.C.); manoel.rios@hotmail.com (M.R.); jpvb@fade.up.pt (J.P.V.-B.); ricfer@fade.up.pt (R.J.F.)

[2] Porto Biomechanics Laboratory (LABIOMEP-UP), Faculty of Sport, University of Porto, 4200-450 Porto, Portugal; pedro.labiomep@fade.up.pt

[3] Faculty of Dental Medicine, University of Porto, 4200-393 Porto, Portugal; pinhojc53@gmail.com

[4] Institute of Science and Innovation in Mechanical and Industrial Engineering (INEGI), Faculty of Engineering, University of Porto, 4200-465 Porto, Portugal

[5] Research Institute for Sport & Exercise, University of Canberra, Canberra 2617, Australia; david.pyne@canberra.edu.au

* Correspondence: up201402398@edu.fade.up.pt or anafg.cardoso@hotmail.com

Abstract: We investigated the acute biophysical responses of changing the mandibular position during a rowing incremental protocol. A World-class 37-year-old male rower performed two 7 × 3 min ergometer rowing trials, once with no intraoral splint (control) and the other with a mandibular forward repositioning splint (splint condition). Ventilatory, kinematics and body electromyography were evaluated and compared between trials (paired samples t-test, $p \leq 0.05$). Under the splint condition, oxygen uptake was lower, particularly at higher exercise intensities (67.3 ± 2.3 vs. 70.9 ± 1.5 mL·kg^{-1}·min^{-1}), and ventilation increased during specific rowing protocol steps (1st–4th and 6th). Wearing the splint condition led to changes in rowing technique, including a slower rowing frequency ([18–30] vs. [19–32] cycles·min^{-1}) and a longer propulsive movement ([1.58–1.52] vs. [1.56–1.50] m) than the control condition. The splint condition also had a faster propulsive phase and a prolonged recovery period than the control condition. The splint reduced peak and mean upper body muscle activation, contrasting with an increase in lower body muscle activity, and generated an energetic benefit by reducing exercise cost and increasing rowing economy compared to the control condition. Changing the mandibular position benefited a World-class rower, supporting the potential of wearing an intraoral splint in high-level sports, particularly in rowing.

Keywords: occlusal splints; mandibular repositioning; elite sport; oxygen uptake; biomechanics; electromyography

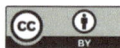

1. Introduction

Rowing is a sport characterized by both strength and endurance where performance is influenced by factors such as aerobic and anaerobic power, physical strength and rowing technique [1]. Given that rowers must develop several skills and capacities to achieve success, multimodal measurement systems are often required to simultaneously evaluate performance, physiology and mechanics in rowing [2]. Notably, during a prominent rowing competition such as the 2000 m race, a rower predominantly relies on aerobic metabolism (~80%) [3–5], underscoring the critical role of aerobic performance in this sport. Given this importance, forwarding the mandibular position using an occlusal splint during rowing may prove beneficial since these intraoral splints have been associated with enhanced gas exchange during exercise [6–8]. Indeed, the effectiveness of mandibular advancement in enlarging upper airway dimensions is well-documented in the treatment of sleep apnoea [8], sparking considerable interest in its potential applications in the field of sport.

The mandibular protruding position and its related effects on the upper airway, such as increased airflow and decreased airway resistance, have been debated regarding their potential to enhance aerobic exercise performance [7,8]. Nevertheless, although the ventilatory effects of wearing a mandibular protruding splint during exercise have recently gained attention and garnered debate, research on its impact on physiology and performance remains limited. Investigations into how a mandibular forward repositioning splint may enhance performance have primarily focused on recreational and trained individuals during submaximal and maximal running [6–8], with less emphasis on other sports and elite athletes. Therefore, we investigated the acute biophysical effects of using a mandibular forward repositioning splint in a World-class rower during a progressive incremental rowing ergometer test.

2. Materials and Methods

2.1. Participant

A World-class male rower (2012 and 2016 Olympic Games finalist, 2022 European and 2019 and 2021 World Rowing Champion), aged 37 years, with height of 1.87 m and body mass of 79.9 kg, gave his written informed consent to participate after explanation of the project aims, methods, benefits and risks (unconditional withdrawal was possible at any point). The local University Ethics Committee approved the study according to the Declaration of Helsinki.

2.2. Design

The rower performed an incremental intermittent protocol in a rowing ergometer (Concept II model D, fixed, Morrisville, VT, USA) in two sessions 24 h apart, once without the use of an intraoral splint (control) and the other wearing a mandibular forward repositioning splint (splint condition). Ventilatory, kinematic and body-surface electromyography (EMG) variables were recorded throughout. The rower was familiarized with the intraoral splint prior to the corresponding testing session without being informed of its potential biophysical effects.

2.3. Methodology

The rower completed a low-intensity 10 min warm-up on the rowing ergometer at a self-selected frequency before each test. The incremental protocol consisted of 7×3 min rowing steps, interspersed with 30 s intervals for blood sampling collection [9,10]. The initial workload was set at 180 W and increased to 30 W between consecutive steps. The 7th step power was based on the individual 2000 m rowing ergometer performance [11], and six power increments were subtracted to calculate the 1st step power output.

Breath-by-breath data were continuously collected (K5, Cosmed, Rome, Italy), and 3D kinematic variables were recorded at 100 Hz (Miqus, Qualisys AB, Göteborg, Sweden) between the 60 and 120 s interval within each step. Biceps brachii, posterior deltoid and rectus femoris EMG were assessed constantly (right hemibody) by the Trigno Avanti sensors (Delsys, Natick, MA, USA). Muscle surface preparation and sensor placement followed the SENIAM recommendations [12]. A 5 µL sample of capillary blood for lactate concentrations ([La-]) assessment was taken from the earlobe (Lactate Pro2; Arkay, Inc., Kyoto, Japan) at rest intervals between steps and at the end of the protocol [13].

2.4. Data Analysis

Oxygen uptake (VO_2) and ventilation were averaged and compared every 10 s of the last minute of exercise [14], and kinematics were obtained using Theia Markerless software (v2023.1.0.3161_ P14, Theia Markerless Inc., Kingston, ON, Canada). EMG signals were processed in MATLAB R2023b (The MathWorks Inc., Natick, MA, USA), including a band-pass filtration (25–450 Hz), full-wave rectification and linear envelope calculation with a 2nd-order Butterworth low-pass filter (6 Hz). Peak and mean amplitudes were expressed as a percentage relative to the initial value (defined as the EMG mean value during the 1st step) [11], being the instant of peak amplitude normalized to the duration of the propulsive phase (drive). Kinematic and EMG data were examined across ten consecutive rowing cycles in each step performed [15]. The energy expenditure was computed by adding the net VO_2 values and converting net [La-] into oxygen equivalents [5,13]. The energy cost was determined as the slope of a regression line between energy expenditure and the corresponding power [10], and rowing economy was calculated as the ratio between the power generated and the energy expenditure for each step [14].

2.5. Statistical Analysis

Statistical comparisons between control and splint conditions were performed for physiological and biomechanical variables using the paired samples *t*-test in SPSS (version 28.0.1.0, IBM Corp., Armonk, NY, USA). Bioenergetic data were only presented and interpreted as raw (rather than standardized) differences. Cohen's d (d) was computed to indicate the magnitude of effects (small ≥ 0.2, medium ≥ 0.5 and large ≥ 0.8). Significance was set to 5%.

3. Results

Ventilatory and kinematic variables for both experimental conditions are displayed in Figure 1. VO_2 values were similar except for the 7th step, where a lower VO_2 was observed for the splint condition (67.3 ± 2.3 vs. 70.9 ± 1.5 mL·kg^{-1}·min^{-1}). Moreover, there was a tendency toward a lower VO_2 at the 5th and 6th steps with the splint compared with the control condition ($p = 0.08$ and 0.06, $d = -0.89$ and -0.99, respectively). The splint condition also exhibited increased ventilation in between the 1st and 4th steps ([76.6–125.6] vs. [70.6–116.4] L·min^{-1}) and at the 6th step (154.4 ± 1.5 vs. 142.6 ± 7.8 L·min^{-1}).

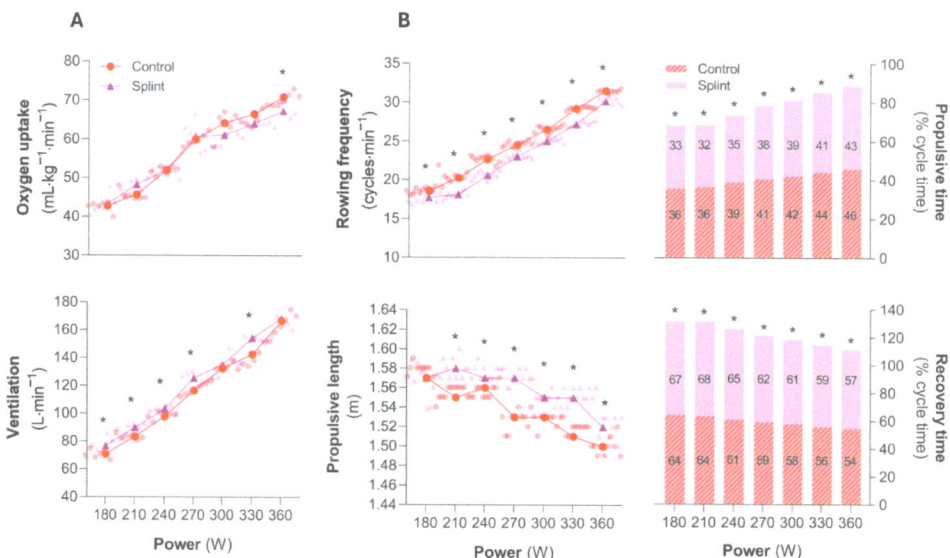

Figure 1. Physiological and kinematic variables (panels (**A**) and (**B**), respectively) assessed during the rowing incremental protocol for the two experimental conditions tested (control vs. splint). * indicates differences between control and splint conditions ($p \leq 0.05$).

When compared to the control condition, kinematic analysis revealed that rowing frequency was lower ([18–30] vs. [19–32] cycles·min^{-1}) and propulsive length was higher ([1.58–1.56] vs. [1.52–1.50] m) for the splint condition along the protocol. Furthermore, shortened propulsive time and extended recovery phases were observed throughout the protocol with the splint. The splint condition exhibited a lower peak and mean biceps brachii and posterior deltoid activation, contrasting with increased rectus femoris activity (Figure 2). The instant of peak activation for the posterior deltoid (except for the 5th step) and rectus femoris consistently occurred later along the propulsive phase in the splint condition, unlike the biceps brachii, where the respective instant occurred earlier (2nd step).

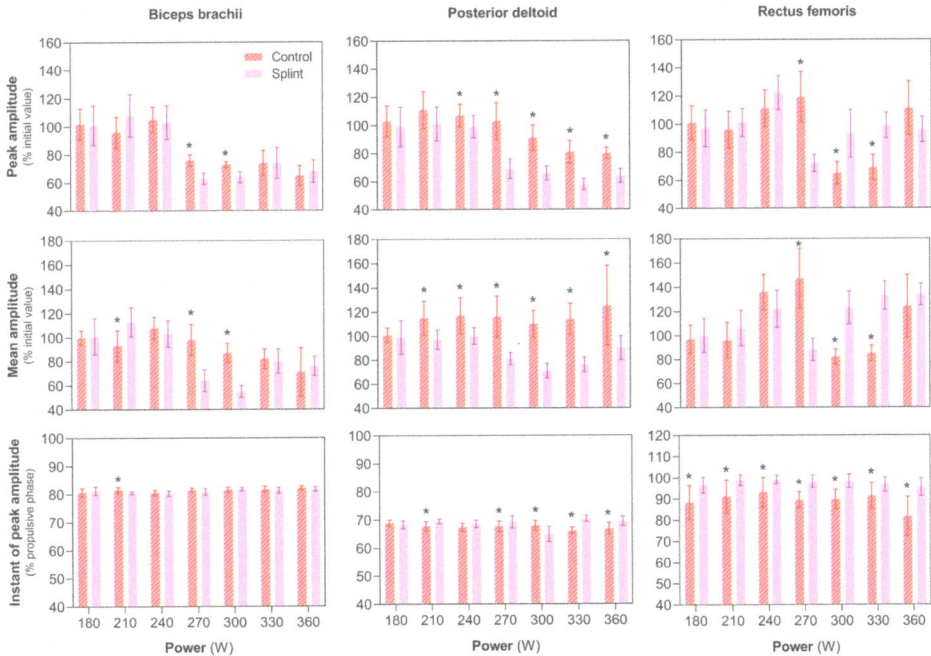

Figure 2. Normalized electromyography for biceps brachii, posterior deltoid and rectus femoris along the rowing incremental protocol for control and splint conditions. The onset and the end of the rowing propulsive phase were 0 and 100%, respectively. * indicates differences between control and splint conditions ($p \leq 0.05$).

The relationships between energy expenditure, rowing economy and the relative energy systems contributions along the protocol are illustrated in Figure 3. A lower slope was observed for the splint condition (0.17 vs. 0.21), indicating a lower exercise energy cost when the mandible was advanced. Moreover, the rowing economy was higher in the splint rather than in the control condition. In both incremental protocol trials, the aerobic and anaerobic energy systems accounted for ~87–99% and 1–13% (respectively) of the energy provided. However, the splint condition showed higher aerobic and lower anaerobic relative contributions than the control condition.

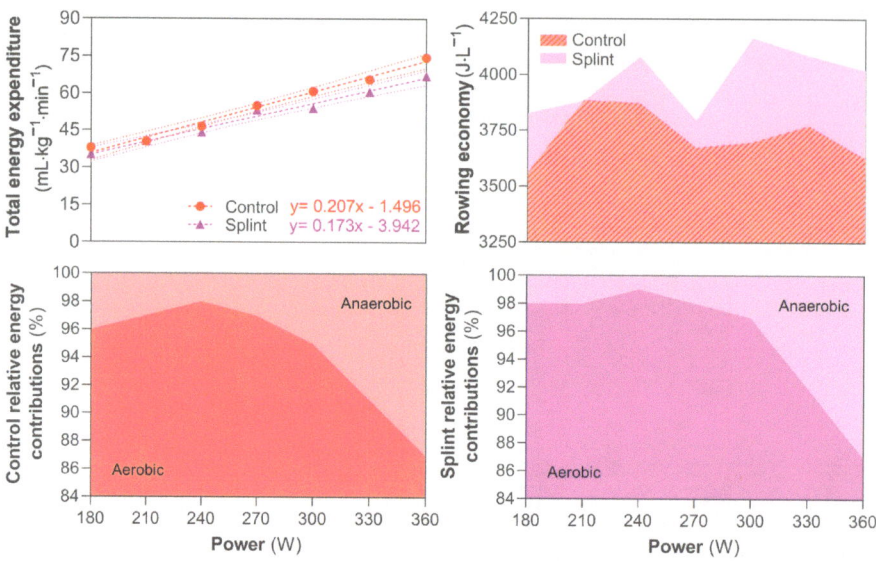

Figure 3. Energetic profile during rowing incremental protocol for control and splint conditions.

4. Discussion

At higher intensities, where respiratory muscles may require ~15% of the whole-body VO_2, the lower VO_2 observed by wearing the mandibular forward repositioning splint suggests a reduced requirement to support the respiratory muscle demands compared to the control condition [16]. Moreover, as a significant portion of ventilation occurs orally during exercise, reducing the effort of breathing or mouth airflow resistance with a mandibular forward repositioning splint likely enhances ventilation, as supported by our results. Although conflicting VO_2 responses are evident while wearing mandibular repositioning splints during exercise [7,8,17], there have been consistent reports of increased ventilation even when different subjects and methodologies were employed [6,8].

Kinematic changes have also been reported while running using splints that modify the mandibular position [6,18]. However, it remains uncertain whether these modifications are a direct consequence or mediated by the ergogenic physiological effects. Our results showed a slower and longer rowing movement, accompanied by a high rowing economy in the splint condition. Indeed, elite rowers may potentially improve performance by slightly lowering their rowing rate (consequently decreasing physiological demands), compensating with increased propulsive force [14]. Given the critical importance of synchronizing breathing with rowing mechanics, the potential reduction in respiratory work and a probable perceived "easier" breathing with the splint might enhance the rowing kinematic pattern.

Rowing is a complex movement that engages multiple muscle groups; however, the activation patterns of the biceps brachii and rectus femoris are frequently investigated when evaluating rowing technique [2]. Although explanations on how intraoral appliances might potentiate strength are inconclusive, certain studies suggest a link between altered occlusal vertical dimension and body muscular activity [19]. These ergogenic strength effects are primarily described for upper body musculature [20,21], with few reports indicating effects on lower limb performance [22,23]. Our data only align with prior research regarding the use of intraoral splints in lower body musculature, although differences in study design and the specific splint tested warrant consideration. Hence, future research should investigate how minor changes resulting from shifts in the lower jaw position may affect muscle activation, potentially leading to a more symmetrical or balanced force production.

The reduced energy cost and enhanced rowing economy noted for the splint condition support an improved rowing efficiency in comparison to the control condition. Furthermore, the observed decrease in anaerobic relative contributions may potentially have delayed the onset of fatigue when the splint was worn. The current ventilatory and energetic findings align with data from a highly trained triathlete who wore an advancement splint during a running incremental protocol [6]. Although the current study is pioneering in demonstrating the effects of mandibular forward repositioning in a high-level performance rower, our findings may not be easily generalized to other athletes or sports, given our small sample size. Additionally, our investigation only assessed the acute response to wearing a mandibular forward repositioning splint during rowing. Therefore, future research should explore the potential chronic effects of using such splints over extended training sessions or an entire competitive season.

5. Conclusions

In World-class rowing events, medal rankings are often decided by mere fractions of a second, underscoring the importance of any competitive advantage. Our findings highlight the potential beneficial impact of wearing a mandibular repositioning splint in rowing, a sport where such effects have not been previously explored. Testing a unique subject, as an Olympic finalist and World Champion, highlights the utility of employing a case study design to "open the door" for further investigation into wearing mandibular forward repositioning splints within high-level sport. An altered mandibular position induced by an intraoral splint elicited favourable biophysical and energetic advantages during an incremental rowing test in a Word-class rower.

Author Contributions: Conceptualization, F.C., R.C., J.C.P., D.B.P. and R.J.F.; methodology, F.C., R.C., P.F., J.P.V.-B. and R.J.F.; formal analysis, F.C., R.C., P.F. and M.R.; investigation, F.C., R.C., P.F. and M.R.; resources, F.C., J.P.V.-B., J.C.P. and R.J.F.; writing—original draft preparation, F.C., R.C., P.F. and M.R.; writing—review and editing, F.C., J.P.V.-B., J.C.P., D.B.P. and R.J.F.; visualization, F.C.; supervision, J.C.P., D.B.P. and R.J.F.; project administration, F.C., J.P.V.-B., J.C.P., D.B.P. and R.J.F.; funding acquisition, F.C., J.P.V.-B. and R.J.F. All authors have read and agreed to the published version of the manuscript.

Funding: This work was supported by Fundação para a Ciência e a Tecnologia, I.P. (FCT) and European Union (EU) by project reference UIDB/05913/2020 and DOI identifier 10.54499/UIDB/05913/2020, and doctoral grants award to Filipa Cardoso (reference 2020.05012.BD and DOI identifier https://doi.org/10.54499/2020.05012.BD), Ricardo Cardoso (2021.04976.BD and DOI identifier https://doi.org/10.54499/2021.04976.BD) and Manoel Rios (2021.04701.BD and DOI identifier https://doi.org/10.54499/2021.04701.BD).

Institutional Review Board Statement: The study was conducted in accordance with the Declaration of Helsinki and approved by the Institutional Review Board of the Faculty of Sport of the University of Porto (protocol code CEFADE282020, approved in 2020).

Informed Consent Statement: Informed consent was obtained from the subject involved in the current study.

Data Availability Statement: All data were contained within the manuscript.

Acknowledgments: The authors would like to acknowledge the rower and collaborators who participated in this study.

Conflicts of Interest: The authors declare no conflicts of interest.

References

1. Mäestu, J.; Jürimäe, J.; Jürimäe, T. Monitoring of Performance and Training in Rowing. *Sports Med.* **2005**, *35*, 597–617. [CrossRef] [PubMed]

2. Hohmuth, R.; Schwensow, D.; Malberg, H.; Schmidt, M. A Wireless Rowing Measurement System for Improving the Rowing Performance of Athletes. *Sensors* **2023**, *23*, 1060. [CrossRef] [PubMed]
3. Pripstein, L.P.; Rhodes, E.C.; McKenzie, D.C.; Coutts, K.D. Aerobic and anaerobic energy during a 2-km race simulation in female rowers. *Eur. J. Appl. Physiol. Occup. Physiol.* **1999**, *79*, 491–494. [CrossRef]
4. Secher, N.H. Physiological and biomechanical aspects of rowing. Implications for training. *Sports Med.* **1993**, *15*, 24–42. [CrossRef] [PubMed]
5. de Campos Mello, F.; de Moraes Bertuzzi, R.C.; Grangeiro, P.M.; Franchini, E. Energy systems contributions in 2,000 m race simulation: A comparison among rowing ergometers and water. *Eur. J. Appl. Physiol.* **2009**, *107*, 615–619. [CrossRef]
6. Cardoso, F.; Coelho, E.P.; Gay, A.; Vilas-Boas, J.P.; Pinho, J.C.; Pyne, D.B.; Fernandes, R.J. Case study: A jaw-protruding dental splint improves running physiology and kinematics. *Int. J. Sports Physiol. Perform.* **2022**, *17*, 791–795. [CrossRef]
7. Garner, D.P.; Dudgeon, W.D.; Scheett, T.P.; McDivitt, E.J. The effects of mouthpiece use on gas exchange parameters during steady-state exercise in college-aged men and women. *J. Am. Dent. Assoc.* **2011**, *142*, 1041–1047. [CrossRef]
8. Schultz Martins, R.; Girouard, P.; Elliott, E.; Mekary, S. Physiological responses of a jaw-repositioning custom-made mouthguard on airway and their effects on athletic performance. *J. Strength Cond. Res.* **2020**, *34*, 422–429. [CrossRef]
9. Fleming, N.; Donne, B.; Mahony, N. A comparison of electromyography and stroke kinematics during ergometer and on-water rowing. *J. Sports Sci.* **2014**, *32*, 1127–1138. [CrossRef]
10. Sousa, A.; Figueiredo, P.; Zamparo, P.; Pyne, D.B.; Vilas-Boas, J.P.; Fernandes, R.J. Exercise modality effect on bioenergetical performance at VO_{2max} intensity. *Med. Sci. Sports Exerc.* **2015**, *47*, 1705–1713. [CrossRef]
11. Martinez-Valdes, E.; Wilson, F.; Fleming, N.; McDonnell, S.J.; Horgan, A.; Falla, D. Rowers with a recent history of low back pain engage different regions of the lumbar erector spinae during rowing. *J. Sci. Med. Sport* **2019**, *22*, 1206–1212. [CrossRef]
12. Hermens, H.J.; Freriks, B.; Disselhorst-Klug, C.; Rau, G. Development of recommendations for SEMG sensors and sensor placement procedures. *J. Electromyogr. Kinesiol.* **2000**, *10*, 361–374. [CrossRef]
13. Cardoso, R.; Rios, M.; Carvalho, D.; Monteiro, A.S.; Soares, S.; Abraldes, J.A.; Gomes, B.B.; Vilas-Boas, J.P.; Fernandes, R.J. Mechanics and Energetic Analysis of Rowing with Big Blades with Randall Foils. *Int. J. Sports Med.* **2023**, *44*, 1043–1048. [CrossRef] [PubMed]
14. Kane, D.A.; Mackenzie, S.J.; Jensen, R.L.; Watts, P.B. Effects of stroke resistance on rowing economy in club rowers post-season. *Int. J. Sports Med.* **2013**, *34*, 131–137. [CrossRef]
15. Held, S.; Siebert, T.; Donath, L. Electromyographic activity of the vastus medialis and gastrocnemius implicates a slow stretch-shortening cycle during rowing in the field. *Sci. Rep.* **2020**, *10*, 9451. [CrossRef]
16. Harms, C.A.; Wetter, T.J.; St Croix, C.M.; Pegelow, D.F.; Dempsey, J.A. Effects of respiratory muscle work on exercise performance. *J. Appl. Physiol.* **2000**, *89*, 131–138. [CrossRef] [PubMed]
17. Cardoso, F.; Monteiro, A.S.; Vilas-Boas, J.P.; Pinho, J.C.; Pyne, D.B.; Fernandes, R.J. Effects of wearing a 50% lower jaw advancement splint on biophysical and perceptual responses at low to severe running intensities. *Life* **2022**, *12*, 253. [CrossRef] [PubMed]
18. Maurer, C.; Stief, F.; Jonas, A.; Kovac, A.; Groneberg, D.A.; Meurer, A.; Ohlendorf, D. Influence of the lower jaw position on the running pattern. *PLoS ONE* **2015**, *10*, e0135712. [CrossRef]
19. Cesanelli, L.; Cesaretti, G.; Ylaitė, B.; Iovane, A.; Bianco, A.; Messina, G. Occlusal Splints and Exercise Performance: A Systematic Review of Current Evidence. *Int. J. Environ. Res. Public Health* **2021**, *18*, 10338. [CrossRef]
20. Abdallah, E.F.; Mehta, N.R.; Forgione, A.G.; Clark, R.E. Affecting Upper Extremity Strength by Changing Maxillo-Mandibular Vertical Dimension in Deep Bite Subjects. *CRANIO®* **2004**, *22*, 268–275. [CrossRef]
21. Dias, A.; Redinha, L.; Vaz, J.R.; Cordeiro, N.; Silva, L.; Pezarat-Correia, P. Effects of occlusal splints on shoulder strength and activation. *Ann. Med.* **2019**, *51*, 15–21. [CrossRef] [PubMed]
22. Buscà, B.; Morales, J.; Solana-Tramunt, M.; Miró, A.; García, M. Effects of Jaw Clenching While Wearing a Customized Bite-Aligning Mouthpiece on Strength in Healthy Young Men. *J. Strength Cond. Res.* **2016**, *30*, 1102–1110. [CrossRef] [PubMed]
23. Maurer, C.; Heller, S.; Sure, J.J.; Fuchs, D.; Mickel, C.; Wanke, E.M.; Groneberg, D.A.; Ohlendorf, D. Strength improvements through occlusal splints? The effects of different lower jaw positions on maximal isometric force production and performance in different jumping types. *PLoS ONE* **2018**, *13*, e0193540. [CrossRef] [PubMed]

Disclaimer/Publisher's Note: The statements, opinions and data contained in all publications are solely those of the individual author(s) and contributor(s) and not of MDPI and/or the editor(s). MDPI and/or the editor(s) disclaim responsibility for any injury to people or property resulting from any ideas, methods, instructions or products referred to in the content.